Primer of Dermatopathology

Primer of dermatopathology

Primer of Dermatopathology

Third Edition

Antoinette F. Hood, M.D.

Professor of Dermatology and Pathology
Eastern Virginia Medical School
Norfolk, Virginia

Theodore H. Kwan, M.D.

Pathologist, Department of Anatomic Pathology
Lahey Clinic
Burlington, Massachusetts

Martin C. Mihm, Jr., M.D.

Clinical Professor of Pathology
Harvard Medical School
Senior Dermatopathologist
Massachusetts General Hospital
Boston, Massachusetts

Thomas D. Horn, M.D.

Chairman, Department of Dermatology
Professor of Pathology and Dermatology
University of Arkansas for Medical Sciences and
Central Arkansas Veterans Administration Health System
Little Rock, Arkansas

Bruce R. Smoller, M.D.

Vice Chair, Department of Pathology
Professor of Pathology and Dermatology
Chief, Dermatopathology Division
University of Arkansas for Medical Sciences
Little Rock, Arkansas

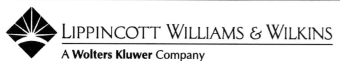

LIPPINCOTT WILLIAMS & WILKINS
A **Wolters Kluwer** Company
Philadelphia • Baltimore • New York • London
Buenos Aires • Hong Kong • Sydney • Tokyo

Acquisitions Editor: Beth Barry
Developmental Editor: Grace Caputo
Production Editor: Rakesh Rampertab
Manufacturing Manager: Benjamin Rivera
Cover Designer: Mark Lerner
Compositor: TechBooks
Printer: Maple Press

© 2002 by LIPPINCOTT WILLIAMS & WILKINS
530 Walnut Street
Philadelphia, PA 19106 USA
LWW.com

Printed in the USA

Library of Congress Cataloging-in-Publication Data

Primer of dermatopathology / Antoinette F. Hood ... [et al.].—3rd ed.
    p. ; cm.
  Includes bibliographical references and index.
  ISBN 0-7817-3236-0
  1. Skin—Diseases. 2. Skin—Pathophysiology. I. Hood, Antoinette F.
  [DNLM: 1. Skin Diseases—pathology. 2. Skin Diseases—pathology—
Atlases. WR 140 P953 2002]
  RL96 .P75 2002
  616.5—dc21   2002066116

10 9 8 7 6 5 4 3 2 1

Contents

Preface

In preparing to write this preface, we were surprised to realize that the *Primer of Dermatopathology* is 18 years old. One could say that as an entity it has come of age, reached maturity. We believe that the continued success of the *Primer* in a world with many excellent dermatopathology textbooks is because the book has remained true to its original intent: to serve as a simple introduction to an area in pathology that can be difficult and perplexing to a novice. The third edition of the *Primer* continues that tradition by providing an easy to use, unambiguous, affordable introduction to the wonders of dermatopathology.

The third edition introduces a new author to the team, Bruce R. Smoller, M.D. On a historical note, Drs. Smoller, Hood, Kwan, and Horn all trained directly or indirectly with our senior author and mentor, Martin C. Mihm, Jr., making us family of a sort. Dr. Smoller, an internationally renowned dermatopathologist with expertise in cutaneous tumors and immunohistochemical techniques, has provided invaluable contributions in the revision of the text and in the addition of new disease entities.

We continue to take pride in keeping the cost of the *Primer* in a price range affordable to residents in dermatology and pathology. Because printing the third edition with color photomicrographs would have been prohibitively expensive, we struck what we thought was an appropriate compromise by including a CD-ROM with the book. The CD-ROM contains approximately 2,000 color images that are accessible by chapter or disorder, and 35 self-assessment quizzes. Credit for the technical development of the CD-ROM goes to Ryan P. Christy, Brent D. Gann, Karen J. Miller, and Jean A. Siders, part of the Pathology Multimedia Education Group at Indiana University. We sincerely thank them for their hard work and perseverance in what at times seemed to be a never-ending task. Our thanks are also extended to John N. Eble, M.D., Chairman of the Department of Pathology and Laboratory Medicine, Indiana University, for the use of departmental resources, and for ongoing encouragement and support.

If you are a first-time user of the *Primer*, we recommend that you begin by reviewing the section entitled, "Guide to the Use of This Book and CD-ROM" on page xi. This brief introduction explains the format of the book, how to use the text to sort through diagnostic dilemmas, and how to use the accompanying CD-ROM optimally.

As noted in the preface to the first two editions, we remind the reader that *The Primer of Dermatopathology* is really meant to be an introduction to dermatopathology, an introduction that we hope inspires further reading and study in a field that we dearly love.

AFH
THK
MCM
TDH
BRS

Preface to the First Edition

Looking at a skin biopsy under the microscope can be a bewildering and frustrating experience for inexperienced dermatology and pathology residents and practitioners alike. This book was conceived from that frustration. When Dan Burnes was rotating through dermatopathology as a dermatology resident at the Massachusetts General Hospital, he frequently complained that there should be a logical and systematic way to look at and evaluate a skin biopsy. The textbooks available at that time were all traditionally organized by pathogenesis, which was useful only if you knew the answer in advance. Challenged by the problem, Dan sat down and outlined dermatopathologic disorders according to (1) their location in the skin—from the stratum corneum to the panniculus—and (2) "reaction patterns" of disease. The latter organization he had learned from Martin Mihm, Jr., who had learned it from Wally Clark, who learned it from heaven knows whom. Encouraged by Dr. Thomas Fitzpatrick, who loves a logical approach to disease, Dan's outline was filled in and expanded, and line drawings and photographs were added. Many revisions later, *Primer of Dermatopathology* became a functional entity.

We deliberately called this book a primer to identify its purpose. It is an introduction to dermatopathology, an expanded outline of diseases according to the anatomic location and the pattern of changes observed. It attempts to simplify and clarify a complex situation in order to get people involved in making a (differential) diagnosis from a piece of tissue on a slide.

This book includes most of the diseases seen by dermatology or pathology residents during their years of training. It is not, however, all-inclusive, and for completeness, the reader should have ready access to at least one (inclusive) major textbook, such as those written by Walter Lever, James Graham, and Elson Helwig, and, for inflammatory disorders, that of A. Bernard Ackerman.

AFH
THK
DCB
MCM

Guide to the Use of This Book and CD-ROM

Primer of Dermatopathology is designed to assist dermatologists and pathologists (in training or in practice) in the microscopic diagnosis of skin disease. By emphasizing a systematic approach to the examination of a skin biopsy, we hope to enable even the relatively uninitiated individual to locate and identify the abnormal histologic features present in a given lesion, to generate a differential diagnosis, and to establish a definitive diagnosis.

To use this book most effectively, we recommend an initial reading of the introductory section. In it, the normal histology of the skin is briefly reviewed, and an illustrated glossary provides an introduction to common pathologic alterations (for example, parakeratosis, dyskeratosis) and to the terminology used in dermatopathology. A brief histochemistry chapter provides important background information on special tissue stains and immunohistochemistry.

A skin biopsy should be examined first with the unaided eye and then with the lowest-power objective on the microscope. Simple appreciation of the type of biopsy submitted can give valuable insight into the questions being asked by the referring physician. For example, trephine (punch) biopsies are usually obtained from inflammatory lesions, whereas shave biopsies and elliptical excisions are usually from neoplastic lesions.

While still using low power, identify the anatomic site of the major pathologic change (that is, the epidermis, dermis, appendages, or panniculus), turn to that section of the book, and note the chapter headings. Determine the predominant abnormality (vesicles, perivascular inflammation, dermal hyperplasia, for example), refine your impressions at medium power (intraepidermal vesicles, perivascular lymphocytic infiltrate, intradermal vascular proliferation), and turn to the corresponding chapter heading. Some chapters, such as Chapter 23, Cysts in the Dermis, will require perusal of the entire contents to generate a diagnosis, whereas others, such as Chapter 9, Disorders of the Melanocyte, are further subdivided. For example, if low-power examination of a skin biopsy reveals that the most prominent change is a perivascular infiltrate in the reticular dermis, turn to Part IV (Reticular Dermis), Chapter 16 (Predominantly Perivascular Infiltrate of the Reticular Dermis). To further classify the lesion, at medium- or high-power magnification, determine the cellular composition of the infiltrate and whether there is vascular damage or thrombosis. Then a chapter subdivision can be selected and a specific diagnosis generated.

Cutaneous biopsies of inflammatory lesions often show histologic changes in more than one anatomic area of the skin. A lesion of lupus erythematosus, for example, may exhibit epidermal atrophy, basal vacuolization, a perivascular mononuclear cell infiltrate, or appendageal infiltration. The diagnosis may be established by looking at any one of those features in the following chapters: Chapter 8 (Atrophic Processes of the Epidermis), Chapter 11 (Subepidermal Clefting, Blister, or Pustule Formation), Chapter 12 (Bandlike Infiltrate at the Dermoepidermal Junction), Chapter 16 (Predominantly Perivascular Infiltrate of the Reticular Dermis), or Chapter 24 (Disorders of the Pilosebaceous Unit).

In this book, the disease entities are listed in the left column, and the histologic criteria for diagnosis are given in the center column, with the most important or distinguishing histologic features emphasized with bold type. The right column is used for differential diagnoses, helpful hints, and clinical information when appropriate. Often, specific histologic findings may be seen in several different diseases. The differential diagnoses of *specific histologic findings*, such as Pautrier microabscesses or hypogranulosis, are also found in the right column; they are set in boxes for emphasis.

Suggested readings are given at the end of each chapter to provide additional information for the curious and inquiring student of dermatopathology.

Characteristic histologic features of individual disorders are illustrated in the textbook with black and white photomicrographs and schematic drawings whenever possible. Approximately 2,000 additional full-color photomicrographs are found on the accompanying CD-ROM. These photomicrographs are categorized by diagnosis, chapter, or sections within the chapters. Each photomicrograph has a legend describing the diagnostic features shown. Accompanying Chapters 4 to 26 are a series of multiple-choice questions that can be used for self-study and self-assessment. There are also 12 bonus quizzes with randomly selected questions from various chapters.

If you are using the *Primer* as a study guide, we recommend that you first review a chapter, or a section of a chapter in the text, then view the supplementary photomicrographs for that section on the CD-ROM, and finally use the quiz to assess your retention of information and to identify areas of strength and weakness.

July 1, 2002
AFH

Primer of Dermatopathology

Part **I**

Introduction

Chapter 1

Normal Histology
of the Skin

A basic knowledge of cutaneous histology is easily attained by a systematic approach. The skin can be considered by anatomic levels: epidermis, dermoepidermal junction, dermis, and subcutis (Fig. 1-1). Traversing the dermis and subcutis are the peripheral branches of the vascular and nervous systems, as well as the epidermal appendages (pilosebaceous, apocrine, and eccrine units). Regional variations in the skin correlate with marked differences in epidermal thickness, dermal thickness, elastic fiber content, and presence or absence of hair follicles and sebaceous, apocrine, or eccrine glands.

Epidermis

The epidermis is composed of four types of cells: keratinocytes, melanocytes, Langerhans cells, and Merkel cells. These cells vary markedly in structure, function, and place of origin. *Keratinocytes* constitute the major cell population of the epidermis (80%). Keratinocytes are subclassified by their location in the epidermis (Fig. 1-2). The *basal layer* consists of a single layer of cuboidal cells located next to the dermoepidermal junction. These cells have a relatively large nuclear-cytoplasmic ratio and slightly basophilic cytoplasm. The *spinous layer*, named for its prominent intercellular connections, which allegedly resemble spines, is located above the basal layer. Usually several cells thick, the spinous layer consists of polygonal cells, which exhibit cytoplasmic eosinophilia reflecting increased keratinization. The *granular layer* is one to five cells thick and consists of flattened cells with coarse, deeply basophilic cytoplasmic granules, called *keratohyaline granules*. These structures contain profilaggrin, which is cleaved to form filaggrin, a molecule aiding keratin organization. The *cornified layer* (stratum corneum), the most superficial layer of the epidermis, is composed of extremely flattened, anucleate keratinocytes arranged in a pattern sometimes described as "basketweave." The cornified layer appears dense and thickened on surfaces subject to friction, such as the palms and soles. Keratinocytes—particularly basal cells—also may contain small, brown pigment (melanin) granules. The degree of epidermal melanization varies with genetic and enviromental factors.

Melanocytes have a variable appearance, which sometimes makes definitive identification difficult in routine hematoxylin–eosin (H&E)-stained sections. Melanocytes are located in the basal layer and usually appear as cuboidal cells with clear cytoplasm and eccentrically placed, crescent-shaped nuclei. The function of these neural crest-derived cells is to synthesize melanin within membrane-bound melanosomes, with subsequent transfer to adjacent keratinocytes via dendritic projections. Pigment production in these cells and their true dendritic shape are infrequently appreciated without special stains. The ratio of melanocytes to basal cells is 1 : 4 to 1 : 9 and varies with anatomic location on the body (but not with race).

Langerhans cells have an appearance similar to that of melanocytes but are located at any level of the epidermis. Reliable identification can be made with gold chloride-stained sections, immunohistochemistry, or electron microscopy. Ultrastructural cytoplasmic organelles called *Birbeck granules* (said to resemble tennis rackets) are characteristic of Langerhans cells. Langerhans cells have many features of monocytes and macrophages and are bone marrow derived.

Merkel cells, located in the basal layer, are also difficult to visualize in H&E-stained sections. They are identified by distinctive ultrastructural

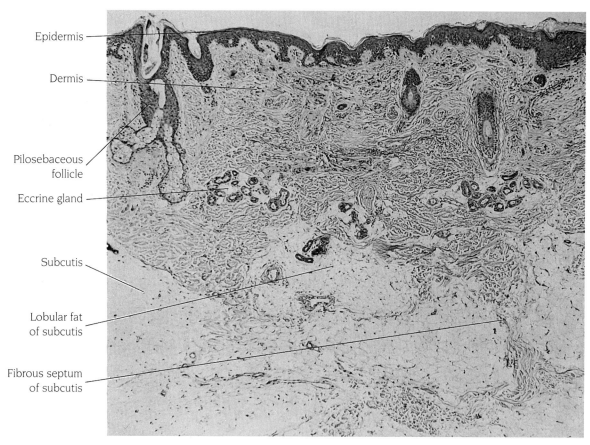

Epidermis

Dermis

Pilosebaceous
follicle

Eccrine gland

Subcutis

Lobular fat
of subcutis

Fibrous septum
of subcutis

Fig. **1-1.** *The skin. The three anatomic layers of the skin are the epidermis, dermis, and subcutis. The epidermal appendages, including pilosebaceous units and eccrine glands, extend into the dermis. The subcutis is subdivided into lobular and septal areas.*

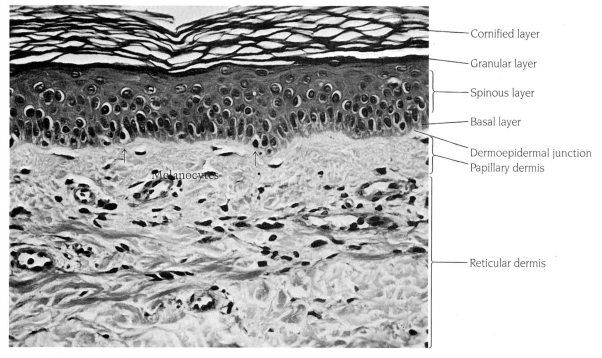

Cornified layer

Granular layer

Spinous layer

Basal layer

Dermoepidermal junction
Papillary dermis

Melanocytes

Reticular dermis

Fig. **1-2.** *Subdivisions of the epidermis and dermis.*

membrane-bound granules similar to those found in neuroendocrine tissues. The function of Merkel cells is not understood.

Dermoepidermal Junction

The dermoepidermal junction in H&E-stained sections appears as a fine (1–2 μm) band of slightly condensed eosinophilic material (see Fig. 1-2). This basement membrane zone consists of a glycoprotein matrix in which are embedded collagen, reticulin, and fine elastic fibers (Fig. 1-3). Periodic acid–Schiff (PAS) stain highlights this area. The basement membrane zone continues around all the epidermal appendages.

The lower border of the epidermis on most parts of the body has numerous undulating downward projections called *rete ridges* (when seen in three dimensions, these form a netlike, or rete, pattern). The corresponding and interdigitating upward elevations of the dermis are called *dermal papillae*.

Dermis

The dermis is divided into two parts: a thin superficial portion known as the *papillary dermis* and a wider, deep area known as the *reticular dermis* (Fig. 1-2). Both the papillary and reticular dermis contain collagen, reticulin, and elastic fibers embedded within a matrix of glycoproteins. Type I collagen, the major component of the dermis, is readily visualized in H&E-stained sections as eosinophilic fibers of regular diameter that are gathered into bundles of varying size. Collagen fibers are birefringent in polarized light. Reticulin fibers (type III collagen) are small collagen fibers and are best visualized with special reticulin stains. Elastic fibers are wavy, eosinophilic, and slightly refractile, and they vary markedly in diameter and length. They are easily visualized with stains such as the Verhoeff–van Gieson. The fine elastic fibers of the uppermost dermis are called elaunin and oxytalan. The glycoprotein matrix of the dermis cannot be visualized in H&E-stained sections. In normal skin and in certain

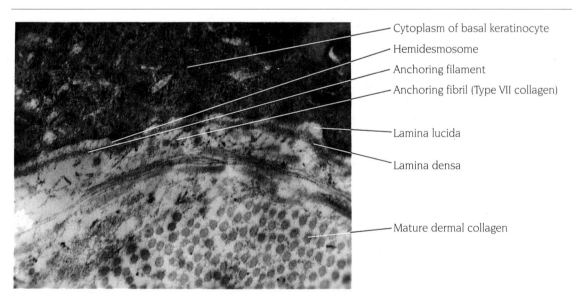

Cytoplasm of basal keratinocyte

Hemidesmosome

Anchoring filament

Anchoring fibril (Type VII collagen)

Lamina lucida

Lamina densa

Mature dermal collagen

Fig. **1-3.** *Transmission electron micrograph of basement membrane zone.*

pathologic states characterized by excessive production of acid mucopolysaccharides, these materials can be identified by alcian blue stain.

The papillary dermis is recognized microscopically as a thin (40–100 μm) zone of connective tissue located below the dermoepidermal junction and above the reticular dermis. The small collagen bundles of the papillary dermis are easily distinguished from the larger collagen bundles of the reticular dermis. The papillary dermis surrounds all the appendageal structures as they extend downward into the dermis and subcutis. This periadnexal papillary dermis is called the *adventitial* (outermost) *dermis*. The dermis contains a population of dendritic cells of bone marrow origin, probably active in certain immunologic functions.

The reticular (netlike) dermis is easily distinguished from the papillary dermis by the presence of large (12–25 μm) collagen bundles. These bundles, which appear to be oriented in every possible plane, are mingled with reticulin and elastic fibers to form a closely knit net.

Subcutis

The subcutis (panniculus adiposus, subcutaneous fat) is composed of lobules of lipocytes separated by fibrous connective-tissue septa. The thickness of the subcutis varies with the sex and nutritional status of the individual and with anatomic location. Vessels, nerves, and appendages pass into and through the subcutis. Below the subcutis, muscle and/or fascia can be found.

Vessels: Arteriovenous and Lymphatic

The arteriovenous framework of the skin can be visualized as follows. Arteries traverse the septa of the subcutis and form a *deep plexus* in the region of the junction of the subcutis and dermis. From this deep plexus, smaller arteries pass upward to the junction of the reticular and papillary dermis, where they form the *superficial plexus*. From these arterioles, capillary-venules form superficial vascular loops, which ascend into and descend from the dermal papillae. Capillary-venules are so named because the flow of blood may be arterial to venous, or vice versa. The venous return in the skin follows a reverse, and frequently more variable, course. The arteriovenous system of the skin, therefore, consists of deep and superficial plexuses with communicating vessels and, most distally, capillary vascular loops (Fig. 1-4).

Given this framework, considerable regional variation exists with regard to the density and caliber of these vessels. Furthermore, there are numerous arteriovenous shunts, particularly on distal extremities. These arteriovenous shunts are controlled by *glomus cells*, abundantly innervated by adrenergic fibers. Glomus cells are modified smooth muscle cells and are recognized by their round nuclei, polygonal shape, and tendency to group around vessels (Fig. 1-5).

The microscopic structure of cutaneous vessels is similar to that of visceral vessels. Surrounding a lumen, endothelial cells rest on a PAS-positive basement membrane zone, which in turn is surrounded by smooth muscle cells, pericytes, and/or connective tissue. The cellular layers vary with the size and type of vessel.

Mast cells in varying numbers (up to five per sectioned vessel) are present around superficial vessels and, to a lesser extent, throughout the dermis. In H&E-stained sections, mast cells have densely basophilic nuclei and opaque, violet cytoplasm. Their characteristic and identifying cytoplasmic granules are metachromatic blue-purple with Giemsa stain.

Fig. **1-4.** *Arteriovenous system. ART, artery; SM ART/A, small artery/ arteriole; SAP, superficial arterial plexus; SCV, superficial capillary venule; SVP₁ and SVP₂, components of superficial vascular plexus. (Reprinted with permission from M. C. Mihm et al., J. Invest. Dermatol. 67:306, 1976. Copyright © 1976, The Williams & Wilkins Co., Baltimore).*

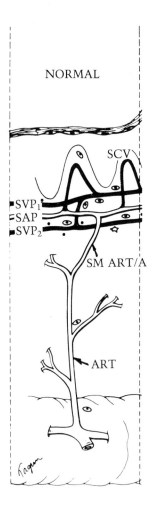

NORMAL

SCV

SVP₁
SAP
SVP₂

SM ART/A

ART

Fig. **1-5.** *Glomus body. Numerous glomus cells surround arteriovenous anastomoses. Glomus bodies are numerous in nailfolds, toes, fingerpads, and the pinnae.*

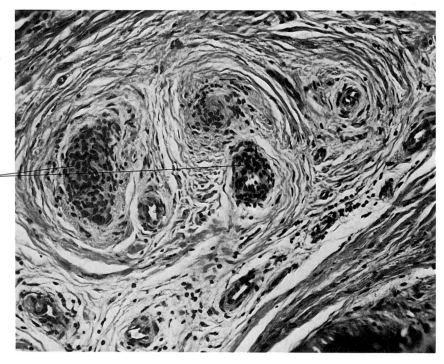

Glomus cells

The lymphatics of the skin consist of a blind-ended vascular system that flows from the superficial dermis to the subcutis and then more centrally. The most distal tributaries in the papillary dermis are lined by endothelial cells without a basal lamina. The thicker-walled, more proximal portions of the system contain valves. Thin walls and valves are the features that distinguish lymphatics from the other vessels. Probably because they are collapsed, lymphatic channels are observed infrequently in normal skin.

Nerves

The cutaneous nerves comprise a system of nerve plexuses and branches that roughly parallels the vascular system. Cutaneous nerves function in sensory (afferent) and autonomic (efferent) modes. Sensory impulses, generated from encapsulated (Meissner and Vater–Pacini corpuscles) and nonencapsulated ("end organs" ramifying about hair follicles and in dermal papillae and ending in Merkel cell–neurite complexes) receptors, pass to the dorsal root ganglia and centrally. By a presumed process of summation and integration, there is perception of particular sensations described as touch, pressure, temperature, pain, itch, and location. Motor impulses, which in the skin are autonomic, originate in the sympathetic nervous system and pass to glomus bodies and smooth muscles of vessels (affecting peripheral flow), to hair follicle–associated smooth muscle (causing gooseflesh), and to apocrine and eccrine glands (causing sweating).

In H&E-stained sections, sensory fibers cannot be distinguished from autonomic fibers, and one appreciates little more than small nerve branches and Meissner and Vater–Pacini corpuscles. Nerve branches have the same structure as elsewhere in the peripheral nervous system. Larger nerves of the subcutis exhibit epineurium, perineurium, and endoneurium (Fig. 1-6). Small nerve branches in the superficial dermis lack these layers. Individual nerve fibers with Schwann cells measure 3 to 5 μm

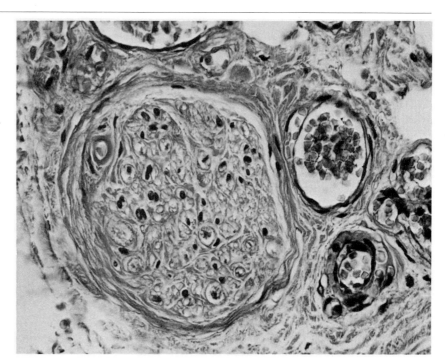

Fig. **1-6.** *Peripheral nerve. A thin fibrous capsule, the perineurium, surrounds the bundle of myelinated nerve axons. Endoneurium refers to the delicate collagen fibers surrounding nerve trunks within the perineurium. Schwann cell nuclei can be identified, but nerve axons are difficult to visualize. Two capillaries also are present in this field.*

Fig. **1-7.** *Meissner corpuscle. Tucked within the dermal papilla, this neuro-receptor resembles a ball of string wound about a spindle. Portions of an intraepidermal eccrine duct are present at left.*

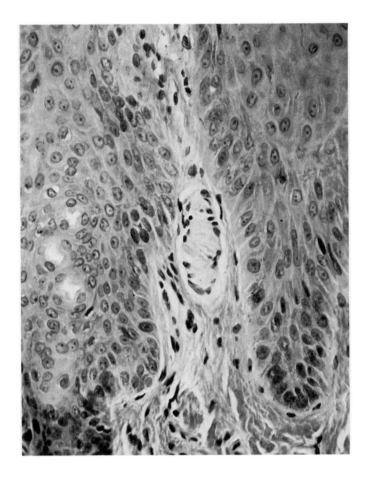

Fig. **1-8.** *Pacinian corpuscles. The rounded forms of these concentric lamellated structures in the subcutis are characteristic.*

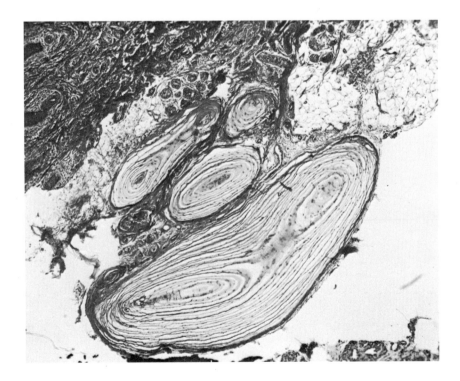

in diameter. The small size of these fibers helps one to distinguish them from smooth muscle. Meissner corpuscles are said to play a role in mediation of the sensation of touch. Located in the dermal papillae, each of these encapsulated ellipsoid structures (20–50 μm) has the appearance of string wound about a spindle (Fig. 1-7). The Vater–Pacini corpuscles, which mediate the sensation of pressure, are located in the subcutis, appearing as a large (up to 1 mm) oval encapsulated body with a distinctive internal structure of concentric lamellae (Fig. 1-8). Vater–Pacini bodies are most numerous on the palms and soles.

Special stains are necessary to demonstrate nonencapsulated receptors and autonomic innervation.

Pilosebaceous Unit

Hair is present everywhere on the body except the palms, soles, and mucocutaneous junctions. The fine, almost imperceptible hairs that cover most of the body are called *lanugo*, or *vellus hairs*. The larger hairs such as those of the scalp and eyebrows are called *terminal hairs*. The pilosebaceous unit makes hair and an oily, fatty emollient; moreover, it is equipped for sensory and motor functions. The components of the pilosebaceous follicle include the hair shaft, hair follicle, sebaceous gland, sensory end organ, and arrector pili.

The Hair and Hair Follicle

The hair shaft is composed of densely layered keratin rich in cysteine cross-links and is the product of cellular differentiation occurring within the follicle. The hair shaft and hair follicle are first described longitudinally and then in cross section. Finally, the histologic changes associated with phases of growth, involution, and rest are described briefly.

Viewed in its long axis, the hair follicle can be divided into three parts:

1. The *infundibulum* (funnel) extends from the surface to the opening of the sebaceous duct into the follicle. On certain areas of the body, the duct of the apocrine gland also opens into the infundibulum near the epidermis.
2. The *isthmus* (by definition, a contracted anatomic part connecting two larger structures) joins the portion from the opening of the sebaceous duct to the insertion of the arrector pili.
3. The *inferior portion* consists of the hair follicle below the insertion of the arrector pili.

Hair formation begins within the bulb, or rounded extremity of the inferior portion. The bulb contains the hair *matrix*, a group of undifferentiated epithelial cells with vesicular nuclei and intensely basophilic cytoplasm. The matrix cells in association with melanocytes sit astride the dermal *papilla* of the hair, a specialized mesenchymal tissue continuous with the papillary dermis. Under the influence of the dermal hair papilla, matrix cells give rise to the hair shaft, as well as the inner and outer root sheaths. The hair shaft forms by keratinization of matrix cells and derives its pigment from the melanocytes of the matrix. The mature hair shaft in cross section exhibits a central *medulla* (absent in vellus hairs) surrounded by *cortex* and covered by a *cuticle*, which somewhat resembles overlapping shingles. Concentric and external to the matrix are the *inner and outer root sheaths* (Fig. 1-9), these two keratinizing layers form a support for the growing hair. Keratinization in the inner root sheath occurs with the production of eosinophilic *trichohyaline* granules. Surrounding the outer root sheath are the *vitreous*, an eosinophilic band continuous with but thicker than the epidermal basement membrane zone; the *fibrous root sheath*; and the *periadnexal adventitial dermis*.

In the hair follicle, cycles of growth, involution, and rest (anagen, catagen, and telogen, respectively) correlate with the following histologic features. During telogen, the inferior portion of the hair follicle resides at upper dermal levels. With the onset of anagen, the inferior portion, apparently under the influence of the dermal papilla, elongates and forms a bulb that contains proliferating matrix cells. The papilla during anagen exhibits metachromasia. Loss of metachromasia signals the onset of catagen. In catagen, individually necrotic cells appear within the bulb, the inner and outer root sheaths condense to form a hyalin band, and the inferior portion retreats to the region of attachment of the arrector pili, leaving in its wake a pleated collagen streamer (stela).

Sensory End Organ and Arrector Pili

The sensory end organ consists of distal, apparently unencapsulated, ramifications of sensory nerves present about the isthmus and inferior portions of the follicle. These receptors and nerves apparently convey information about the movement of hair follicles. These sensory end organs are not apparent in H&E-stained sections but can be demonstrated by special techniques.

Fig. **1-9.** *Hair follicle.*

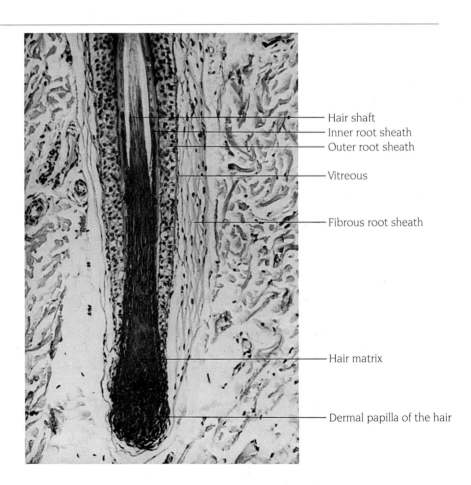

- Hair shaft
- Inner root sheath
- Outer root sheath
- Vitreous
- Fibrous root sheath
- Hair matrix
- Dermal papilla of the hair

Arrector pili muscles are associated with hair follicles and are composed of bundles of smooth-muscle fibers. The arrector pili, which inserts into the follicle below the sebaceous gland duct, extends obliquely upward to the superficial dermis. Contraction of the arrector pili (mediated by autonomic nerves) causes the hair to be pulled from its normally angled position to a more perpendicular position. This action results in cutis anserina, or goosebumps.

Sebaceous Gland

Sebaceous glands produce oily, lipid-rich secretions that function as emollients for the hair and skin. These glands frequently are associated with hairs, but the hairs may be inapparent. Present everywhere except on the palms and soles, sebaceous glands are most numerous on the face, chest, and back, they are also found frequently on the buccal mucosa and lip (Fordyce spots), areola (Montgomery's tubercles), labia minora, prepuce (Tyson's glands), and even in the parotids and on the tongue and cervix. The Meibomian glands of the eyelid are also sebaceous. Hormonal factors probably regulate the holocrine secretions of these glands.

The sebaceous gland can be multilobular or unilobular. Cuboidal cells with basophilic cytoplasm located at the periphery of the lobule differentiate into large, vacuolated lipid-laden cells (Fig. 1-10), which disintegrate as they reach the sebaceous duct. This short duct, composed of squamous epithelium, conveys the cellular contents to the infundibulum of the follicle or, less frequently, directly to the skin surface. As with all other appendages, a basement membrane zone and adventitial dermis surround the sebaceous gland.

Fig. **1-10.** *Sebaceous glands. Basophilic cells at the periphery of each lobule give rise to the central cell with foamy cytoplasm. These glands are usually associated with a hair.*

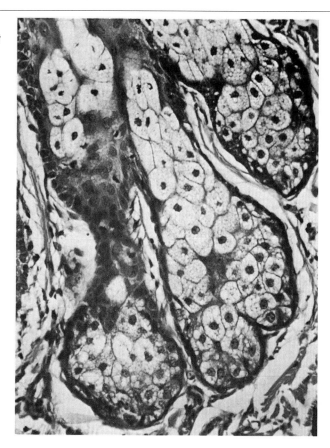

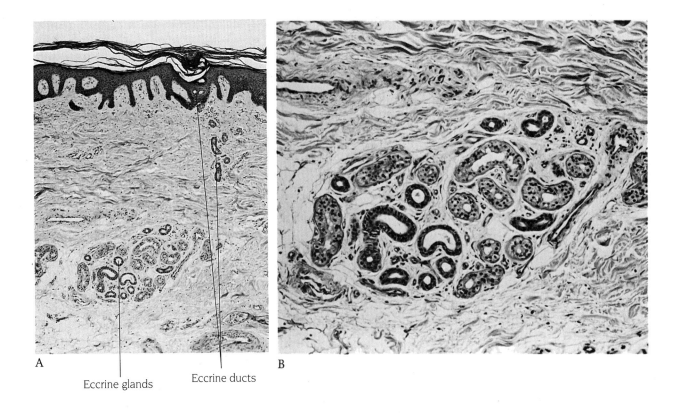

A

B

Eccrine glands   Eccrine ducts

Fig. **1-11.**

A. *Eccrine gland and duct (with overlying lentigo). Two cell layers line the entire system; an inner secretory cell adjacent to the lumen is ensheathed by an outer myoepithelial cell.*

B. *Eccrine gland. Note the normal investment of the gland by loose connective tissue and lipocytes. The cytoplasm of these cells is clear to amphophilic.*

C. *Eccrine duct within the dermis and epidermis. Two cell layers with a PAS-positive cuticle lining the lumen are characteristic.*

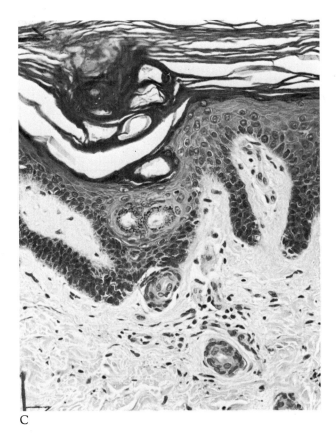

C

Eccrine Glands and Ducts

Eccrine glands produce an isotonic to hypertonic secretion that is modified by the ducts and emerges on the skin surface as sweat. Especially numerous on the palms, soles, forehead, and axillae, eccrine glands are found everywhere on the skin except the mucocutaneous junctions, earlobes, and nailbeds.

The eccrine unit can be divided into the secretory gland, intradermal duct, and intraepidermal duct (Fig. 1-11A). The coiled secretory gland is located in the area of the deep dermis and subcutis (see Fig. 1-11B). Adjacent to the lumen (20-μm diameter) are two types of cells: cells with clear cytoplasm that contain glycogen and cells with dark (basophilic) cytoplasm that contain mucopolysaccharides. These secretory cells overlie a basal lamina that is surrounded by myoepithelial cells and periadnexal dermis (see Fig. 1-11C). Nonmyelinated cholinergic and adrenergic fibers innervate the gland. The intradermal duct coils just before beginning its relatively direct ascent through the dermis. Adjacent to the duct lumen is a PAS-positive eosinophilic cuticle that is produced by the basophilic duct cells. The duct is surrounded also by myoepithelial cells and periadnexal dermis. The intraepidermal duct follows a spiral course through the epidermis to the surface (see Fig. 1-11C). The lumen in this portion of the duct is lined by cells that undergo keratinization independently of adjacent epidermal keratinocytes. The intraepidermal duct cells do not contain melanin granules.

Apocrine Glands and Ducts

Apocrine glands produce secretions that are rendered odoriferous by bacteria. They are most numerous in the axillae and groin but can also be found on the scalp, forehead, and areolae, as well as in the periumbilical region. Also considered to be of apocrine derivation are the mammary glands of the breast, the ceruminous glands of the external auditory canal, and Moll's glands in the eyelid. Apocrine secretions have been difficult to isolate and study because of the proximity of their duct openings to those of sebaceous glands. In animals, apocrine secretions act as pheromones and in thermoregulation, but their function in humans is unclear.

The apocrine unit consists of a secretory coil and an intradermal duct ending in follicular epithelium. The secretory coil is located in the subcutis and has a large (up to 200-μm) lumen surrounded by columnar to cuboidal cells with eosinophilic cytoplasm. The latter often show apical budding for which the glands are named (apocrine means "to separate") (Fig. 1-12). Cytoplasmic granules are present and are best visualized with PAS or iron stains. These secretory cells rest on a basal lamina and are surrounded by elongated myoepithelial cells and periadnexal dermis. Response to cholinergic and adrenergic stimulation, as well as to circulating catecholamines, has been proposed. The intradermal duct ascends in a relatively straight course to the hair follicle, where it opens above the sebaceous duct orifice. The duct also may open directly to the skin surface. The intradermal duct closely resembles its eccrine counterpart. Surrounding the lumen is a double layer of cells with basophilic cytoplasm resting on a basal lamina. The basal lamina is surrounded by myoepithelial cells and periadnexal dermis. The portion of the apocrine duct that traverses the epithelium of the follicle or of the epidermis is less well characterized than that of the eccrine unit.

Fig. **1-12.** *Apocrine gland. The cells appear larger and more eosinophilic than eccrine gland cells (which have clear or amphophilic cytoplasm). Note the appearance of apical budding in some of these cells. Myoepithelial cells are situated external to the glandular epithelium.*

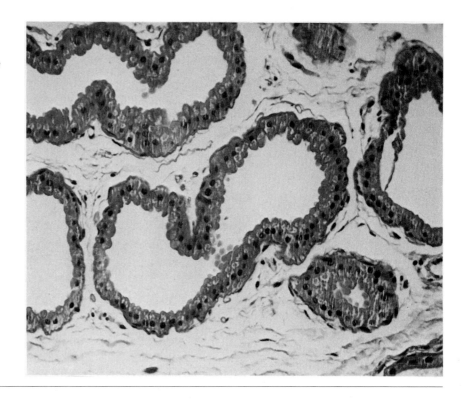

Examples of specialized epidermal structures and regional variation are given in Figure 1-13.

Some disorders exhibit such subtle histologic changes that at first inspection the skin appears normal (see table, inside front cover). Closer examination and/or special stains in the light of the clinical history often yield diagnostic clues.

Fig. **1-13.**
A. *Nail. The nailplate is formed within the nail matrix, the area of indentation. The nail fold lies above the matrix and nail. The structure at the lower left portion of the field is bone with artifactual loss of medulla.*

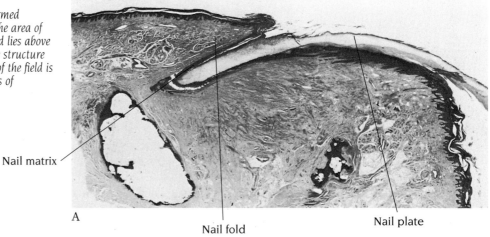

Nail matrix

A

Nail fold

Nail plate

B. Nipple. Primary as well as accessory nipple tissue contains numerous smooth-muscle bundles within the dermis

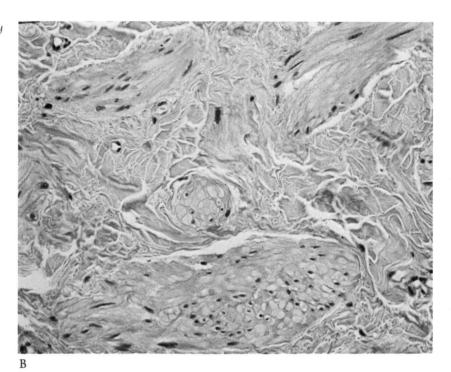

B

C. Scrotal tissue. Many small smooth-muscle bundles and numerous thin-walled vessels are typical of scrotal skin.

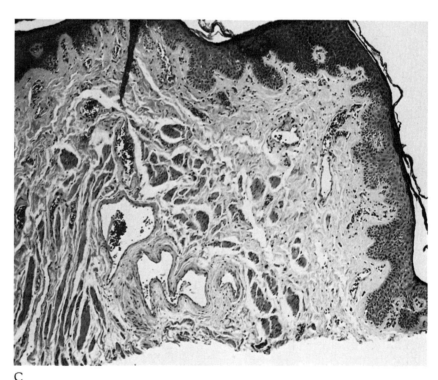

C

Suggested Reading

General

Ackerman, A. B. Skin: Structure and Function. In H*istologic Diagnosis of Inflammatory Skin Diseases.* Philadelphia: Lea & Febiger, 1978.

Lever, W. F., and Schaumberg-Lever, G. Histology of the Skin. In H*istopathology of the Skin* (6th ed.). Philadelphia: Lippincott, 1983.

Mihm, M. C., Soter, N. A., Dvorak, H. F., et al. The structure of normal skin and the morphology of atopic eczema. J. *Invest. Dermatol.* 67:305, 1976.

Pinkus, H., and Mehregan, A. H. Normal Structure of Skin. In Pinkus, H. (Ed.), A *Guide to Dermatohistopathology* (3d ed.). New York: Appleton-Century-Crofts, 1981.

Stenn, K. S., and Bhawan, J. The Normal Histology of the Skin. In Farmer, E. R., and Hood, A. F. (Eds.), *Pathology of the Skin.* Norwalk, CT: Appleton and Lange, 1990.

Urmacher, C. Histology of normal skin. A*m. J. Surg. Pathol.* 14:671, 1990.

Epidermis

Keratinocytes

Dale, B. A. Filaggrin, the matrix protein of keratin. A*m. J. Dermatopathol.* 7:65, 1985.

Fukuyama, K., Inone, N., Suzuki, H., et al. Keratinization. *Int. J. Dermatol.* 15:474, 1976.

Lavker, R. M., and Sun, T-T. Heterogeneity in epidermal basal keratinocytes: Morphological and functional correlations. *Science* 215:1239, 1982.

Montagna, W., and Lobiz, W. C., Jr. (Eds.). *The Epidermis.* New York: Academic, 1964.

Wessels, W. K. Differentiation of epidermis and epidermal derivatives. N. *Engl. J. Med.* 277:21, 1967.

Melanocytes

Montagna, W., and Hu, F. (Eds.). *Advances in Biology of Skin.* Vol. 8. *The Pigmentary System.* New York: Pergamon, 1967.

Langerhans Cells

Basset, F., Soler, P., and Hance, A. J. The Langerhans' cell in human pathology. *Ann. N.Y. Acad. Sci.* 465:324, 1986.

Katz, S. I. The skin as an immunologic organ. J. *Am. Acad. Dermatol.* 13:530, 1985.

Katz, S. I., Tamaki, K., and Sachs, D. H. Epidermal Langerhans cells are derived from cells originating in bone marrow. N*ature* 282:324, 1979.

Stingl, G., Katz, S. I., Clement, L., et al. Immunologic functions of Ia-bearing epidermal Langerhans cells. J. *Immunol.* 121:2005, 1978.

Streilein, J. W., Toews, G. B., and Bergstresser, P. R. Langerhans cells: Functional aspects revealed by *in vivo* grafting studies. J. *Invest. Dermatol.* 75:17, 1980.

Merkel Cells

Gould, V. E., Moll, R., Moll, I., Lee, I., and Franke, W. Neuroendocrine (Merkel) cells of the skin: Hyperplasias, dysplasias and neoplasms. *Lab. Invest.* 52:334, 1985.

Winkelmann, R. K. The Merkel cell system and a comparison between it and the neurosecretory or APUD cell system. J. *Invest. Dermatol.* 69:41, 1977.

Dermoepidermal Junction

Briggaman, R. A., and Wheeler, C. E. The epidermal–dermal junction. J. *Invest. Dermatol.* 66:71, 1975.

Caughman, S. W., Kreig, T., Timpl, R., Hintner, H., and Katz, S. I. Nidogen and heparan sulfate proteoglycan: Detection of newly isolated basement membrane components in normal and epidermolysis bullosa skin. J. *Invest. Dermatol.* 89:547–550, 1987.

Fine, J-D. The skin basement membrane zone. *Adv. Dermatol.* 2:283–303, 1987.

Hodge, S., and Freeman, R. G. The basal lamina in skin disease. *Int. J. Dermatol.* 17:261, 1978.

Katz, S. I. The epidermal basement membrane zone—structure, ontogeny, and role in disease. J. A*m. Acad. Dermatol.* 11:1025, 1984.

Murray, J. C., Stingl, G., Kleinman, H. K., et al. Epidermal cells adhere preferentially to type IV (basement membrane) collagen. J. *Cell Biol.* 80:197, 1979.

Sakai, L. Y., Keene, D. R., Morris, N. P., and Burgeson, R. E. Type VII collagen is a major structural component of anchoring fibrils. *Cell. Biol.* 103:1577–1586, 1986a.

Dermis

Cotta-Pereira, G., Rodrigo, F. G., and Bittencourt-Sampaio, S. Oxytalan, elaunin, and elastic fibers in the human skin. J. Invest. Dermatol. 66:143–148, 1976.

Jarrett, A. (Ed.). The Physiology and Pathophysiology of the Skin. Vol. 3. The Dermis and the Dendrocytes. New York: Academic, 1974.

Kasper, C. S., and Tharp, M. D. Quantification of cutaneous mast cells using morphometric point counting and a conjugated avidin stain. J. Am. Acad. Dermatol. 16:326–331, 1987.

Prockop, D. J., Kivirikko, K. I., Tuderman, L., et al. The biosynthesis of collagen and its disorders. N. Engl. J. Med. 301:13, 77, 1979.

Sandberg, L. B., Suskel, N. T., and Leslie, J. G. Elastin structure, biosynthesis and relation to disease states. N. Engl. J. Med. 304:566, 1981.

Silbert, J. E. Structure and metabolism of proteoglycans and glycosaminoglycans. J. Invest. Dermatol. 79:31s–37s, 1982.

Weber, L., Kirsch, E., Muller, P., and Krieg, T. Collagen type, distribution, and macromolecular organization of connective tissue in different layers of human skin. J. Invest. Dermatol. 82:156–160, 1984.

Blood Vessels

Braverman, I. M., and Keh-Yen, A. Ultrastructure of the human dermal microcirculation. IV. Valve containing collecting veins at the dermal-subcutaneous junction. J. Invest. Dermatol. 81:438–442, 1983.

Braverman, I. M., and Yen, A. Ultrastructure of the human dermal microcirculation II. The capillary loops of the dermal papillae. J. Invest. Dermatol. 68:44–52, 1977.

Moretti, G. The Blood Vessels of the Skin. In O. Gans and G. K. Steigleder (Eds.), Handbuch der Haut-und Geschlechtskrankheiten. Vol. 1., Berlin: Springer-Verlag, 1968, Pp. 491–623.

Ryan, T. J. Structure, Pattern, and Shape of the Blood Vessels of the Skin. In A. Jarrett (Ed.), The Physiology and Pathophysiology of the Skin. Vol. 2. London: Academic, 1973.

Ryan, T. J., Mortimer, P. S., and Jones, R. L. Lymphatics of the skin. Neglected but important. Int. J. Dermatol. 25:411–419, 1986.

Yen, A., and Braverman, I. M. Ultrastructure of the human dermal microcirculation: The horizontal plexus of the papillary dermis. J. Invest. Dermatol. 66:131–142, 1976.

Mast Cells

Bloom, G. D. Structural and biochemical characteristics of mast cells. In B. W. Q. Zwerbach, L. Grant, and R. J. McCluskey (Eds.), The Inflammatory Process. New York: Academic, 1965.

Eady, R. A. J. The mast cells: Distribution and morphology. Clin. Exp. Dermatol. 1:313, 1976.

Lagunoff, D., and Chi, E. Y. Mast cell secretion: Membrane events. J. Invest. Dermatol. 71:81, 1978.

Nerves

Cauna, N. Fine morphological characteristics and microtopography of the free nerve endings of the human digital skin. Anat. Rec. 198:643–656, 1980.

Kenshalo, D. R. (Ed.). International Symposium on the Skin Senses, Second, Florida State University, 1978. New York: Plenum, 1979.

Montagna, W., and Brookhart, J. M. (Eds.). Proceedings of the 26th Annual Symposium on the Biology of Skin: Cutaneous innervation and modalities of cutaneous sensibility. J. Invest. Dermatol. 69:3, 1981.

Pilosebaceous Unit

Hair

Headington, J. T. Transverse microscopic anatomy of the human scalp. Arch. Dermatol. 120:449, 1984.

Johnson, E. Cycles and Patterns of Hair Growth. In A. Jarrett (Ed.), The Physiology and Pathophysiology of the Skin. Vol. 4. New York: Academic, 1977.

Snell, B. S. An electron microscopic study of melanin in the hair and hair follicles. J. Invest. Dermatol. 38:218, 1972.

Spearman, R. I. C. Hair Follicle Development, Cyclical Changes and Hair Form. In A. Jarrett (Ed.), The Physiology and Pathophysiology of the Skin. Vol. 4. New York: Academic, 1977.

Spearman R. I. C. The Structure and Function of the Fully Developed Follicle. In A. Jarrett (Ed.), The Physiology and Pathophysiology of the Skin. Vol. 4. New York: Academic, 1977.

Sebaceous Gland

Montagna, W., Ellis, R. A., and Silver, A. F. (Eds.). *Advances in Biology of Skin*. Vol. 4. *The Sebaceous Glands*. New York: Pergamon, 1963.

Strauss, J. S., and Pochi, P. E. Histology, Histochemistry, and Electron Microscopy of Sebaceous Glands in Man. In O. Gans and G. K. Steigleder (Eds.), *Handbuch der Haut-und Geschlechtskrankheiten*. Berlin: Springer-Verlag, 1968.

Eccrine Glands

Dobson, R. L., and Sato, K. The secretion of salt and water by the eccrine sweat gland. *Arch. Dermatol.* 105:366, 1972.

Ellis, R. A. Eccrine Sweat Glands: Elektron [sic] Microscopy; Cytochemistry and Anatomy. In O. Gans and G. K. Steigleder (Eds.), *Handbuch der Haut-und Geschlechtskrankheiten*. Vol. 1. Berlin: Springer-Verlag, 1968, Pp. 224–266.

Munger, B. L. The ultrastructure and histophysiology of human eccrine sweat glands. *J. Biophys. Biochem. Cytol.* 11:385, 1961.

Apocrine Glands

Hurley, H. J., and Shelley, W. B. *The Human Apocrine Gland in Health and Disease*. Springfield, IL: Thomas, 1960.

Shehadeh, N. H., and Kligman, A. M. Bacteria responsible for axillary odor. II. *J. Invest. Dermatol.* 41:3, 1963.

Chapter 2

Glossary

This glossary introduces the terminology used in dermatopathology. Common pathologic alterations and definitions are listed in the left column. Some diseases in which these alterations can occur are listed on the right.

acantholysis Rounding and loss of cohesion between epidermal cells or adnexal keratinocytes owing to loss of intercellular cement substances or faulty formation of desmosomes (Fig. 2-1).

Pemphigus
Benign familial pemphigus (Hailey–Hailey disease)
Keratosis follicularis (Darier's disease)
Herpes infections

acanthosis Increased thickness of the epidermis caused by hyperplasia or hypertrophy of the spinous layer.

Psoriasis
Squamous cell carcinoma
Pseudoepitheliomatous hyperplasia

apoptosis The process by which dyskeratotic keratinocytes, which form in the epidermis, fall into the papillary dermis.

Lupus erythematosus
Lichen planus
Localized amyloidoses
Graft-versus-host reaction

asteroid body Stellate inclusions with macrophages and multinucleated giant cells; may be found in any chronic granulomatous inflammation.

Sarcoidosis

atrophy Decreased thickness of epidermis and/or dermis.

Lupus erythematosus
Lichen sclerosus
Atrophoderma

ballooning degeneration Epidermal changes characterized by cytoplasmic swelling and vacuolization.

Viral infections (herpes simplex and varicella-zoster)
Epidermolytic hyperkeratosis

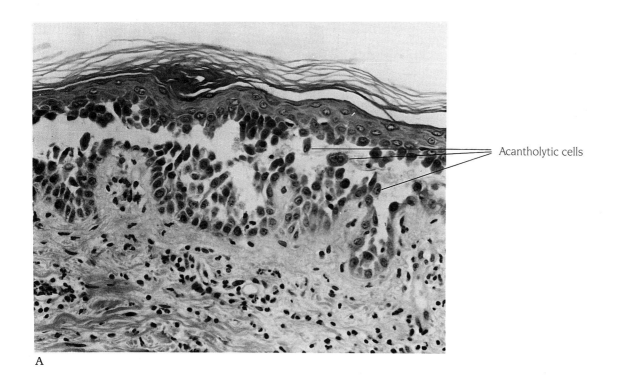

Acantholytic cells

A

Fig. **2-1.**
A. *Acantholysis in a lesion of pemphigus vulgaris at low magnification.*
B. *Acantholysis from a biopsy of benign familial pemphigus (Hailey–Hailey disease).*

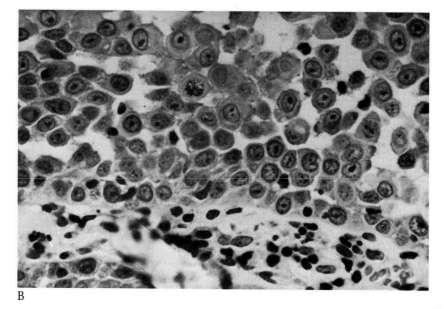

B

birefringence Having the power of double refraction. When examined with polarized light, certain materials "light up." In dermatopathology the most commonly encountered birefringent materials are collagen fibers, hair, silica, amyloid, and uric acid crystals (Fig. 2-2).

Amyloidosis

bulla A blister. The blister cavity and fluid may be located within the epidermis (subcorneal, intraepidermal, suprabasilar) or beneath the epidermis (subepidermal) (Fig. 2-3).

See Chs. 6, 11

caseation Tissue necrosis characterized by eosinophilic, amorphous degeneration of collagen and dermal structures.

Tuberculosis
Lupus miliaris disseminatus faciei
Syphilis

Civatte bodies Homogeneous, eosinophilic round structures seen in the epidermis and upper papillary dermis in various diseases. These structures are altered (dyskeratotic) keratinocytes; they may drop into the dermis (apoptosis) and may evolve into amyloid. Also called colloid, or hyaline bodies.

Lichen planus
Lupus erythematosus

colloid bodies *See* Civatte bodies.

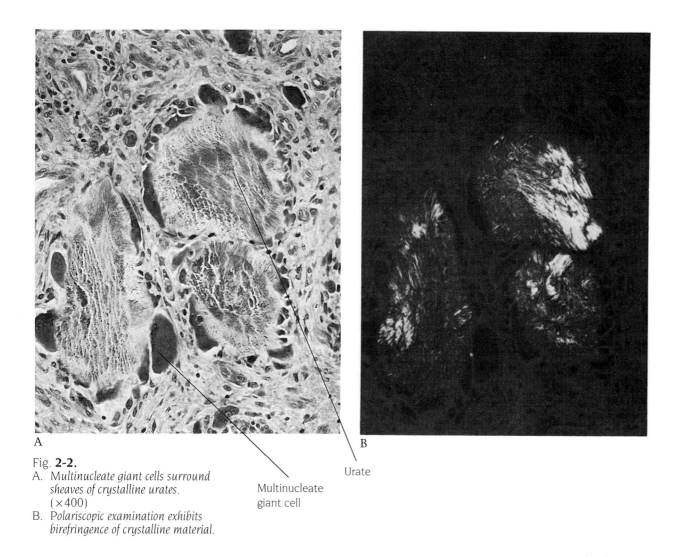

A

B

Fig. **2-2.**
A. *Multinucleate giant cells surround sheaves of crystalline urates. (×400)*
B. *Polariscopic examination exhibits birefringence of crystalline material.*

Urate

Multinucleate giant cell

Fig. **2-3.** Bullous (and vesicular) disorders are classified according to the location of the cleft. (Reprinted with permission from T. H. Kwan and M. C. Mihm. The Skin. In S. L. Robbins and R. S. Cotran (Eds.), Pathologic Basis of Disease (2nd ed.). Philadelphia: Saunders, 1979.)

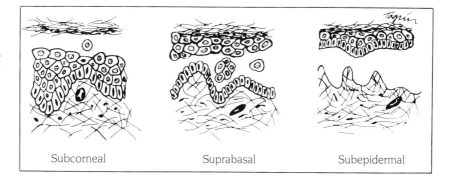

Subcorneal   Suprabasal   Subepidermal

cornoid lamella Wedge-shaped column of parakeratosis sometimes arising in an epidermal invagination. Underlying epidermis often thinned, with few dyskeratotic cells (Fig. 2-4).

Porokeratosis
Seborrheic keratosis
Verruca vulgaris
Actinic keratosis
Squamous cell carcinoma *in situ*
Basal cell carcinoma

corps grains; corps ronds Dyskeratotic, acantholytic basophilic epidermal cells, which may be oval (corps grains) or round (corps ronds). The latter usually have perinuclear halos.

Keratosis follicularis (Darier's disease)
Warty dyskeratoma
Transient acantholytic disease

curvilinear bodies *See* Farber body.

decapitation secretion Term used to describe the mechanism of apocrine secretion whereby the apical portion of the cell is "pinched off" and released into the lumen of the gland (see Fig. 1-12).

Donovan body Ovoid structures in granuloma inguinale displaying bipolar highlights within a capsule; best seen with Giemsa or silver stains. These bodies are intracytoplasmic inclusions within macrophages.

dyskeratosis Abnormal, imperfect, or incomplete keratinization of individual keratinocytes. Histologically dyskeratotic cells are shrunken and intensely eosinophilic and may contain a small, dense basophilic nuclear remnant (Fig. 2-5). Dyskeratosis also refers to densely basophilic cytoplasmic change (as in Darier's disease).

exocytosis A term used to indicate leukocytes and erythrocytes that are "out of place," i.e., in the epidermis instead of the dermis or blood vessels.

Mycosis fungoides
Pityriasis lichenoides et varioliformis acuta
Eczematous dermatitis

Fig. **2-4.** *Cornoid lamella. The column of parakeratotic cells, typical of porokeratosis, rests within an epidermal invagination and overlies an area of hypogranulosis and dyskeratosis.*

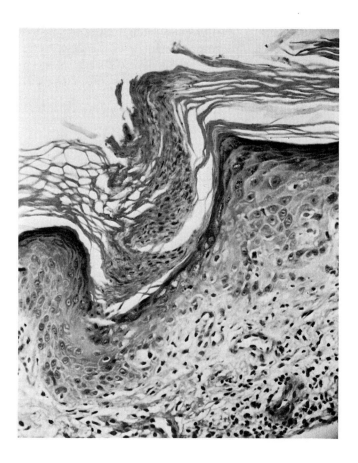

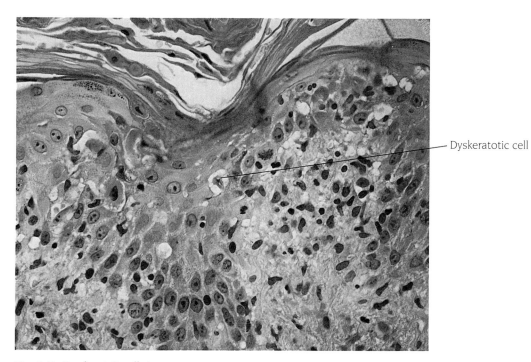

—Dyskeratotic cell

Fig. **2-5.** *Dyskeratotic cells in erythema multiforme.*

Farber body Inclusions that
assume the shape of a comma
and are present within vacuoles
of fibroblasts and macrophages,
also known as curvilinear
bodies. Visible with electron
microscopy.

Farber's disease
  (lipogranulomatosis)

**fibrinoid necrosis of blood
vessels** Deposition of
eosinophilic fibrin in and
around vessel walls (Fig. 2-6).

Necrotizing vasculitis

foam cell Lipid-laden macrophage
with pale vacuolated or "foamy"
cytoplasm and a round to oval
dark-staining nucleus.

Xanthomas
Juvenile xanthogranuloma

ghost cell (shadow cell) Pale,
faintly eosinophilic cell with
central unstained area where the
nucleus was located (Fig. 2-7).

Pilomatrixoma

giant cell Large, multinucleate
cell that may be seen in the
epidermis or dermis. Epidermal
multinucleate keratinocytes are seen
in a variety of situations; when
associated with viral infections
such as herpes simplex and
measles, characteristic nuclear
inclusions and cytopathic effects
can be observed. Multinucleate
giant cells in the dermis may be
derived from *nevocellular nevus cells*
or histiocytes. Histiocytic giant
cells with nuclei arranged in a
horseshoe at the periphery are
known as *Langhans-type* giant
cells. *Touton-type* histiocytic giant
cells characteristically have a
ring of nuclei arranged around a
central core of cytoplasm; foamy
cytoplasm is seen peripheral to
the nuclei. *Foreign-body*
histiocytic giant cells have
nuclei haphazardly scattered
throughout the cytoplasm.

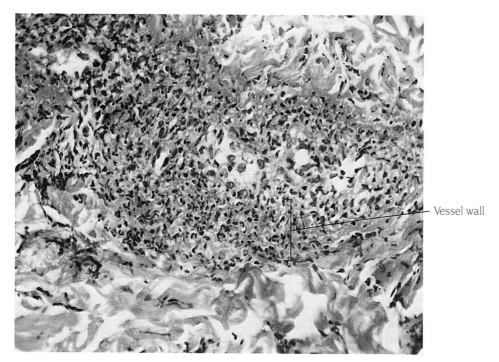

Vessel wall

Fig. **2-6.** Fibrinoid necrosis and
nuclear dust in cutaneous necrotizing
vasculitis.

Fig. **2-7.** Ghost (shadow) cells in
pilomatrixoma.

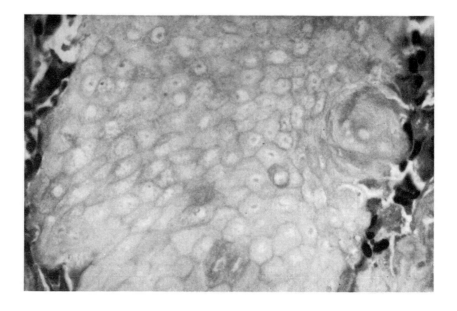

grenz zone A clear area of uninvolved (usually papillary) dermis between the epidermis and inflammatory or neoplastic infiltrate. From the German *Grenze* meaning "border."

Granuloma faciale
Lymphoma cutis, B cell

Guarnieri body Bodies that occur as eosinophilic, intracytoplasmic inclusions within keratinocytes infected with vaccinia or smallpox.

hamartoma An abnormal arrangement and excessive collection of otherwise normal tissue element(s). Nevus sebaceous represents a hamartoma.

Henderson–Patterson body *See* molluscum body.

histiocytic cell Mononuclear cell distinguished from lymphocytes by an oval, pale-staining nucleus, abundant eosinophilic cytoplasm derived from the monocyte–macrophage cell line in the bone marrow. These cells cannot always be distinguished from lymphocytes by light microscopy.

horn cyst Intraepidermal, keratin-filled space resembling a cyst. "Pseudohorn cysts" are formed by obvious epidermal invagination.

Seborrheic keratosis

hyperkeratosis An increase in the thickness of the stratum corneum. The thickened stratum corneum may retain its basketweave pattern, may appear delicately layered (stratified, laminated), or may become dense and compact. The term *hyperkeratosis* is used to describe the thickening of the normal anucleate stratum corneum in contrast to the term *parakeratosis*, which describes the thickened stratum corneum with retained keratinocyte nuclei.

Lamellar ichthyosis and ichthyosis vulgaris
Pityriasis rosea
Psoriasis

Parakeratosis, which infers incomplete keratinization, is seen normally in mucous membranes and abnormally in association with numerous inflammatory and neoplastic processes.

hyperplasia An increase in the number of cells in a given tissue.

hypertrophy An increase in the size of a cell.

Kamino body Eosinophilic globules resembling dyskeratotic keratinocytes within the epidermis in spindle and epithelioid cell nevi. They are also seen in melanoma, although in lesser number.

koilocyte An enlarged epithelial cell, usually in the upper epidermis, containing an eccentrically placed, basophilic, shrunken nucleus surrounded by a clear halo. Deeply basophilic cytoplasmic granules are present, representing altered keratohyalin. Koilocytes are typical of infection with human papillomavirus. Viral inclusions may be identified.

Langhans giant cell *See* giant cell.

melanophage Histiocyte containing phagocytized melanin.

Postinflammatory hyperpigmentation
Lentigo
Cellular blue nevus
Fixed drug eruption

Michaelis–Gutman body Small basophilic bodies present within macrophages in malakoplakia. Special stains for calcium may identify those Michaelis–Gutman bodies invested with laminated material.

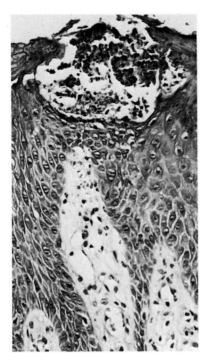

Fig. **2-8.** *Munro microabscess in psoriasis.*

molluscum body Visible as eosinophilic or basophilic intracytoplasmic inclusions within the spinous layer of the epidermis infected by molluscum contagiosum virus. The inclusions become very large toward the granular layer of the epidermis and often coalesce in epidermal invaginations near the surface. Also known as Henderson–Patterson bodies.

Munro microabscess Neutrophil aggregates within the stratum corneum (Fig. 2-8).

necrobiosis A form of collagen alteration with loss of normal eosinophilia and fibrillar appearance, becoming smudged due to loss of integrity of collagen fibers and bundles, more basophilic in association with deposition of acid mucopolysaccharides, and having loss of fibroblast nuclei with residual nuclear debris.   Necrobiosis lipoidica

nuclear dust Nuclear fragments scattered in the dermis, usually around blood vessels (see Fig. 2-6).   Vasculitis

Odland body An ovoid organelle within spinous layer keratinocytes that fuses with the cytoplasmic membrane, releasing lipid-rich, hydrophobic molecules into the intercellular space. Also known as lamellar bodies, keratinosomes, membrane coating granules, and cementosomes.

papillomatosis Epidermal and papillary dermal proliferation upward in irregular waves or spires (Fig. 2-9).   Seborrheic keratosis, hyperkeratotic type
Verruca

Fig. **2-9.**
A. *Papillomatosis in acanthosis nigricans.*
B. *Papillomatosis in this lesion is flatter.*

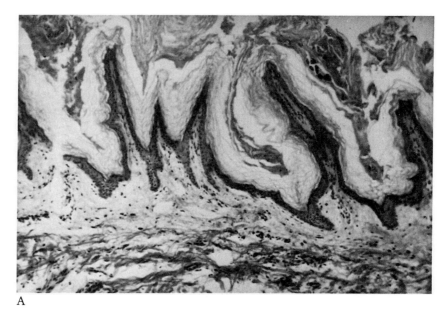

A

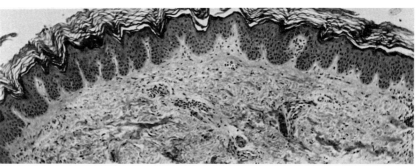

B

Pautrier microabscess A collection of three or more atypical lymphocytes within the epidermis, often surrounded by a clear space, or "halo."

Mycosis fungoides

pigment incontinence Deposition of melanin in the dermis, as either free particles or particles within macrophages (melanophages).

Lentigo
Postinflammatory hyperpigmentation

pleomorphic Variation in cellular and nuclear size and shape.

polymorphous With reference to inflammatory infiltrates, this term connotes a mixed infiltrate, e.g., a mixture of lymphocytes, eosinophils, and plasma cells, in contrast to a purely lymphocytic infiltrate.

Mycosis fungoides
Arthropod bite reaction

psammoma body Inclusion that is a calcified mass with a laminated appearance characteristic of meningioma, thyroid carcinoma, and nevocellular nevi.

pseudoepitheliomatous hyperplasia Reactive process of the epidermis characterized by irregular acanthosis with downward proliferation of the epidermis. Often accompanied by chronic dermal inflammation. The massive degree of proliferation may simulate a well-differentiated squamous cell carcinoma.

Chronic cutaneous ulcers
Fungal and mycobacterial infections
Pyoderma gangrenosum
Pemphigus vegetans
Halogenoderma
Granular cell tumor

pustule Fluid-filled space (usually intraepidermal) containing leukocytes and products of inflammation.

Impetigo
Pustular psoriasis
Erythema toxicum neonatorum
Incontinentia pigmenti, first stage

pustulo-ovoid body of Milian Inclusions that are present as round eosinophilic bodies within the cytoplasm of granular cell tumors.

pyknosis Condensation of nuclear chromatin, producing a dense, shrunken mass.

Usually occurs with cell death

reticular degeneration Intracellular edema of keratinocytes with retention of cell walls, producing a reticular, or netlike, appearance (Fig. 2-10).

Viral infections
Epidermolytic hyperkeratosis
Acute eczematous dermatitis

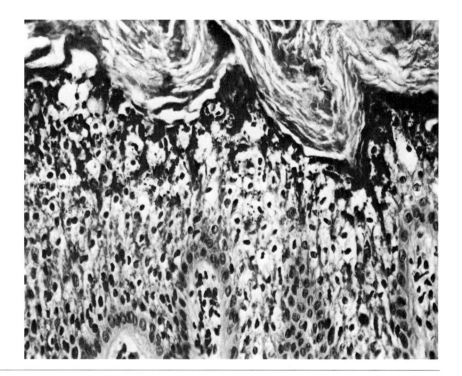

Fig. **2-10.** *Reticular degeneration in epidermolytic hyperkeratosis.*

Russell body Cytoplasmic accumulation of immunoglobulin within plasma cells that appear as refractile, eosinophilic inclusions. Found in any disease with numerous infiltrating plasma cells.

Syphilis

Schaumann body Lamellated, round, calcified inclusions within macrophages and multinucleated giant cells. May be found in any chronic granulomatous inflammation.

Sarcoidosis

spongiform pustule Collections of neutrophils within the epidermis, often surrounded by clear spaces, or "halos," thus somewhat resembling a sponge.

Psoriasis
Reiter's disease
Geographic tongue
Pustular psoriasis

spongiosis Intercellular edema in the epidermis with separation of keratinocytes and stretching of intercellular bridges (Fig. 2-11). Edematous spaces can coalesce, forming spongiotic vesicles.

Acute eczematous dermatitis

squamatization Replacement of normally cuboidal or columnar, slightly basophilic basal cells by polygonal or flattened eosinophilic keratinocytes (Fig. 2-12).

Lichen planus
Lupus erythematosus
Graft-versus-host reaction

squamous eddy A round or whorled focus of keratinized epidermal cells with brightly eosinophilic cytoplasm, surrounded by keratinocytes without notable keratinization.

Squamous cell carcinoma
Inverted follicular keratosis
"Irritated" seborrheic keratosis

storiform Refers to the cartwheel pattern formed by spindle cells, which appear to emanate from a central anucleate area, recalling the spokes of a wheel. This pattern frequently is seen in fibrous histiocytoma and dermatofibrosarcoma protuberans, but other spindle-cell tumors such as leiomyomas can mimic this pattern.

Fibrous histiocytoma
Dermatofibrosarcoma protuberans

Touton giant cell *See* giant cell.

vacuolization Presence of small, clear spaces, or vacuoles, beneath the basilar epidermis.

Lupus erythematosus
Lichen planus
Erythema multiforme
Graft-versus-host disease
Incipient subepidermal blisters
Lichenoid infiltrate

Verocay body Occurs in the Antoni type A tissue of neurilemmomas as parallel arrays of nuclei bordering a zone of eosinophilic fibrillar material.

Neurilemmoma

vesicle Small blister (see Fig. 2-3).

See Chs. 6,11

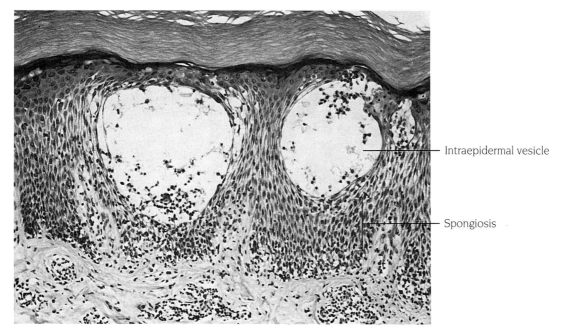

Intraepidermal vesicle

Spongiosis

Fig. **2-11.** *Spongiosis and spongiotic vesicles in a biopsy of nummular eczema.*

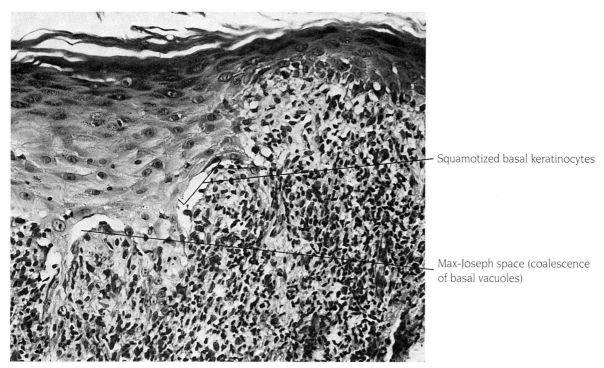

Squamotized basal keratinocytes

Max-Joseph space (coalescence of basal vacuoles)

Fig. **2-12.** *Squamatization in lichen planus.*

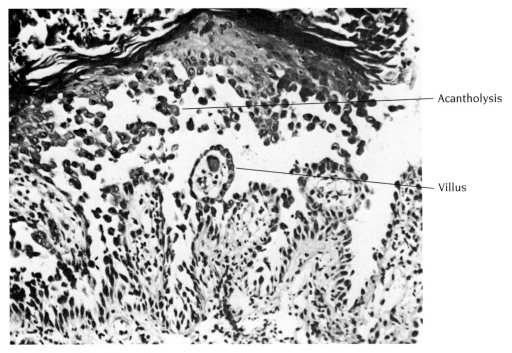

Acantholysis

Villus

Fig. **2-13.** *Villi in a biopsy of
pemphigus vulgaris.*

---

villus Prominent dermal papilla in acantholytic disorders, lined by a row of basal cells, thus resembling "tombstones on a hill" (Fig. 2-13).

Pemphigus
Darier's disease
Warty dyskeratoma

Weibel–Palade body Unique structure identified by electron microscopy that is found within normal endothelial cells. Appears as an electron-dense rodshaped organelle composed of tubules in parallel configuration.

zebra body Resides in endothelial cells as membranous lipid vacuoles. Visible with electron microscopy.

Farber's disease (lipogranulomatosis)

Chapter **3**

Histochemistry

Special Stains

Material to Be Demonstrated	Stains	Results
Actinomyces	Brown–Brenn Gram–Weigert MacCallum–Goodpasture	Organism: blue
Acid mucopolysaccharides (AMPS)	Alcian blue at pH 2.5 and 0.5 Colloidal iron Crystal violet Toluidine blue	AMPS: light blue AMPS: blue to light green AMPS: metachromatic magenta AMPS: metachromatic magenta
Amyloid	Congo red Congo red and polarized light Crystal violet Thioflavin-T	Amyloid: pale pink to red Amyloid: red with green birefringence Amyloid: purplish red (metachromasia) Amyloid: fluoresces with ultraviolet radiation
Bacteria	Brown–Brenn Gram–Weigert MacCallum–Goodpasture	Gram-positive bacteria: blue Gram-negative bacteria: red
Basement membrane	Periodic acid–Schiff (PAS) Jones methenamine silver	Basement membrane: red Basement membrane: black
Blood cells	Giemsa Chloracetate esterase (Leder) neutrophils & mast cells	Erythrocytes: red Leukocytes: cytoplasm, light blue; nucleus, dark blue Granules: red
Blood vessel walls	Verhoeff elastic Periodic acid–Schiff (PAS) Gormori's aldehyde fuchsin	Elastic membrane: black Basement membrane: red Elastic fibers, mucin: deep purple
Calcium	Alizarin red-S Von Kossa	Calcium: orange-red Calcium salts: black
Collagen	Malloy aniline blue Masson trichrome Van Gieson Movat's pentachrome	Collagen: blue Elastic fibers: pale yellow Mature collagen, mucin: green Keratin, nuclei, muscle fibers, nerve fibers: dark red Mature collagen: red Muscle, nerves: yellow Collagen, reticular fibers: yellow Nuclei, elastic fibers: black Muscle: red Ground substance, mucin: blue Fibrinoid: intense red
Cryptococcus	Alcian blue Mucicarmine Periodic acid–Schiff (PAS)	Capsule: blue Capsule: red Cell wall of organism: red
Donovan bodies	Giemsa Warthin-Starry	Organism: blue Organism: black
Elastic fibers	Verhoeff–van Gieson Weigert's resorcin–fuchsin Acid orcein	Elastic fibers: blue-black to black Elastic fibers: violet to purple Elastic fibers: dark brown
Fat	*See* lipids	
Fibrin	Phosphotungstic acid-hematoxylin (PTAH)	Fibrin: deep blue

Material to be Demonstrated	Stains	Results
Fungi	Gomori methenamine silver (GMS) Periodic acid–Schiff (PAS) *See* Cryptococcus, *Histoplasma*	Fungus walls: black Fungus: red
Glycogen	Best's carmine Periodic acid–Schiff with and without diastase digestion	Glycogen: pink to red Glycogen is PAS-positive (pink) before but not after diastase digestion
Hemosiderin	*See* iron	
Histoplasma capsulatum	Giemsa	Organism: reddish blue
Leishmania bodies	Giemsa	Organism: reddish blue
Iron	Perl's potassium ferrocyanide Prussian blue Turnbull blue Gomori's iron reaction	Iron: blue
Lipids: frozen sections of fresh or formalin-fixed tissue	Oil-red O Sudan Black B Scharlack R	Fat: orange to bright red Fat: black Fat: bright red
Mast cells	Giemsa Toluidine blue Naphthol AS-D chloacetate esterase activity (Leder)	Metachromatic granules: magenta and blue
Melanin	Fontana–Masson	Red melanin: black granules
Mucin	Mucicarmine (*See* also acid mucopolysaccharides, mucoprotein)	Mucin: red

Mucoprotein
  With acid mucopolysaccharides
  With neutral mucopolysaccharides
	Alcian blue
	Toluidine blue
	Mucicarmine
	Colloidal iron
	Periodic acid–Schiff (PAS) with diastase digestion
		Mucin: blue
		Mucin: magenta
		Mucin: red
		Mucin: blue to light green
		Mucin: pink; no change after diastase digestion

Muscle	Masson trichrome Phosphotungstic acid–hematoxylin (PTAH)	Muscle: red Collagen: green Muscle: blue to purple

Mycobacteria	Acid-fast stains:
	  Ziehl-Neelsen
	  Putt-Fite
	  Kinyoun's carbol fuchsin
	  Wade-Fite
		Mycobacteria: bright red
		
		This modification is favored for the demonstration of M. *leprae*

Nerve	Bodian Osmium tetroxide	Axons: black Myelin: black

Nocardia	Gram stains:
	  Brown-Brenn
	  Gram-Weigert
	  MacCallum–Goodpasture
	Gomori methenamine silver (GMS)
	Acid-fast stains:
	  Ziehl-Neelsen
	  Putt-Fite
		Organism: irregularly blue
		
		Organism: black
		
		Organism: bright red

Plasma cells	Giemsa	Cytoplasm: blue
	Methyl green–pyronin (MGP)	Cytoplasm: red
Reticulum fibers (type III collagen fibers)	Foot	Reticulum fibers, melanin, nerves: black Collagen: rose red
	Wilder Gridley	} Reticulum fibers: black
Rickettsia	Giemsa	Organism: blue to violet
Spirochetes	Modified Steiner Warthin–Starry Dieterle	} Organism: black

Immunohistochemistry

The use of monoclonal and polyclonal antibodies directed against various antigens found in normal and diseased skin has greatly affected the daily practice of dermatopathology. Application of the antisera to fixed or frozen tissue sections and subsequent procedures designed to promote visualization of bound antibody—for example, the avidin–biotin bridge—aid in determinations of cell type (e.g., anti-cytokeratin for epithelial cells; cellular activity (e.g., anti-intercellular adhesion molecule-1 for keratinocyte "activation" by gamma-interferon), and basement membrane zone structure (e.g., anti–type IV collagen to highlight the basement membrane lined "slits" of Kaposi's sarcoma). Readers are directed to more detailed references regarding the procedures, uses, and interpretation of immunohistology using monoclonal and polyclonal antibodies. Table 3-1 summarizes several commonly used antibodies against antigens stable in formalin-fixed and paraffin-embedded tissue.

Table **3-1.** *Selected Commonly Employed Antibodies in Immunohistochemistry*

Antibody	Specificity in Skin	Comments
1. Anti-S-100	Neural crest derived cells; Langerhans cells, acrosyringium	Decorates both benign and malignant melanocytic lesions
2. Anti-cytokeratin	Keratinocyte; adnexal epithelia	Decorates tumors of keratinocytic origin and metastatic carcinomas
3. Anti-desmin	Smooth and skeletal muscle	Decorates leiomyoma and leiomyosarcoma
4. Anti-vimentin	Cells of mesenchymal origin	Useful in distinguishing carcinoma from sarcoma
5. Anti-carcinoembryonic antigen (CEA)	Eccrine and apocrine apparatus	Useful in identifying tumors with glandular element, primary and metastatic in the skin
6. Anti-epithelial membrane antigen (EMA)	Normal epidermis; eccrine, apocrine, and sebaceous glands	Useful in identifying carcinomas
7. Anti–common leukocyte antigen (CLA)	Inflammatory cells	Helpful in identifying inflammatory and neoplastic infiltrates
8. Anti-alpha-l-chymotrypsin	Fibrohistiocytic cells	Positive staining obtained in atypical fibroxanthoma
9. Anti–type IV collagen	Basement membranes	Aids in identification of Kaposi's sarcoma
10. Anti–factor VIII related antigen	Endothelial cells	Useful in identifying blood vessels, lymphatics, and vascular tumors
11. Anti–factor XIIIa related antigen	Dermal dendritic cells	Decorates dermatofibroma and dermatofibrosarcoma protuberans
12. Anti-cytokeratin 20	Merkel cells	Stains Merkel cell carcinoma
13. MART-1	Melanocytes	Identifying melanoma
14. HMB-45	Melanocytes	Identifying melanoma
15. Anti-CD1a	Langerhans cells	Langerhans cell histiocytosis
16. Anti-CD3	Pan T cell marker	Lymphocyte subsets
17. Anti-CD4	T helper cells	Lymphoma diagnoses
18. Anti-CD8	T cytotoxic suppressors	Lymphoma diagnoses
19. Anti-CD20	Pan B cell marker	Lymphoma diagnoses
20. Anti-CD31	Endothelial cells	Vascular neoplasms
21. Anti-CD34	Endothelial cells dermal spindle cells	Vascular neoplasms, dermatofibrosarcoma
22. Anti-CD43	Pan T cell marker	Lymphoma diagnoses
23. Anti-CD56	NK marker	NK lymphoma marker
24. Anti-CD68	Histiocytes	Useful for xanthogranuloma, lymphoma

Suggested Reading

Bancroft, J. D., and Stevens, A. *Theory and Practice of Histologic Techniques.* New York: Churchill Livingstone, 1977.

Clark, G. *Staining Procedures* (2nd ed.). Baltimore, MD: Williams & Wilkins, 1973.

Doherty, M. J., Russo, G. G., and Jolly, H. W., et al. Immunoenzyme techniques in dermatopathology. *J. Am. Acad. Dermatol.* 20:827–837, 1989.

Graham, J. H., Johnson, W. C., and Helwig, E. B. (Eds.). *Dermal Pathology.* Hagerstown, MD: Harper & Row, 1972.

Jennette, J. C. (ed.). *Immunohistology in Diagnostic Pathology.* Boca Raton, Fl: CRC Press, 1989.

Lillie, R. W. *Histopathologic Technic and Practical Histochemistry* (3rd ed.). New York: McGraw-Hill, 1965.

Luna, L. G. *Manual of Histologic Staining Methods of the Armed Forces Institute of Pathology* (3rd ed.). New York: McGraw-Hill, 1968.

Preece, A. A *Manual for Histologic Technicians* (3rd ed.). London: J&A Churchill, 1972.

Sheehan, D. C., and Hrapchak, B. B. *Theory and Practice of Histotechnology.* St. Louis: Mosby, 1973.

Part **II**

Epidermis

Chapter 4

Hyperkeratosis with or without Alteration of the Granular Layer

    I. Ichthyosis vulgaris
    II. Dominant congenital ichthyosiform erythroderma (*epidermolytic hyperkeratosis*)
    III. Recessive congenital ichthyosiform erythroderma (*lamellar ichthyosis*)
    IV. X-linked ichthyosis
    V. Acquired ichthyosis
    VI. Ichthyoses associated with congenital syndromes
    VII. Superficial fungal and yeast infections

The predominant histologic change demonstrated by the diseases discussed in this chapter is hyperkeratosis, or thickening of the stratum corneum. With the exception of dominant ichthyosiform erythroderma (epidermolytic hyperkeratosis), there is very little alteration in the epidermis or dermis in these diseases; in fact, this change may be subtle and easily overlooked on cursory examination. Many other diseases have hyperkeratosis as a prominent histologic feature, but the hyperkeratosis is associated with other epidermal changes such as hyperplasia, atrophy, and dermal inflammation. These diseases are discussed in subsequent chapters. The absence of a specific histologic finding does not preclude the diagnosis of a specific type of ichthyosis. Diagnosis must be based on clinicopathologic and laboratory correlation.

The Reactive Process and the Disease	Histopathology	Comments
I. Ichthyosis vulgaris	1. Mild to moderate basketweave or compact **hyperkeratosis** 2. Decreased to absent granular layer (**hypogranulosis**) 3. Flattened rete ridges	*Hypogranulosis* may be seen in: Ichthyosis vulgaris Psoriasis Normal mucous membrane Under parakeratotic scale associated with inflammation Nutritional deficiencies such as acrodermatitis enteropathica and pellagra
Pathophysiology: *In familial ichthyosis vulgaris, profilaggrin and filaggrin are reduced or absent. The abnormality correlates with the amount of keratohyalin and clinical severity. Filaggrin is present in keratohyaline granules and plays a role in keratin filament arrangements.*		
	4. Atrophic to absent sebaceous glands	Characteristic histologic changes; of ichthyosis are best seen in areas of maximal involvement. Biopsies obtained from less severely affected areas may be histologically indistinguishable from normal skin
II. Dominant congenital ichthyosiform erythroderma (*epidermolytic hyperkeratosis*) (Fig. 4-1)	1. Marked **compact hyperkeratosis**	Clinical term *epidermolytic hyperkeratosis* is synonymous with dominant congenital ichthyosiform erythroderma; the term also refers to the histologic changes of reticular degeneration and abnormal granule formation seen in other diseases, such as palmar and plantar epidermolytic hyperkeratosis and epidermolytic acanthoma

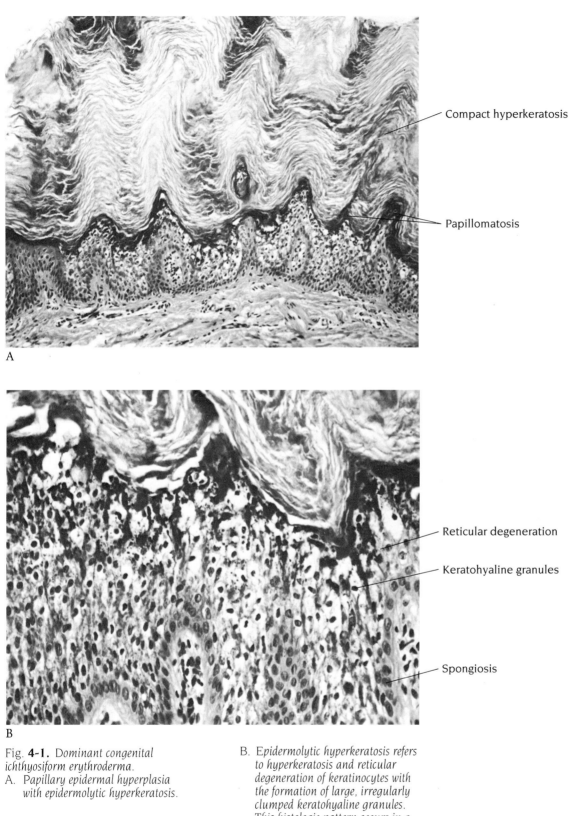

Compact hyperkeratosis

Papillomatosis

A

Reticular degeneration

Keratohyaline granules

Spongiosis

B

Fig. **4-1.** Dominant congenital ichthyosiform erythroderma.
A. Papillary epidermal hyperplasia with epidermolytic hyperkeratosis.

B. Epidermolytic hyperkeratosis refers to hyperkeratosis and reticular degeneration of keratinocytes with the formation of large, irregularly clumped keratohyaline granules. This histologic pattern occurs in a variety of other conditions besides ichthyosis.

2. Prominent granular layer with **reticular degeneration** and abnormal granules (irregular, dark basophilic keratohyaline and eosinophilic trichohyaline-like granules)
3. Intercellular edema of slightly thickened epidermis

Foci of *epidermolytic hyperkeratosis* may be seen in:

Normal skin
Actinic keratosis
Lining of an epidermal cyst
Adjacent to or within squamous cell carcinoma
Seborrheic keratosis
Granuloma annulare
Verruca plana
Dermatofibroma
Systematized linear epidermal nevus

III. Recessive congenital ichthyosiform erythroderma (*lamellar ichthyosis*) (Fig. 4-2).

1. Moderate compact **hyperkeratosis**
2. Focal parakeratosis
3. Normal to increased granular layer

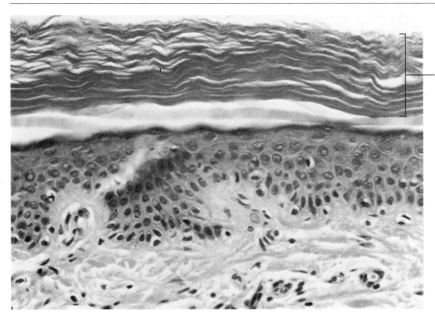

Compact and laminated hyperkeratosis

Fig. **4-2.** *Recessive congenital ichthyosiform erythroderma (lamellar ichthyosis). The stratum spinosum appears unremarkable, but the stratum corneum exhibits compact and laminated hyperkeratosis. Compare this stratum corneum with that of Figure 1-2.*

IV. X-linked ichthyosis

Pathophysiology: *Steroid sulfatase activity is reduced or absent in patients with X-linked ichthyosis. Unregulated cholesterol sulfate in the stratum corneum produces greater cell adhesion and therefore a retention of squames*

1. Moderate compact, laminated, brightly eosinophilic **hyperkeratosis**
2. Parakeratosis
3. Increased granular layer (**hypergranulosis**)
4. Sparse perivascular and periappendageal lymphocytic infiltrate

Hypergranulosis may be seen in any hyperkeratotic lesion but is characteristically seen in:

Epidermolytic hyperkeratosis
X-linked ichthyosis
Prurigo nodularis
Lichen simplex chronicus
Epidermal nevus
Verruca vulgaris
Lichen planus and its variants

V. Acquired ichthyosis

Histology is identical to that of ichthyosis vulgaris

VI. Ichthyoses associated with congenital syndromes

1. Histology is identical to that of ichthyosis in most cases
2. Refsum's syndrome displays basilar and suprabasilar vacuoles

Some syndromes with ichthyosis include Sjögren–Larsson syndrome, Rud's syndrome, Conradi's syndrome, and Netherton's syndrome
In Refsum's syndrome, there is an abnormality of phytanic acid metabolism with accumulation of lipid in the skin and other organs

VII. Superficial fungal and yeast infections (Fig. 4-3)

1. Hyphal or pseudohyphal forms are present in the stratum corneum and sometimes the stratum granulosum (see Fig. 4-3A,B)
2. Yeast forms may be present; yeast forms alone can be seen as a normal commensal
3. Parakeratosis, epidermal hyperplasia, spongiosis, vesiculation, and exocytosis may be variably present
4. Superficial perivascular and interstitial mononuclear cell infiltrates are typical
5. Neutrophilic infiltrates within the epidermis are variable

Special stains (see Ch. 3) such as PAS highlight organisms

Candidiasis exhibits yeast and pseudohyphal forms (see Fig. 4-3C)
Invasive superficial fungi may be seen in immunocompromised states

Fig. **4-3.**
A,B. *Dermatophytosis. PAS stain delineates these septate hyphae within the stratum corneum.*
C. *Candidiasis. Yeast and pseudohyphae are present within the stratum corneum and stratum granulosum.*

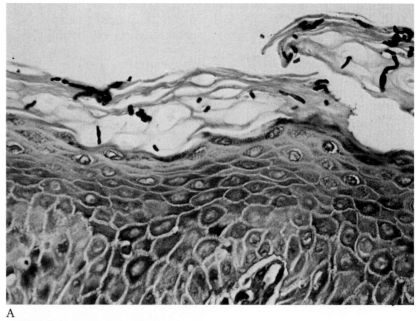

A

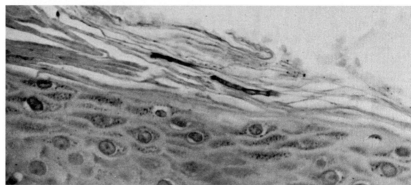

B

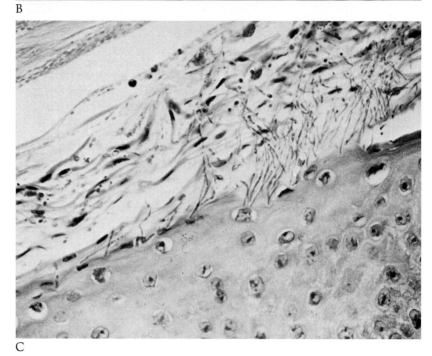

C

Suggested Reading

Ichthyosis

Ackerman, A. B. Histopathologic concept of epidermolytic hyperkeratosis. *Arch. Dermatol.* 102:253, 1970.

Baden, H. P., Hooker, P. A., Kubilus, J., and Tarascio, A. Sulfatase activity of keratinizing tissues in X-linked ichthyosis. *Pediatr. Res.* 14:1347, 1980.

Dykes, P.J., and Mark, R. Acquired ichthyosis: Multiple causes for an acquired generalized disturbance in desquamation. *Br. J. Dermatol.* 97:327, 1977.

Epstein, E. H., Krauss, R. M., and Shackleton, C. H. L. X-linked ichthyosis: Increased blood cholesterol sulfate and electrophoretic mobility of low density lipoprotein. *Science* 214:659, 1981.

Feinstein, A., Ackerman, A. B., and Ziprkowski, L. Histology of autosomal dominant ichthyosis vulgaris and X-linked ichthyosis. *Arch. Dermatol.* 101:524, 1970.

Flint, G. L., Flam, M., and Soter, N.A. Acquired ichthyosis: A sign of nonlymphoproliferative malignant disorders. *Arch. Dermatol.* 111:1446, 1975.

Frost, P. Ichthyosiform dermatoses. *J. Invest. Dermatol.* 60:541, 1973.

Goldsmith, L. A. The ichthyoses. *Prog. Med. Genet.* 1:185, 1976.

Marks, R., and Dykes, P.J. *The Ichthyoses.* New York: S.P. Medical and Scientific Books, 1978.

Sybert, V. P., Dale, B. A., and Holbrook, K. A. Ichthyosis vulgaris: Identification of a defect in synthesis of filaggrin correlated with an absence of keratohyaline granules. *J. Invest. Dermatol.* 84:191, 1985.

Vandersteen, P. R., and Muller, S. A. Lamellar ichthyosis: An enzyme histochemical light, and electron microscopic study. *Arch. Dermatol.* 106:694, 1972.

Van Scott, E. J., and Yu, R. J. "Ichthyosiform dermatoses" by Frost and Van Scott, August 1966. Commentary: Ichthyosis and keratinization. Concepts in transition. *Arch. Dermatol.* 118:846, 1982.

Dermatophytosis

Rebell, G., and Iaplin, D. *Dermatophytes: Their Recognition and Identification* (rev. ed.). Coral Gables, FLa.: University of Miami Press, 1970.

Stretcher, G. S., and Smith, J. G. Diagnosis and treatment of cutaneous fungus diseases. *D.M.* 1–40, September 1975.

Svejgaard, E. Immunologic investigations of dermatophytoses and dermatophytosis. *Semin. Dermatol.* 4:201–221, 1985.

Chapter 5

Psoriasiform Hyperplasia

I. Psoriasiform hyperplasia
   A. Psoriasis
   B. Chronic eczematous dermatitis
      1. Unclassified or nonspecific
      2. Atopic dermatitis or eczema—chronic lichenified plaque
      3. Allergic contact dermatitis, chronic
      4. Lichen simplex chronicus
      5. Prurigo nodularis
      6. Nummular eczema
   C. Seborrheic dermatitis
   D. Exfoliative dermatitis (erythroderma)
   E. Parapsoriasis
   F. Pityriasis rubra pilaris
   G. Incontinentia pigmenti, second stage: verrucous lesions
   H. Inflammatory pityriasis rosea
   I. Inflammatory linear verrucous epidermal nevus (ILVEN)
   J. Necrolytic migratory erythema
   K. Acrodermatitis enteropathica
II. Psoriasiform hyperplasia with pustules
   A. Pustular psoriasis including generalized and localized forms, acrodermatitis continua of Hallopeau, and impetigo herpetiformis
   B. Reiter's syndrome
III. Psoriasiform hyperplasia with polymorphous infiltrate
   A. Arthropod bite reaction
   B. Cutaneous T cell lymphoma, mycosis fungoides variant, plaque stage
   C. Secondary syphilis

Psoriasiform hyperplasia is a term used to describe epidermal hyperplasia with elongation of the rete ridges. The prototype of psoriasiform hyperplasia is psoriasis, but it may be seen in chronic eczematous dermatitis, seborrheic dermatitis, exfoliative dermatitis, parapsoriasis en plaques, pityriasis rubra pilaris, incontinentia pigmenti, and inflammatory pityriasis rosea.

Psoriasiform hyperplasia with pustule formation is seen in pustular psoriasis and its variants, acrodermatitis continua, and impetigo herpetiformis, as well as Reiter's syndrome.

In contrast to the above diseases, psoriasiform hyperplasia may be accompanied by an intense polymorphous inflammatory infiltrate as in mycosis fungoides, arthropod bite reaction, and secondary syphilis.

The Reactive Process and the Disease	Histopathology	Comments
I. Psoriasiform hyperplasia		
A. Psoriasis (Fig. 5-1)	1. Laminated **hyperkeratosis** 2. Confluent or focal **parakeratosis** 3. Focal **hypogranulosis** 4. Thin suprapapillary plate	The granular layer can be seen in early and treated psoriatic lesions

Fig. **5-1.** *Psoriasis.*
A,B. *Psoriasiform hyperplasia and elongated, blunt epidermal rete.*

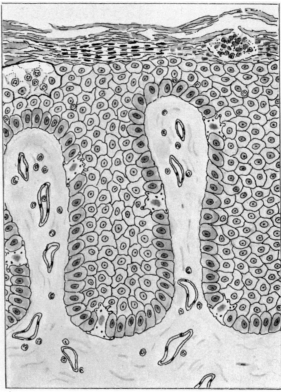

A

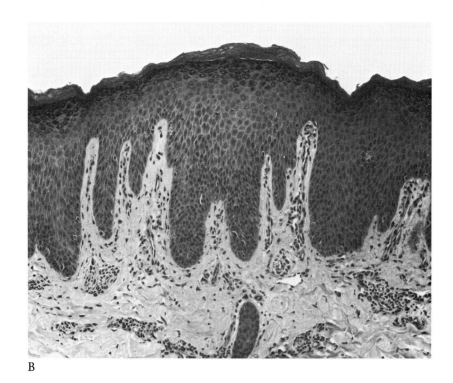

B

C. Psoriasiform hyperplasia, hyperkeratosis, parakeratosis, hypogranulosis, suprapapillary thinning, vascular ectasia, spongiform pustules, and Munro microabscesses are characteristic.

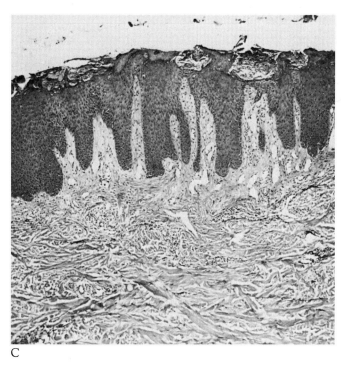

C

Fig. **5-1.** (continued)
D. *Spongiform pustule.*

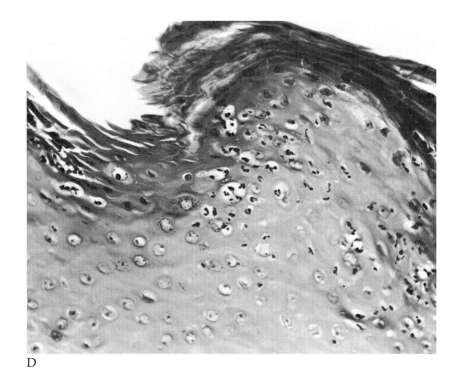

D

E. A *Munro microabscess,
suprapapillary thinning, and
vascular ectasia.*

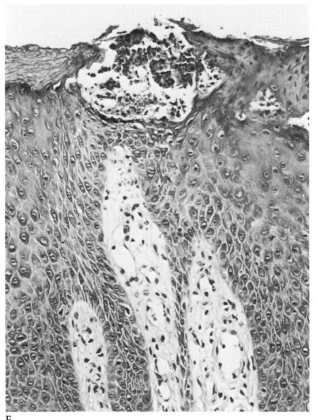

E

5. Relatively regular **psoriasiform hyperplasia** with elongated, club-shaped rete ridges
6. **Spongiform pustule** of Kogoj and/or **Munro microabscess**

In early lesions of psoriasis and in variants such as guttate and pustular psoriasis, epidermal hyperplasia may be minimal

---

Spongiform pustules are present in:

Psoriasis, all types
Subcorneal pustular dermatosis
Reiter's syndrome
Candidiasis and impetigo
Halogenodermas and other pustular drug eruptions
Geographic tongue (Fig. 5-2)

---

7. Elongation and edema of dermal papillae
8. Papillary vessel ectasia, proliferation, and tortuosity
9. Sparse perivascular mononuclear cell infiltrate

In patients with the human immunodeficiency virus-I, the inflammatory infiltrate contains more plasma cells and fewer T lymphocytes than in otherwise healthy persons

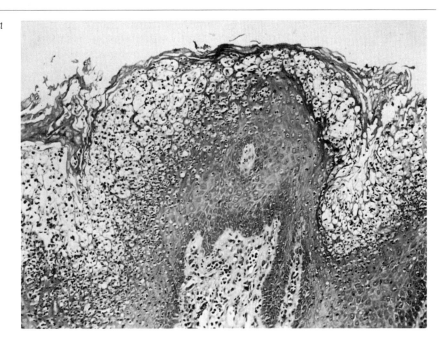

Fig. **5-2.** *Geographic tongue. Location on the tongue, epidermal hyperplasia, and numerous Munro microabscesses are typical of this disorder. A similar pattern can be seen in psoriasis, candidiasis, and Reiter's disease.*

B. Chronic eczematous dermatitis

1. Unclassified or nonspecific

    1. Hyperkeratosis
    2. Focal hypergranulosis
    3. Marked **psoriasiform hyperplasia**
    4. Slight intercellular edema (spongiosis)
    5. Superficial perivascular mononuclear cell infiltrate
    6. Papillary dermal edema and **fibrosis**
    7. Pigment incontinence

Chronic eczematous dermatitis is a general term applied to an end-stage reaction pattern produced by a wide variety of causes

Entities exhibiting the histologic pattern of *chronic eczematous dermatitis* include:

Atopic dermatitis
Nummular eczema
Lichen simplex chronicus
Chronic contact dermatitis
Prurigo nodularis
Dermatophytosis
Pityriasis rubra pilaris
Persistent light eruptions

2. Atopic dermatitis or eczema—chronic lichenified plaque

    1. Irregular hyperkeratosis
    2. Irregular psoriasiform hyperplasia
    3. Slight intercellular edema
    4. Occasional lymphocytes invading epidermis
    5. Papillary dermal fibrosis
    6. Mild to moderate perivascular and interstitial mononuclear cell infiltrate with variable numbers of eosinophils

Mast cell hyperplasia may be prominent in chronic atopic dermatitis

See also Ch. 6, II.C

3. Allergic contact dermatitis, chronic

    1. Hyperkeratosis
    2. Variable psoriasiform hyperplasia
    3. Intercellular edema
    4. Lymphocytes and eosinophils arranged in aggregates about vessels in superficial dermis

Acute forms of contact dermatitis show less epidermal hyperplasia with more intercellular edema and vesicle formation

4. Lichen simplex chronicus (Fig. 5-3)

    1. Hyperkeratosis
    2. **Hypergranulosis**
    3. Psoriasiform hyperplasia with **irregular elongation** of rete ridges
    4. Perivascular infiltrate of lymphocytes and eosinophils
    5. **Lamellar fibrosis** of papillary dermis
    6. Perineural fibrosis

Prominent follicular involvement may be noted in chronic atopic dermatitis and in chronic contact dermatitis

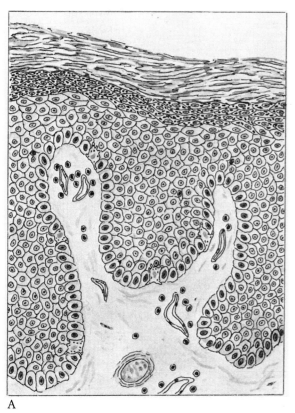

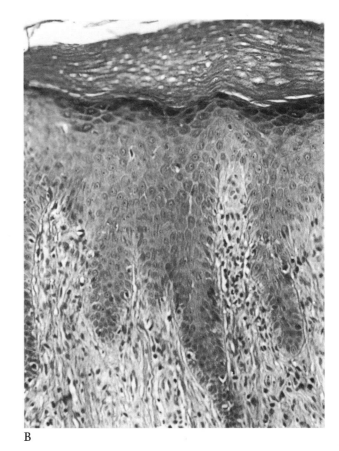

A

B

Fig. **5-3.** (A,B) *Lichen simplex chronicus. Irregular psoriasiform hyperplasia, hypergranulosis, a variable degree of perivascular infiltrate, and papillary dermal fibrosis are commonly seen in this disorder.*

5. Prurigo nodularis

1. **Progressive elongation of rete ridges from edge to center of lesion**
2. Center of lesion may exhibit focal ulceration with fibrin at its base (site of excoriation)
3. **Marked papillary dermal fibrosis and sclerosis**
4. Perineural fibrosis and endoneural hypertrophy, variably observed
5. Blood vessel proliferation and ectasia
6. Variable superficial dermal infiltrate, often containing numerous eosinophils

Epidermal hyperplasia may simulate pseudoepitheliomatous hyperplasia

6. Nummular eczema

1. Hyperkeratosis with scale crust
2. Parakeratosis
3. Psoriasiform hyperplasia
4. Spongiosis and intraepidermal vesicle formation
5. Superficial perivascular lymphocytic sometimes perifollicular and eosinophilic infiltrate

Nummular eczema may resemble acute and chronic contact dermatitis or atopic dermatitis

C. Seborrheic dermatitis

1. Hyperkeratosis
2. Focal parakeratosis
3. Slight to moderate psoriasiform hyperplasia
4. Slight intracellular and inter-cellular edema (**spongiosis**)
5. Mild perivascular mononuclear cell infiltrate
6. Occasional Munro micro-abscess

A differentiating point between psoriasis and seborrheic dermatitis is the presence of spongiosis in seborrheic dermatitis

In immunocompromised individuals, there may be a more prominent neutrophilic infiltration of the epidermis and a more extensive superficial and deep infiltrate of lymphocytes, neutrophils, and plasma cells

D. Exfoliative dermatitis (erythroderma)

1. Hyperkeratosis
2. Parakeratosis
3. Intercellular and intracellular edema
4. Mild psoriasiform hyperplasia
5. Edema of papillary dermis
6. Vascular ectasia
7. Dermal infiltrate of lympho-cytes, plasma cells, and occasional eosinophils
8. Exocytosis of mononuclear cells into epidermis
9. Occasionally, features of one of the entities listed in the box to the right are present

Although most cases are idiopathic, recognized causes of *exfoliative dermatitis* include:

Preexisting cutaneous diseases (psoriasis, atopic eczema, mycosis fungoides, lichen planus, seborrheic dermatitis, pemphigus foliaceus, pityriasis rubra pilaris, stasis dermatitis, ichthyosis)
Systemic diseases (leukemia, lymphoma, carcinoma of the lung or rectum, multiple myeloma, Sézary's syndrome)
Drugs (aspirin, arsenic, barbiturates, codeine, diphenylhydantoin [Dilantin], gold, iodine, isoniazid, mephenytoin, mercury, penicillin, quinacrine, quinadine, sulfonamides, trimethadione)

E. Parapsoriasis

1. Hyperkeratosis
2. **Mounds of parakeratotic** scale either closely adherent to or separated in toto from the underlying epidermis
3. Normal, hyperplastic, or occasionally atrophic epidermis
4. **Infiltration of epidermis by lymphocytes** (exocytosis)

This pattern may be seen in small plaque parapsoriasis

The histologic differential diagnosis includes patch and plaque stage mycosis fungoides and pityriasis lichenoides chronica
See also Ch. 8, II; Ch.12, IX

5. Bandlike or perivascular lymphohistiocytic infiltrate may include eosinophils and plasma cells

F. Pityriasis rubra pilaris

1. Follicular hyperkeratosis and occasionally "shoulder" parakeratosis
2. Focal parakeratosis in horizontal and vertical array
3. Mild psoriasiform hyperplasia
4. Basal vacuolization frequently present
5. Mild lymphocytic perivascular and perifollicular infiltrate

Shoulder parakeratosis describes a column of parakeratotic cells at the edge of the follicular orifice

Pityriasis rubra pilaris may be histologically indistinguishable from chronic eczematous dermatitis

G. Incontinentia pigmenti, second stage: verrucous lesions

1. Hyperkeratosis
2. Papillomatosis
3. Marked psoriasiform hyperplasia
4. **Intraepidermal keratinization in whorls**
5. Individual **dyskeratotic cells** scattered throughout the epidermis
6. Mild dermal infiltrate of mononuclear cells and eosinophils

H. Inflammatory pityriasis rosea (see Fig. 13-2)

1. Focal **mounds of parakeratosis,** sometimes called **skipping scale**
2. Occasional scattered dyskeratotic cells
3. Variable psoriasiform hyperplasia
4. **Exocytosis** of lymphocytes and erythrocytes
5. Intraepidermal microabscesses containing mononuclear cells
6. Vacuolization along the dermal epidermal junction
7. Superficial perivascular mononuclear cell infiltrate
8. Extravasation of erythrocytes variable but may be extensive

See also Ch. 6, II,C; Ch. 13, I.D

I. Inflammatory linear verrucous epidermal nevus (ILVEN)

1. Striking **hyperkeratosis** alternating with parakeratosis
2. Hypogranulosis
3. Psoriasiform hyperplasia with variable papillomatosis
4. Edematous dermal papillae with tortuous vessels, perivascular and interstitial mononuclear cell, and neutrophilic infiltrate

Some cases cannot be distinguished from lichen striatus

J. Necrolytic migratory erythema (Fig. 5-4)

1. Spongiosis and necrosis in upper layers of epidermis
2. Superficial bulla formation without acantholysis
3. Psoriasiform epidermal hyperplasia
4. Mild perivascular lymphocytic infiltrate

Histologically indistinguishable:

Acrodermatitis entheropathica
Cystic fibrosis-associated
  dermatitis
Necrolytic migratory erythema
Pellagra

K. Acrodermatitis enteropathica

1. Confluent parakeratosis
2. Spongiosis and necrosis in upper layers
3. Intraepidermal vacuolar changes with massive ballooning
4. Psoriasiform epidermal hyperplasia
5. Mild lymphohistiocytic infiltrate in dermis

Fig. **5-4.** Necrolytic migratory erythema.

A. Normal stratum corneum overlying necrotic debris, loss of the granular layer, and characteristic pallor of the upper epidermis. Papillary dermal edema and a superficial perivascular infiltrate are also present.

B. Necrotic cellular debris, loss of the granular layer, pallor of individual keratinocytes, and scattered dyskeratotic cells.

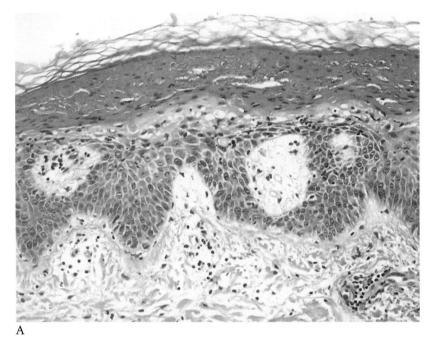

A

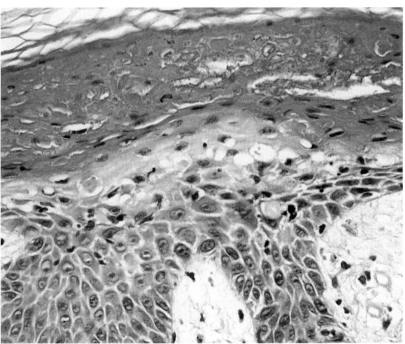

B

II. Psoriasiform hyperplasia
with pustules

A. Pustular psoriasis including generalized and localized forms, acrodermatitis continua of Hallopeau, and impetigo herpetiformis (Fig. 5-5).	1. Discrete, large intraepidermal **pustules** filled with many neutrophils and surrounded by spongiform pustules 2. Variable psoriasiform hyperplasia; other changes characteristic of psoriasis may be absent	In localized forms of pustular psoriasis, the pustules tend to be unilocular (for differential diagnosis of spongiform pustule, see p. 59)
B. Reiter's syndrome	Similar to pustular psoriasis but hyperkeratosis, parakeratosis, and psoriasiform hyperplasia are more prominent	

III. Psoriasiform hyperplasia
with polymorphous infiltrate

A. Arthropod bite reaction (see Fig. 16-2)	1. **Marked psoriasiform hyperplasia** 2. An erosion or ulceration may be present 3. Dense, superficial and deep perivascular and/or diffuse infiltrate of mononuclear cells, plasma cells, and numerous **eosinophils** 4. Endothelial cell swelling and proliferation 5. Inflammatory infiltrate and endothelial proliferation extend deep into the reticular dermis, even into the subcutaneous fat 6. Lymphoid follicles with germinal centers may be present	See also Ch. 16, I.A.2, 19 II: Ch. 12, IV; Ch. 13, I.F; Ch. 16, I.2

Fig. **5-5.** Pustular psoriasis. An intraepidermal pustule with adjacent numerous spongiform pustules on a background of psoriasiform hyperplasia is typical.

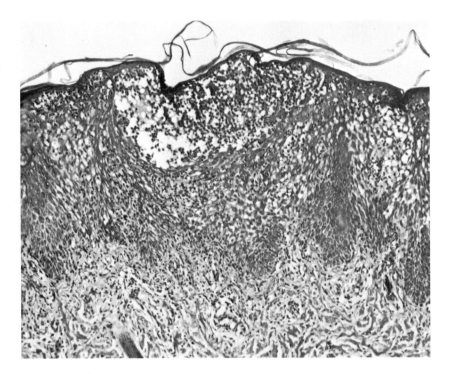

B. Cutaneous T cell lymphoma, mycosis fungoides variant, plaque stage (Fig. 5-6)

1. Psoriasiform hyperplasia
2. Intercellular edema is typically absent, but its presence does not exclude the diagnosis
3. Dermal infiltrate of pleomorphic and variably atypical mononuclear cells admixed with eosinophils and plasma cells. The distribution of the infiltrate may be bandlike and/or perivascular

Mononuclear cell atypia may be difficult to define and to appreciate. Often present are: (1) small, atypical mononuclear cells, 8 to 15 μm in diameter, with hyperchromatic, convoluted nuclei and minimal cytoplasm; and (2) larger atypical hyperchromatic mononuclear cells, measuring up to 20 to 25 μm

The presence of numerous eosinophils in the dermal infiltrate is quite typical of mycosis fungoides

4. **Epidermal invasion by atypical mononuclear cells**
5. **Pautrier microabscess**

Aggregates of mononuclear cells similar to those in mycosis fungoides may be seen in:

Pityriasis rosea
Contact dermatitis
Parapsoriasis
Leukemia cutis (acute myelomonocytic leukemia)
Drug eruptions
Pityriasis lichenoides et varioliformis acuta
Poikiloderma vasculare atrophicans

Follicular mucinosis may occur in lesions of mycosis fungoides

See also Ch. 12, X; Ch. 18, VII.A.2

Fig. **5-6.** *Mycosis fungoides.*
A. *Mycosis fungoides, plaque type. Pautrier's microabscesses and a diffuse dermal infiltrate with mild psoriasiform hyperplasia are characteristic.*
B. *Mycosis fungoides with epidermotropism. An infiltrate of atypical hyperchromatic lymphocytes is present within the lower epidermis.*
C. *Mycosis fungoides. The large cell size and convoluted nuclear outlines of the neoplastic cells (arrowheads) are easier to appreciate in this Giemsa-stained 1-μm Epon-embedded section from the same patient illustrated in B.*

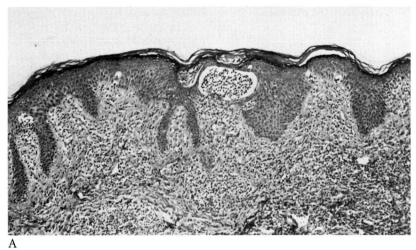

A

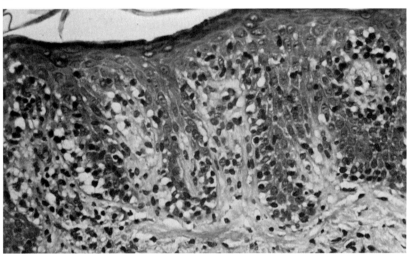

B

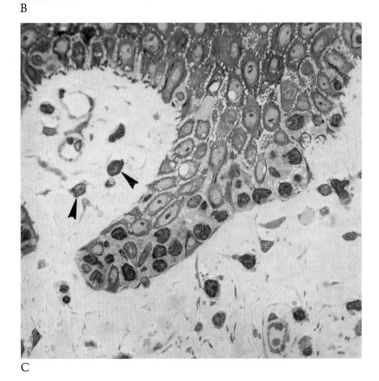

C

C. Secondary syphilis
(Fig. 5-7)

1. Parakeratosis
2. Psoriasiform hyperplasia
3. Exocytosis of mononuclear cells, neutrophils, and occasionally erythrocytes may be prominent
4. Dyskeratosis
5. Basilar vacuolization
6. Edema and occasional fibrosis of papillary dermis
7. Dermal infiltrate
   a. Bandlike infiltrate of lymphocytes and **plasma cells** may obscure the dermoepidermal interface
   b. Superficial and deep perivascular infiltrate of mononuclear cells and **plasma cells**
   c. Epithelioid granulomas admixed with **plasma cells** may be seen
8. **Endothelial cell hypertrophy**
9. Pigment incontinence common

Special silver stains (see Ch. 3) may demonstrate spirochetes within the epidermis or around blood vessels in the upper dermis

---

Plasma cell infiltrates occur in:

Mucosal, paramucosal surfaces, face, scalp, and sundamaged skin
Secondary syphilis
Mycosis fungoides
Folliculitis
Foreign body reaction
Rhinoscleroma
Basal cell and squamous cell carcinoma
Actinic keratosis
Syringocystadenoma papilliferum
Morphea
Necrobiosis lipoidica
Inflammatory cell infiltrates in patients with human immunodeficiency infection

---

See also Ch. 12, XIII; Ch. 13, I.G; Ch. 16, I.A.6

Fig. **5-7.** *Secondary syphilis.*

A. Psoriasiform hyperplasia with vacuolization at the dermoepidermal junction, exocytosis, dyskeratosis, perivascular infiltrate of lymphocytes, plasma cells, and endothelial cell swelling are characteristic. Sometimes (but not here) the infiltrate contains numerous histiocytic cells, forming "shoddy granulomas."

B. Plasma cells (arrowheads) and endothelial changes usually are considered the hallmark of syphilis, but 25% of cases in one series (Abell, Marks, and Wilson-Jones) did not show plasma cells in biopsies. Serologic confirmation should always be obtained.

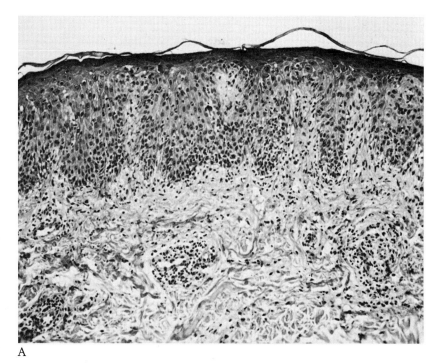

A

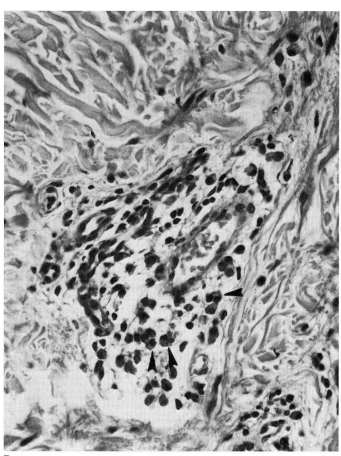

B

Suggested Reading

General Reading

Barr, R. J., and Young, E. M., Jr. Psoriasiform and related papulosquamous disorders. J. *Cutan. Pathol.* 12:412, 1985.

Psoriasis

Baker, H., and Ryan, T. J. Generalized pustular psoriasis. *Br. J. Dermatol.* 80:771, 1968.

Boyd, A. S., and Menter, A. Erythrodermic psoriasis. J. *Am. Acad. Dermatol.* 21:1985–1991, 1989.

Cox, A. J., and Watson, W. Histological variations in lesions of psoriasis. *Arch. Dermatol.* 106:503, 1972.

Gordon, M., and Johnson, W. C. Histopathology and histochemistry of psoriasis. *Arch. Dermatol.* 95:402, 1967.

Pinkus, H., and Mehregan, A. H. The primary histologic lesion of seborrheic dermatitis and psoriasis. J. *Invest. Dermatol.* 46:109, 1966.

Ragaz, A., and Ackerman, A. B. Evolution maturation, and regression of lesions of psoriasis. *Am. J. Dermatopathol.* 1:199, 1979.

Soltani, K., and Van Scott, E. J. Patterns and sequence of tissue changes in incipient and evolving lesions of psoriasis. *Arch. Dermatol.* 106:484, 1972.

Eczematous Dermatitis

Blaylock, W. K. Atopic dermatitis: Diagnosis and pathobiology. J. *Allergy Clin. Immunol.* 57:62, 1976.

Doyle, J. A., Connolly, S. M., Hunziker, N., and Winkelmann, R. K. Prurigo nodularis: A reappraisal of the clinical and histologic features. J. *Cutan. Pathol.* 6:392, 1979.

Dvorak, H. F., Mihm, M. C., Jr., Dvorak, A. M., et al. Morphology of delayed type hypersensitivity reactions in man. I. Quantitative description of inflammatory response. *Lab. Invest.* 31:111, 1974.

Hanifin, J. M., and Lobitz, W. C. Newer concepts of atopic dermatitis. *Arch. Dermatol.* 113:663, 1977.

Mihm, M. C., Jr., Soter, N. A., Dvorak, H. F., and Austen, K. F. The structure of normal skin and the morphology of atopic eczema. J. *Invest. Dermatol.* 67:305, 1976.

Norins, A. L. Atopic dermatitis. *Pediatr. Clin. North Am.* 18:801, 1971.

Shaffer, B., and Beerman, H. Lichen simplex chronicus and its variants. *Arch. Dermatol. Syphilol.* 64:340, 1951.

Seborrheic Dermatitis

Ackerman, A. B. Histopathologic differentiation of eczematous dermatitides from psoriasis and seborrheic dermatitis. *Cutis* 20:619, 1977.

Pinkus, H., and Mehregan, A. H. The primary histologic lesion of seborrheic dermatitis and psoriasis. J. *Invest. Dermatol.* 46:109, 1966.

Exfoliative Dermatitis

Nicolis, G. D., and Helwig, E. B. Exfoliative dermatitis: A clinicopathologic study of 135 cases. *Arch. Dermatol.* 108:788, 1973.

Exfoliative Erythroderma

Horn, T. D., Altomonte, V., Vogelsang, G., and Kennedy, M. J. Erythroderma after autologous bone marrow transplantation modified by administration of cyclosporine and interferon gamma for breast cancer. J. *Am. Acad. Dermatol.* 34:413–417, 1996.

Parapsoriasis

Bonvalet, D., et al. The different forms of parapsoriasis en plaques. A report of 90 cases. *Acta Derm. Venereol.* (Stockh.) 104:18, 1977.

Hu, C.-H., and Winkelmann, R. K. Digitate dermatosis. A new look at symmetrical, small plaque parapsoriasis. *Arch. Dermatol.* 107:65, 1973.

Wood, G.-S., Hu, C.-H. Parapsoriasis in I. M. Freedberg et al (Eds), *Fitzpatrick's Dermatology in Medicine* (5th ed.). New York: McGraw-Hill, 1999.

Samman, P. D. Survey of reticuloses and premycotic eruptions. *Br. J. Dermatol.* 76:1, 1964.

Sanchez, J. F., and Ackerman, A. B. The patch stage of mycosis fungoides. Criteria for histologic diagnosis. *Am. J. Dermatopathol.* 1:5, 1979.

Pityriasis Rubra Pilaris

Griffiths, W. A. D. Pityriasis rubra pilaris. *Clin. Exp. Dermatol.* 5:105, 1980.

Niemi, K. M., Kousa, M., Storgards, K., et al. Pityriasis rubra pilaris. *Dermatologica* 152:109, 1976.

Soeprono, F. F. Histologic criteria for the diagnosis of pityriasis rubra pilaris. Am. J. Dermatopathol. 8:277, 1986.

Incontinentia Pigmenti

Carney, R. G. Incontinentia pigmenti: A world statistical analysis. Arch. Dermatol. 112:535–542, 1976.

Carney, R. G., and Carney, R. G., Jr. Incontinentia pigmenti. Arch. Dermatol. 102:157, 1970.

Epstein, S., Vedder, J. S., and Pinkus, H. Bullous variety of incontinentia pigmenti (Bloch–Sulzberger). Arch. Dermatol. Syphilol. 65:557, 1952.

O'Brien, J. E., and Feingold, M. Incontinentia pigment: A longitudinal study. Am. J. Dis. Child. 139:711–712, 1985.

Wiklund, D. A., and Weston, W. L. Incontinentia pigmenti. A four-generation study. Arch. Dermatol. 116:701, 1980.

Pityriasis Rosea

Bunch, L. W., and Tilley, J. C. Pityriasis rosea: A histologic and serologic study. Arch. Dermatol. 84:79, 1961.

Lipman Cohen, E. Pityriasis rosea. Br. J. Dermatol. 79:533, 1967.

Inflammatory Linear Verrucous Epidermal Nevus (ILVEN)

Adrian, R. M., and Baden, H. P. Analysis of epidermal fibrous protein in inflammatory linear verrucous epidermal nevus. Arch. Dermatol. 116:1179, 1970.

Dupre, A., and Christol, B. Inflammatory verrucose epidermal nevus: A pathological study. Arch. Dermatol. 113:767, 1977.

Golitz, L. E., and Weston, W. L. Inflammatory linear verrucose epidermal nevus. Arch. Dermatol. 115:1208, 1979.

Pustular Psoriasis

Baker, H., and Ryan, T. J. Generalized pustular psoriasis. Br. J. Dermatol. 80:771, 1968.

Kingery, F. A. J., Chinn, H. D., and Saunders, T. S. Generalized pustular psoriasis. Arch. Dermatol. 84:912, 1961.

Reiter's Syndrome

Duvic, M., Johnson, T. M., Rapini, R. P., Freese, T., Brewton, G., and Rios, A. Acquired immunodeficiency syndrome-associated psoriasis and Reiter's syndrome. Arch. Dermatol. 123:1622–1632, 1987.

Perry, H. O., and Mayne, J. G. Psoriasis and Reiter's syndrome. Arch. Dermatol. 92:129, 1965.

Arthropod Bite Reaction

Fernandez, N., Torres, A., and Ackerman, A. B. Pathologic findings in human scabies. Arch. Dermatol. 113:320, 1977.

Goldman, L., Rockwell, E., and Richfield, D. F., III. Histopathological studies on cutaneous reactions to the bites of various arthropods. Am. J. Trop. Med. Hyg. 1:514, 1952.

Horen. W. P. Insect and scorpion sting. J.A.M.A. 221:894, 1972.

Larrivee, D. H., Benjamini, E., Feingold, B. F., et al. Histologic studies of guinea pig skin: Different stages of allergic reactivity to flea bites. Exp. Parasitol. 15:491, 1964.

Steffen, C. Clinical and histopathologic correlation of midge bites. Arch. Dermatol. 117:785, 1981.

Thomson, J., Cochran, T., Cochran, R., and McQueen, A. Histology simulating reticulosis in persistent nodular scabies. Br. J. Dermatol. 90:241, 1974.

Mycosis Fungoides

Brehmer-Andersson, E. Mycosis fungoides and its relation to Sézary's syndrome, lymphomatoid papulosis, and primary cutaneous Hodgkin's disease. Acta Derm. Venereol. (Stockh.) 75:(Suppl. 56):9, 1976.

Degreef, H., Holvoet, C., Van Vloten, W. A., et al. Woringer–Kolopp disease. An epidermotropic variant of mycosis fungoides. Cancer 38:2154, 1976.

Jimbow, K., Chiba, M., and Horikoshi, T. Electron microscopic identification of Langerhans cells in the dermal infiltrates of mycosis fungoides. J. Invest. Dermatol. 78:102, 1982.

Lutzner, M., Edelson, R., Schein, P., et al. Cutaneous T-cell lymphomas: The Sézary syndrome, mycosis fungoides and related disorders. Ann. Intern. Med 83:534, 1975.

Smoller, B. R., Bishop, K., Glusac, E. J., Kim, Y. H., and Hendrickson, M. R. Re-evaluation of histologic parameters in diagnosing mycosis fungoides. Am. J. Surg. Pathol. 19:1423–1430, 1995.

Waldorf, D. S., Ratner, A. C., and Van Scott, E. J. Cells in lesions of mycosis fungoides lymphoma following therapy. Changes in number and type. *Cancer* 21:264, 1968.

Winkelmann, R. K., and Caro, W. A. Current problems in mycosis fungoides and Sézary syndrome. *Annu. Rev. Med.* 28:251, 1977.

Secondary Syphilis

Abell, E., Marks, R., and Wilson-Jones, E. Secondary syphilis: A clinicopathological review. *Br. J. Dermatol.* 93:53, 1975.

Carbia, S. G., Lagodin, C., Abbruzzese, M., Sevinsky, L., Casco, R., Casas, J., and Woscoff, A. Lichenoid secondary syphilis. *Int. J. Dermatol,* 38:53–55, 1999.

Engelkens, H. J., ten Kate, F. J. Vuzevski, V. D., van der Sluis, J. J., and Stolz, E. Primary and secondary syphilis: A histopathological study. *Int. J. STD AIDS,* 2:280–284, 1991.

Jeerapaet, P., and Ackerman, A. B. Histologic patterns of secondary syphilis. *Arch. Dermatol.* 107:373, 1973.

Lawrence, P., and Saxe, N. Bullous secondary syphilis. *Clin. Exp. Dermatol.* 17:44–46, 1992.

Chapter 6

Vesicles, Pustules, and Bullae

I. Intracorneal or subcorneal
   A. Pemphigus foliaceus and pemphigus erythematosus
   B. Staphylococcal scalded skin syndrome
   C. Impetigo
   D. Cutaneous candidiasis
   E. Subcorneal pustular dermatosis (Sneddon-Wilkinson)
   F. Transient neonatal pustular melanosis
   G. Acropustulosis of infancy
   H. Erythema toxicum neonatorum
   I. Miliaria crystallina
   J. Acute generalized exanthematous pustulosis
II. Intraepidermal
   A. Epidermolysis bullosa simplex
   B. Friction blisters
   C. Eczematous dermatitis—acute and subacute
   D. Incontinentia pigmenti, first stage: vesicular lesions
   E. Herpesvirus infections: herpes simplex, herpes varicella-zoster
   F. Picornavirus infections: hand-foot-and-mouth disease
   G. Miliaria rubra
   H. Dominant congenital ichthyosiform erythroderma (epidermolytic hyperkeratosis)
   I. Bullous dermatosis of diabetes mellitus and uremia
   J. Coma bulla (pressure necrosis) and sweat gland necrosis
   K. Pustular psoriasis
   L. Erythema multiforme
   M. IgA pustular dermatosis
III. Suprabasilar
   A. Pemphigus vulgaris
   B. Pemphigus vegetans
      1. Early
      2. Late
   C. Benign familial pemphigus (Hailey–Hailey disease)
   D. Darier's disease (keratosis follicularis)
   E. Transient acantholytic dermatosis (Grover's disease)
IV. Subepidermal vesicles (see Ch. 11)

Students learning dermatopathology are always frustrated, and often overwhelmed, by the vesiculopustular disorders. Simple classification is hampered by the large number of diseases with vesicles and/or pustules as part of their clinical spectrum, and the wide diversity of mechanisms producing blisters. When dealing with a vesiculopustular disease microscopically, the sorting process should begin with certain basic determinations:

1. Location of the vesicle or pustule (see Fig. 2-3): intracorneal, subcorneal, intraepidermal, suprabasilar, subepidermal, intraappendageal
2. Presence or absence of inflammation
3. Compositon of infiltrate
4. Presence of dyskeratosis or epidermal necrosis
5. Mechanism of lesion formation: aggregates of cells, intercellular edema (spongiosis), intracellular edema (reticular degeneration), acantholysis, basal vacuolization

With this limited information, the various diseases can be categorized (Table 6-1). No classification, of course, is failproof, but it does provide a structure to help differentiate these entities. Accurate diagnosis of a blistering disease is dependent on adequate sampling of a representative, fully formed lesion. Older lesions often develop histologic changes that obscure the characteristic and diagnostic features.

This chapter examines diseases characterized by vesicles that are formed within the stratum corneum and epidermis; vesicles, pustules, and bullae that are located beneath the epidermis are discussed in Chapter 11.

The Reactive Process and the Disease	Histopathology	Comments
I. Intracorneal or subcorneal		
A. Pemphigus foliaceus and pemphigus erythematosus (Fig. 6-1) *Pathophysiology: Desmoplakins (intracellular) and desmogleins (transmembrane) are glycoproteins active in keratinocyte adhesion in association with desmosomes. Desmoglein 1 is the pemphigus foliaceos antigen.*	1. **Subcorneal, intragranular, or upper epidermal clefts** 2. **Acantholysis** 3. Dyskeratotic acantholytic cells in granular cell layer 4. Perivascular infiltrate often with **eosinophils** 5. Exocytosis of eosinophils in a spongiotic epidermis	Histologic changes are often subtle; serial sections may be required to demonstrate changes *Spongiosis with epidermal invasion by eosinophils is seen in:* Pemphigus foliaceus and vulgaris Allergic contact dermatitis Urticarial and/or eczematous lesions of bullous pemphigoid and herpes gestationis Epidermolysis bullosa acquisita Incontinentia pigmenti Erythema/toxicum neonatorum Scabies infestation

Table **6-1.** *Characteristics of Intraepidermal Vesicles*

Specific Attribute	Location			
	Intracorneal	Subcorneal	Intraspinous	Suprabasilar
Noninflammatory	Miliaria crystallina	Miliaria crystallina Staphylococcal scalded skin syndrome	Epidermolysis bullosa of the hands and feet Epidermolysis bullosa simplex Friction blisters	
Spongiotic			Eczematous dermatitis	
Acantholytic	Pemphigus foliaceus	Pemphigus foliaceus	Herpex virus infection Benign familial pemphigus (Hailey–Hailey) Acantholytic dermatosis Pemphigus vulgaris	Pemphigus vulgaris Darier's disease Acantholytic dermatosis
Neutrophil	Impetigo Candidiasis Dermatophytosis	Subcorneal pustular dermatosis Pustular psoriasis	IgA pustular dermatosis	
Eosinophil	Pemphigus foliaceus		Incontinentia pigmenti Contact dermatitis Insect bite reaction	Pemphigus vulgaris
Lymphocyte			Eczematous dermatitis Miliaria rubra	

Fig. **6-1.** *Pemphigus foliaceus. The cleavage is intraepidermal, just below or within the granular layer. Many granulocytes are in the blister cavity.*

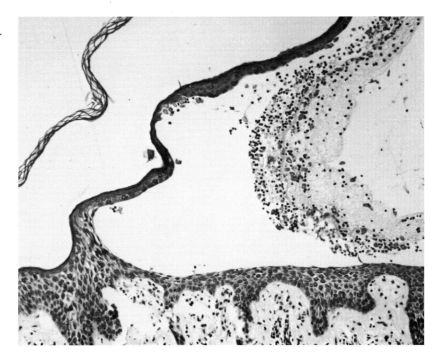

Drugs that may induce *pemphigus* or *pemphigus-like disease* include:

Penicillamine
Captopril
Piroxicam
Pyritinol
Thiopromine
Thiamazole

Superinfection of vesicles may obscure the basic underlying process with superficial crust/neutrophilic infiltrate.

B. Staphylococcal scalded skin syndrome

1. Subcorneal cleavage
2. Rare acantholytic granular layer cells
3. Dermal infiltrate minimal to absent

Characteristically seen in infants and adults with impaired renal function

Pathophysiology: *The mechanism underlying the staphylococcal scalded skin syndrome involves the production of an epidermal toxin by pathogenic staphylococci, phage group II. This toxin mediates a subcorneal or intragranular layer cleft.*

C. Impetigo (Fig. 6-2)

1. Subcorneal pustule filled with **neutrophils** and an occasional acantholytic cell

Differential diagnosis of *subcorneal pustules*:

Impetigo
Subcorneal pustular dermatosis
Fungal infection
Pustular psoriasis
Geographic tongue
Acute generalized exanthematous pustulosis

2. Spongiosis
3. Neutrophilic exocytosis
4. Moderately intense inflammatory infiltrate (neutrophils, lymphocytes) in the papillary dermis

Special stains may demonstrate organism (see Ch. 3)

D. Cutaneous candidiasis

Subcorneal pustule filled with neutrophils

Special stains demonstrate organisms within the stratum corneum (see Ch. 3)

E. Subcorneal pustular dermatosis (Sneddon-Wilkinson) (Fig. 6-3)

1. Subcorneal pustules containing neutrophils and occasional eosinophils
2. Intercellular epidermal edema (spongiosis)
3. Spongiform pustules may be present adjacent to subcorneal pustule

Occasional acantholytic cells may be seen within the pustule
Special stains to exclude an infectious etiology are requisite

Fig. **6-2.** *Impetigo (nonbullous). A subcorneal pustule is evident here. Neutrophils infiltrating through the epidermis are also noted. Gram's stain often shows gram-positive cocci in the pustule.*

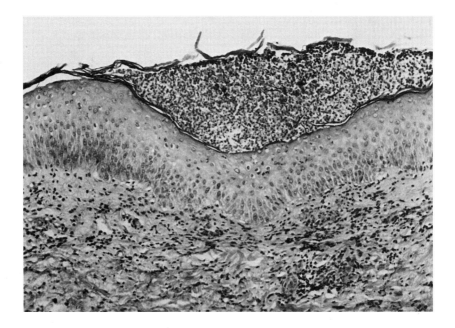

Fig. **6-3.** *Subcorneal pustular dermatosis (Sneddon–Wilkinson disease). The subcorneal neutrophils are associated with spongiosis, occasional acantholysis, and a dermal infiltrate of neutrophils, lymphocytes, and occasional eosinophils. Inflammatory cells can be seen within the epidermis as well.*

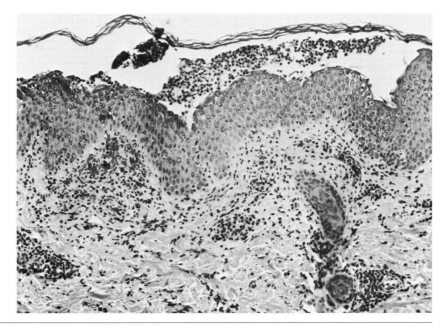

4. Slight leukocytic exocytosis
5. Perivascular infiltrate of neutrophils, eosinophils, and mononuclear cells

F. Transient neonatal pustular melanosis

1. Subcorneal pustule filled with neutrophils
2. Melanin incontinence in older lesions

G. Acropustulosis of infancy

Subcorneal pustule filled with neutrophils

Clinicopathologic correlation is required to differentiate from transient neonatal pustular melanosis

H. Erythema toxicum
neonatorum

Perifollicular subcorneal **pustules**
filled with **eosinophils**

I. Miliaria crystallina
(Fig. 6-4)

1. Intracorneal or subcorneal
vesicles in direct
communication with an
underlying sweat duct
2. Spongiotic microvesicle may
be present

Multiple sections may be required
to demonstrate ductal
communication

See also Ch. 25, II.A.1

J. Acute generalized
exanthematous
pustulosis

1. Epidermis of normal thickness
with overlying parakeratosis
2. Spongiform superficial
epidermal pustules
3. Papillary dermal edema
4. Mixed dermal inflammatory
infiltrates with eosinophils
5. Focal necrosis of keratinocytes
in occasional cases

Leukocytoclastic vasculitis is
observed affecting the vessels of
the superficial vascular plexus in
about 25% of cases

II. Intraepidermal

A. Epidermolysis bullosa
simplex (see Fig. 11-3)

1. Disruption of basal
keratinocytes with apparent
subepidermal bulla formation

2. Variable degeneration of cells
in stratum spinosum

3. Occasional dyskeratosis

Epidermolysis bullosa of the
hands and feet is a form of
epidermolysis bullosa simplex
with dishesion of keratinocytes
in the spinous layers
In the several types of
epidermolvsis bullosa, the
blisters form in different regions
of the epidermis (Fig. 6-5)
Clinically normal skin in a patient
with epidermolysis bullosa
simplex characteristically shows
basement membrane zone
microvesiculation

B. Friction blisters

1. High- to mid-intraepidermal
cleavage often present
2. Dermal infiltrate sparse to
absent

Histologic changes and location of
blister vary according to age of
lesion

Fig. **6-4.** *Miliaria crystallina. An intraepidermal vesicle is present in association with an eccrine duct. Notice the paucity of inflammation.*

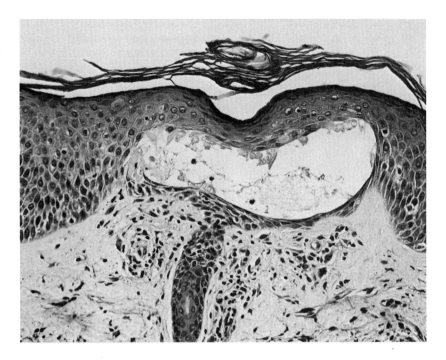

Fig. **6-5.** *Epidermolysis bullosa.*
a. *Epidermolysis bullosa of the hands and feet. Cytolysis and dyskeratosis occur in the mid to upper epidermis.*
b. *Epidermolysis bullosa, junctional (or letalis) type. The vesicle forms at the dermoepidermal junction, and the PAS-positive basement membrane zone is present at the base of the vesicle.*
c. *Epidermolysis bullosa, simplex type. Cleft formation is the result of vacuolation and degeneration of basal cells.*
d. *Epidermolysis bullosa dystrophica (dominant and recessive type) and epidermolysis bullosa acquisita. Vacuolation at the dermoepidermal junction occurs early, but the fully developed vesicle occurs within the superficial papillary dermis.*

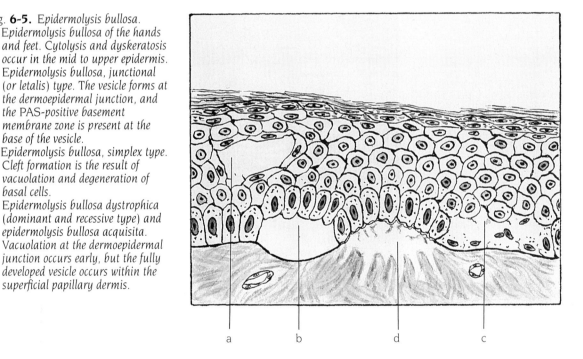

C. Eczematous dermatitis—acute and subacute (Fig. 6-6)

1. Focal parakeratosis
2. **Spongiosis and spongiotic vesicles** occurring in lower two-thirds of epidermis

Spongiosis and presence of the granular layer help differentiate eczematous dermatitis from psoriasis

Fig. **6-6.** (A, B) *Acute eczematous dermatitis. An intraepidermal vesicle is present, with surrounding spongiosis and exocytosis of lymphocytes. The thickness of the stratum corneum and stratum Malpighii is characteristic of acral sites, such as the hand.*

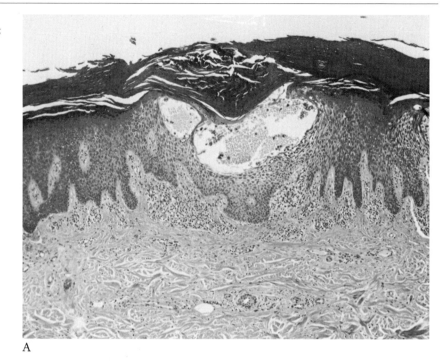

A

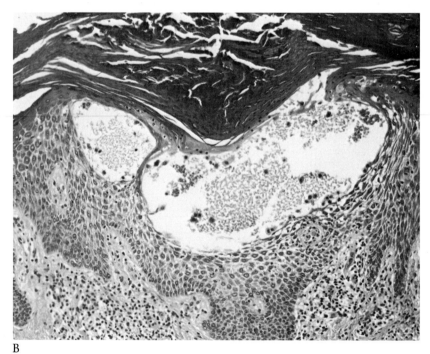

B

Fig. **6-6.** (C, D) *Subacute eczematous dermatitis. Psoriasiform hyperplasia, spongiosis, and perivascular lymphocytic infiltrate are present.*

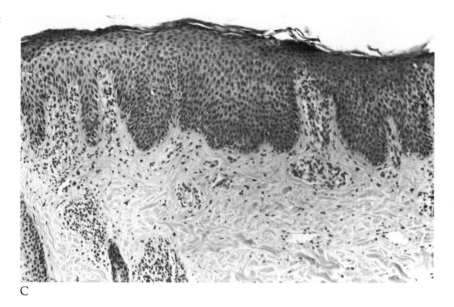

C

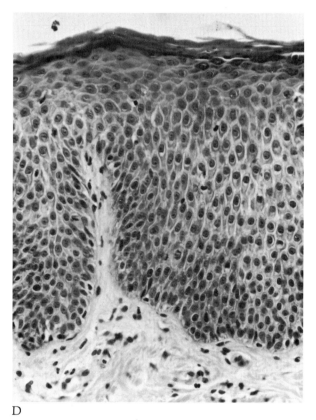

D

3. Superficial, predominantly perivascular infiltrate of mononuclear cells and occasional eosinophils

> *Spongiotic vesicles* may be seen in:
>
> Acute and subacute eczematous dermatitis, including atopic, nummular, dyshidrotic, photoinduced, and contact dermatitis
> Pityriasis rosea
> Miliaria crystallina and rubra
> Dermatophytosis and candidiasis
> Erythema annulare centrifugum

D. Incontinentia pigmenti, first stage: vesicular lesions (Fig. 6-7)

1. Spongiosis
2. Vesicles containing **eosinophils**
3. Eosinophils within epidermis
4. Dyskeratosis observed, often in association with eosinophils
5. Mild, superficial perivascular and diffuse infiltrate of lymphocytes and eosinophils

> *Epidermal invasion by eosinophils* may be seen in:
>
> Bullous pemphigoid
> Pemphigus vulgaris and foliaceus
> Arthropod bite reaction
> Allergic contact dermatitis
> Incontinentia pigmenti

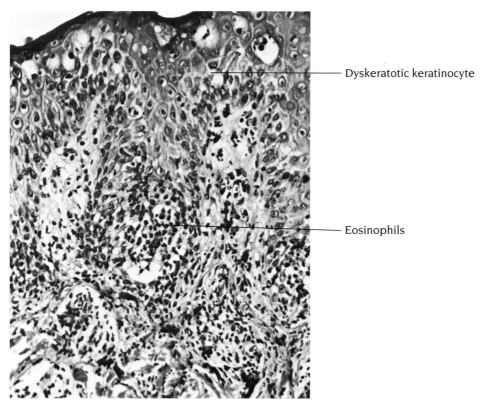

Dyskeratotic keratinocyte

Eosinophils

Fig. **6-7.** *Incontinentia pigmenti. Epidermal hyperplasia, intraepidermal eosinophilic microabscesses* (center), *and melanin-laden macrophages in the upper dermis are hallmarks of this disorder.*

E. Herpesvirus infections: herpes simplex, herpes varicella-zoster (Fig. 6-8)

1. **Balloning and reticular degeneration** of epidermis
2. **Acantholytic keratinocytes** with homogeneous cytoplasm
3. Large, irregular or **multinucleate keratinocytes**
4. Nuclear margination of chromatin with violet "ground glass" appearance

5. Intranuclear eosinophilic inclusion body surrounded by a faint, clear halo

6. Perivascular infiltrate of mononuclear cells and neutrophils may extend into deep reticular dermis
7. Leukocytoclastic vasculitis with fibrinoid necrosis may be present

Differential diagnosis of *ballooning degeneration*:

Herpes varicella-zoster
Herpes simplex
Epidermolytic hyperkeratosis
Verruca vulgaris
Orf
Smallpox (variola)
Vaccinia

Many viruses affecting the epidermis have cytopathic effects, sometimes resulting in blisters or leading to epidermal hyperplasia

Nuclear inclusions may be seen in hair appendages and endothelial cells as well as in epidermis

In early lesions of zoster or herpetic folliculitis, changes may be restricted to follicular epithelium

Dermal inflammatory changes may be absent in immuno-suppressed individuals

Herpes simplex and herpes zoster are histologically indistinguishable

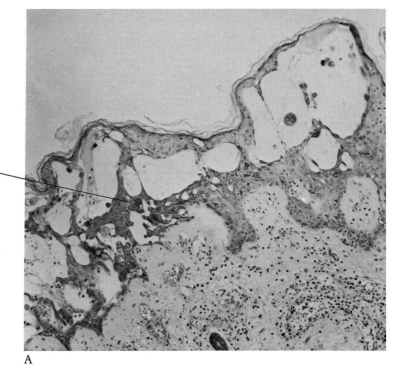

Fig. **6-8.** *Herpes virus infection. A. Reticular degeneration with multinucleate giant cells.*

Giant multinucleate cell

A

B. Older lesion caused by a herpesvirus with cytopathic effect throughout the epidermis.
C. Characteristic multinucleated and acantholytic keratinocytes.

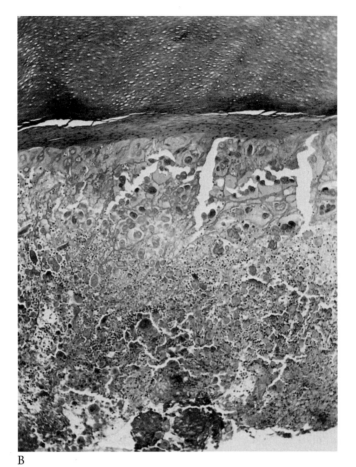

B

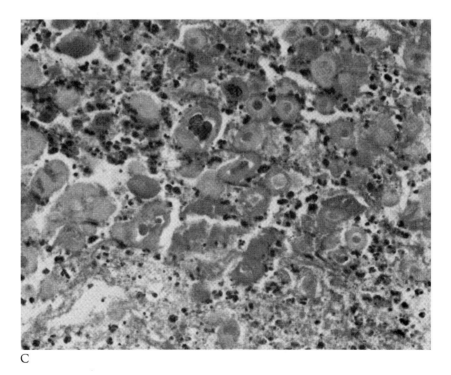

C

F. Picornavirus infections: hand-foot-and-mouth disease (Fig. 6-9)

1. Massive reticular degeneration of keratinocytes abruptly demarcated from the normal epidermis
2. Ballooning degeneration of deep spinous cells
3. Superficial perivascular lymphocytic infiltrate
4. Late lesions show exocytosis of neutrophils and lymphocytes

Focal loss of the basal cell layer in older lesions results in a subepidermal vesicle

G. Miliaria rubra

1. Intraepidermal spongiotic vesicles in direct communication with a sweat duct
2. Mononuclear cells within vesicles and in subjacent dermis

See also Ch. 25, II.A.2

H. Dominant congenital ichthyosiform erythroderma (epidermolytic hyperkeratosis) (see Fig. 4-1)

1. Massive, compact hyperkeratosis
2. Reticular and ballooning degeneration of granular layer and upper epidermis

See also Ch. 4, II

I. Bullous dermatosis of diabetes mellitus and uremia

1. Intraepidermal and subepidermal vesicles and bullae
2. Mild superficial perivascular mononuclear cell infiltrate

See also Ch. 11, I.F–G
Clinical–pathologic correlation is necessary for diagnosis
The presence of diabetic vasculopathy, specifically vessel wall thickening, is helpful in diagnosis

J. Coma bulla (pressure necrosis) and sweat gland necrosis (see Fig. 25-1)

1. Intraepidermal and subepidermal blisters
2. Epidermal necrosis
3. **Eccrine duct and gland necrosis**
4. Variable infiltrate of neutrophils and mononuclear cells in and around necrotic eccrine glands
5. Predominantly neutrophilic infiltrate in and around pilosebaceous structures; focal follicular necrosis may be seen
6. Dermal hemorrhage
7. Focal areas of necrosis, edema, and acute inflammation in the subcutaneous tissue

See also Ch. 25, II.C

K. Pustular psoriasis (see Fig. 5-5)

See also Ch. 5, II.A

L. Erythema multiforme (see Fig. 11-8)

Intraepidermal vesicles occasionally may occur in erythema multiforme (see also Ch. 10, I; Ch. 11, II.I)

Fig. **6-9.** *Hand-foot-and-mouth disease. Ballooning degeneration within the epidermis results in the microvesicle formation and dyskeratosis seen here. A specific cytopathic effect is absent.*

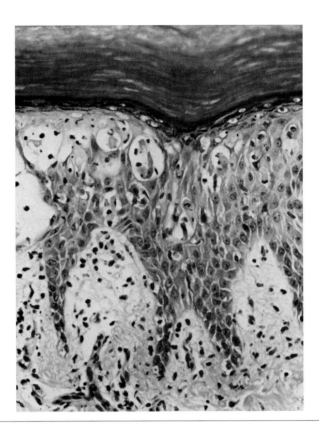

M. IgA pustular dermatosis

1. Large mid-intraepidermal neutrophilic aggregates in spongiotic vesicle
2. Exocytosis of neutrophils
3. Perivascular lymphocytes and neutrophils
4. Papillary dermal edema variable
5. Neutrophils variably present in papillary dermis

Immunofluorescence findings are diagnostic: Intraepidermal (intercellular) granular IgA deposition

III. Suprabasilar

    A. Pemphigus vulgaris (Fig. 6-10)

1. Eosinophils with apparent spongiosis in lower epidermis
2. **Suprabasilar clefts**
3. **Acantholysis**
4. Roof of bulla is composed of intact epidermis
5. Base of bulla composed of basal cell layer on prominent dermal papillae (so-called **villi**)
6. Scant perivascular inflammatory infiltrate composed of lymphocytes and eosinophils, and occasional neutrophils, or plasma cells

> Differential diagnosis of *acantholysis* includes:
>
> Pemphigus, all forms
> Darier's disease (keratosis follicularis)
> Benign familial pemphigus (Hailey–Hailey disease)
> Transient acantholytic dermatosis (Grover's disease)
> Focal acantholytic dermatosis
> Viral vesicles (herpesvirus infections)
> Squamous cell carcinoma
> Actinic keratosis
> Impetigo
> Warty dyskeratoma
> Staphylococcal scalded skin syndrome
> Subcorneal pustular dermatosis

Suprabasilar acantholysis combined with the loss of intercellular attachments between basal cells gives a "tombstone" appearance to the basal layer

    B. Pemphigus vegetans

        1. Early

1. **Suprabasilar cleft** formation
2. **Acantholysis**
3. Bullae are filled with eosinophils
4. **Epidermal hyperplasia**
5. Perivascular papillary and upper reticular dermal infiltrate composed predominantly of eosinophils

> *Intraepidermal eosinophilic abscesses* may be seen in:
>
> Pemphigus vegetans
> Incontinentia pigmenti
> Bromoderma and iododerma
> Erythema toxicum neonatorum
> Scabies infestation

        2. Late

1. Epidermal hyperplasia with hyperkeratosis and papillomatosis
2. Acantholysis may be absent at this stage
3. A dense, diffuse infiltrate of eosinophils, lymphocytes, and plasma cells in the papillary and upper reticular dermis

Fig. **6-10.** (A, B) *Pemphigus vulgaris. Acantholysis with suprabasilar cleft formation is the hallmark of pemphigus vulgaris. The prominent dermal papillae ("villi") also are characteristic. Notice the presence of acantholytic cells, i.e., keratinocytes with round shapes resulting from the loss of intercellular connections.*

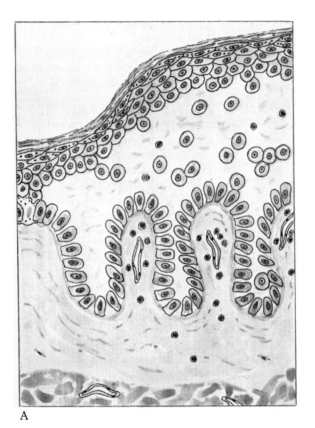

A

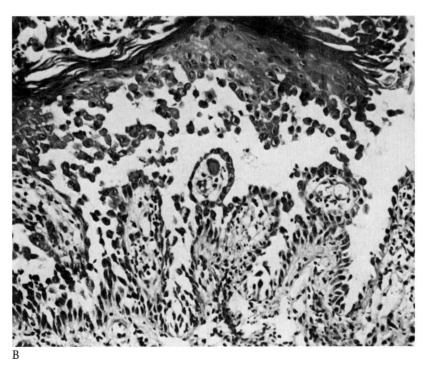

B

C. Benign familial
pemphigus
(Hailey–Hailey disease)
(Fig. 6-11)

1. Suprabasilar clefts
2. Acantholysis
3. Partial acantholysis throughout the epidermis, giving the appearance of a **dilapidated brick wall**
4. Dyskeratosis, with basal cell shrinkage and alteration in staining of cytoplasm (brightly eosinophilic in color)
5. Elongated papillae may form villi, which protrude into vesicle
6. Superficial perivascular lymphocytic infiltrate with occasional eosinophils

D. Darier's disease
(keratosis follicularis)
(Fig. 6-12)

1. **Hyperkeratosis**
2. Epidermal hyperplasia, and, rarely, pseudoepitheliomatous hyperplasia have been noted
3. Acantholytic dyskeratosis resulting in **corps ronds** (granular layer and upper epidermis) and **corps grains** (within cleft and parakeratotic stratum corneum)
4. **Suprabasilar acantholysis** with formation of clefts
5. Irregular upward proliferation of dermal papillae with formation of villi
6. Sparse lymphocytic perivascular infiltrate in the upper dermis

See Ch. 2 for definition of corps ronds and corps grains

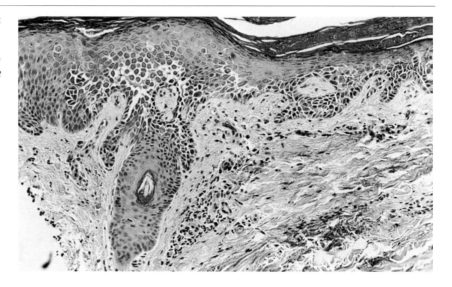

Fig. **6-11.** *Benign familial pemphigus (Hailey–Hailey disease). Acantholysis results in the "dilapidated brick wall" appearance, a feature that is commonly observed in this disorder. More complete acantholysis, resulting in suprabasal cleft formation, is also present.*

Fig. **6-12.** (A, B) *Darier's disease (keratosis follicularis). Suprabasal cleft formation with corps ronds (arrows, cells with apparent perinuclear halos) and corps grains (arrowheads, cells with small, dark oval nuclei resembling millet grains) are typical.*

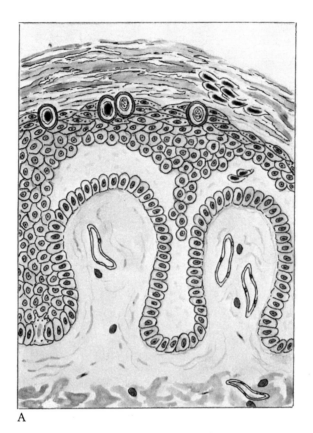

A

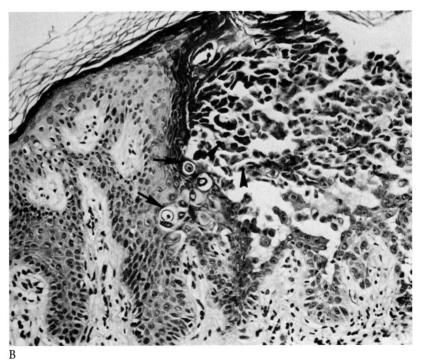

B

E. Transient acantholytic dermatosis (Grover's disease) (Fig. 6-13)

1. Lesion very focal; entire lesion usually contained within one high-power field
2. Compact orthohyperkeratosis and parakeratosis
3. Acantholysis at any level of the epidermis
4. Spongiosis may be prominent
5. Focal suprabasilar clefts and vesicles
6. Occasional corps ronds and corps grains
7. Perivascular and interstitial lymphocytic infiltrate

Differential diagnosis:
Pemphigus vulgaris and foliaceus
Benign familial pemphigus
Darier's disease

The clue to diagnosis is the focality of histologic changes and mixture of acantholytic patterns

These changes may be observed incidentally in normal skin, where the condition is referred to as *focal acantholytic dyskeratosis*

Most of the entities included in this category are primarily disorders of the papillary dermis and basement membrane zone and are described in Chs. 10, 11

IV. Subepidermal vesicles (see Ch. 11)

A. Cell poor
1. Porphyria cutanea tarda
2. Epidermolysis bullosa
3. Toxic epidermal necrolysis
4. Graft-versus-host reaction (GVHR), acute
5. Acute radiodermatitis
6. Bullous dermatosis of diabetes mellitus
7. Bullous dermatosis of renal failure
8. Electrical burn
9. Thermal burn

B. With inflammation
1. Bullous pemphigoid
2. Herpes gestationis
3. Dermatitis herpetiformis
4. Bullous lupus erythematosus
5. Linear IgA dermatosis
6. Chronic bullous disease of childhood
7. Focal embolic lesions in gonococcemia and acute meningococcemia
8. Epidermolysis bullosa acquisita

9. Erythema
   multiforme
10. Fixed drug eruption
11. Bullous lichen
    planus
12. Lichen sclerosus et
    atrophicus
13. Bullous drug
    eruption
14. Light eruption
15. Mastocytosis

Fig. **6-13.** (A, B) *Transient acantholytic dermatosis (Grover's disease). Dyskeratotic cells, corps ronds, and suprabasal clefts with spongiosis, as well as focal parakeratosis and papillary dermal lymphocytic infiltrates, are typical. These histologic changes resemble those of a poorly formed Darier's disease.*

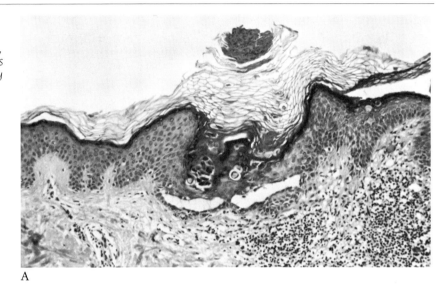

A

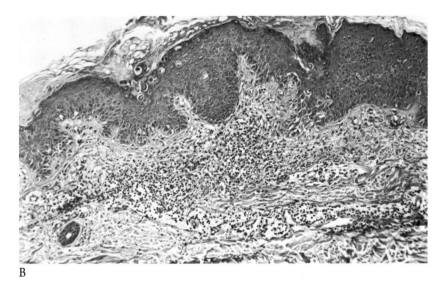

B

Suggested Reading

General

Beutner, E. H., Chorzelski, T. P., and Kumar, V. (Eds.). *Immunopathology of the Skin* (3rd ed.). New York: Wiley & Sons, 1987.

Pearson, R. W. Advances in the Diagnosis and Treatment of Blistering Diseases: A Selective Review. In F. D. Malkinson and R. W. Pearson (Eds.), *Year Book of Dermatology*. Chicago: Year Book, 1977.

Farmer, E. R. Intraepidermal bullous diseases. J. *Cutan. Pathol.* 12:313, 1985.

Intracorneal or Subcorneal

Pemphigus Foliaceus

Furtado, T. A. Histopathology of pemphigus foliaceus. *Arch. Dermatol.* 80:66, 1959.

Mutasim, D. F., Pelc, N. J., and Anhalt, G. J. Paraneoplastic pemphigus, pemphigus vulgaris, and pemphigus foliaceus. *Clin. Dermatol,* 11:113–117, 1993.

Perry, H. O., and Brunsting, L. A. Pemphigus foliaceus. Further observations. *Arch. Dermatol.* 91:10, 1965.

Staphylococcal Scalded Skin

Elias, P. M., Fritsch, P., and Epstein, E. H., Jr. Staphylococcal scalded skin syndrome: Clinical features, pathogenesis, and recent microbiological and biochemical developments. *Arch. Dermatol.* 113:207, 1979.

Gemmell, C. G. Staphylococcal scalded skin syndrome. J. *Med. Microbiol.* 43:318–327, 1995.

Hardwick, N., Parry, C. M., and Sharpe, G. R. Staphylococcal scalded skin syndrome in an adult. Influence of immune and renal factors. *Br. J. Dermatol.* 132:468–471, 1995.

Lyell, A. Toxic epidermal necrolysis (the scalded skin syndrome): A reappraisal. *Br. J. Dermatol.* 100:69, 1979.

Melish, M. E., Glasgow, L. A., and Turner, M. D. The staphylococcal scalded skin syndrome: Isolation and partial characterization of the exfoliative toxin. J. *Infect. Dis.* 125:129, 1972.

Impetigo

Darmstadt, G. L., and Lane, A. T. Impetigo: An overview. *Pediatr. Dermatol.* 11:293–303, 1994.

Dillon, H. C., Jr. Impetigo contagiosa: Suppurative and non-suppurative complications: I. Clinical, bacteriologic, and epidemiologic characteristics of impetigo. *Am. J. Dis. Child.* 115:530–541, 1968.

Jordan, W. E., Montes, L. F., and Pittillo, R. F. Microscopic features of pustule formation in experimental impetigo of guinea pig. J. *Cutan. Pathol.* 1:54, 1974.

Peter, G., and Smith, A. L. Group A streptococcal infections of the skin and pharynx. (First of two parts). *N. Engl. J. Med.* 297:311, 1977.

Subcorneal Pustular Dermatosis

Johnson, S. A. M., and Cripps, D. J. Subcorneal pustular dermatosis in children. *Arch. Dermatol.* 109:73, 1974.

Sneddon, I. B., and Wilkinson, D. S. Subcorneal pustular dermatosis. *Br. J. Dermatol.* 100:61, 1979.

Wilkinson, D. S. Pustular dermatoses. *Br. J. Dermatol.* 81 (Suppl. 3):38, 1969.

Transient Neonatal Pustular Melanosis

Barr, R. J., Globerman, L. M., and Seeber, F. A. Transient pustular melanosis. *Int. J. Dermatol.* 18:636, 1979.

Acropustulosis of Infancy

Lucky, A. W., and McGuire, J. S. Infantile acropustulosis with eosinophilic pustulosis. J. *Pediatr.* 100:428, 1982.

Newton, J. A., Salisburg, J., Marsden, A., and McGibbon, D. H. Acropustulosis of infancy. *Br. J. Dermatol.* 115:735–739, 1986.

Vignon-Pennamen, M. D., and Wallach, D. Infantile acropustulosis: A clinico-pathologic study of six cases. *Arch. Dermatol.* 122:1155–1160, 1986.

Erythema Toxicum Neonatorum

Freeman, R. G., Spiller, R., and Knox, J. M. Histopathology of erythema toxicum neonatorum. *Arch. Dermatol.* 82:586, 1960.

Luders, D. Histologic observations in erythema toxicum neonatorum. *Pediatrics* 26:219, 1960.

Miliaria Crystallina
Shelley, W. B., and Horvath, P. N. Experimental miliaria in man. II. Production of sweat retention anidrosis and miliaria crystallina by various kinds of injury. J. Invest. Dermatol. 14:9, 1950.

Intraepidermal   *Epidermolysis Bullosa Simplex*
Marinkovich M. P., et al. Hereditary Epidermolysis Bullosa in I. M. Freedberg et al. (Eds) Fitzpatrick's *Dermatology in General Medicine* (5th ed.). New York: McGraw-Hill, 1999.
Bergman, R. Immunohistopathologic diagnosis of epidermolysis bullosa. Am. J. Dermatopathol. 21:185–192, 1999.
Fine, J.-D., Bauer, E. A., Briggman, R. A., Carter, D. M., Eady, R. A. J., Esterly, N. B., Holbrook, K. A., et al. Revised clinical and laboratory criteria for subtypes of inherited epidermolysis bullosa. J. Am. Acad. Dermatol. 24:119–135, 1991.

Friction Blisters
Braun-Falco, O. The Pathology of Blister Formation. In A. W. Kopf and R. Andrade (Eds.), *The Year Book of Dematology*. Chicago: Year Book, 1969.
Sulzberger, M. B., Cortese, T. A., Fishman, L., and Wiley, H. S. Studies on blisters produced by friction. J. Invest. Dermatol. 47:456, 1966.

Eczematous Dermatitis
Blaylock, W. K. Atopic dermatitis: Diagnosis and pathobiology. J. *Allergy Clin. Immunol.* 57:62, 1976.
Doyle, J. A., Connolly, S. M., Hunziker, N., and Winkelmann, R. K. Prurigo nodularis: A reappraisal of the clinical and histologic features. J. Cutan. Pathol. 6:392, 1979.
Dvorak, H. F., et al. Morphology of delayed type hypersensitivity reactions in man. I. Quantitative description of inflammatory response. Lab. Invest. 31:111, 1974.
Hanifin, J. M., and Lobitz, W. C. Newer concepts of atopic dermatitis. Arch. Dermatol. 113:663, 1977.
Mihm, M. C., Jr., Soter, N. A., Dvorak, H. F., and Austen, K. F. The structure of normal skin and the morphology of atopic eczema. J. Invest. Dermatol. 67:305, 1976.
Norins, A. L. Atopic dermatitis. Pediatr. Clin. North Am. 18:801, 1971.
Shaffer, B., and Beerman, H. Lichen simplex chronicus and its variants. Arch. Dermatol. Syphilol. 64:340, 1951.

Incontinentia Pigmenti
Caputo, R., Gianotti, F., and Innocenti, M. Ultrastructural findings in incontinentia pigmenti. Int. J. Dermatol. 14:46, 1975.
Carney, R. G., and Carney, R. G., Jr. Incontinentia pigmenti. Arch. Dermatol. 102:157, 1970.
Epstein, S., Vedder, J. S., and Pinkus, H. Bullous variety of incontinentia pigmenti (Bloch–Sulzberger). Arch. Dermatol. Syphilol. 65:557, 1952.
Wiklund, D. A., and Weston, W. L. Incontinentia pigmenti. A four-generation study. Arch. Dermatol. 116:701, 1980.

Herpes Virus Infections
Corey, L., and Spear, P. G. Infections with herpes simplex viruses. N. Engl. J. Med. 314:686–691, 749, 1986.
Kapan, A. S. *The Herpes Viruses*. New York: Academic, 1973.
McSorley, J., Shapiro, L., Brownstein, M. H., and Hsu, K. Simplex and varicella-zoster: Comparative cases. Int. J. Dermatol. 13:69, 1974.
Strano, A. J. Light microscopy of selected viral disease (morphology of viral inclusion bodies). Pathol. Annu. 11:53, 1976.

Picornavirus Infections
Higgins, P. G., and Warin, R. P. Hand, foot, and mouth disease: A clinically recognizable virus infection seen mainly in children. Clin. Pediatr. 6:373, 1967.

Kimura, A., Abe, N., and Nakato, T. Light and electron microscopic study of skin lesions of patients with the hand, foot, and mouth disease. *Tohoku J. Exp. Med.* 122:237, 1977.

Miliaria Rubra
Shelley, W. B., and Horvath, P. N. Experimental miliaria in man. *J. Invest. Dermatol.* 14:193, 1950.

Bullous Dermatosis of Diabetes Mellitus
Allen, G. E., and Hadden, D. R. Bullous lesions of the skin in diabetes (bullosis diabeticorum). *Br. J. Dermatol.* 82:216, 1970.
Bernstein, J. E., Medenica, M., Soltani, K., and Griem, S. F. Bullous eruption of diabetes mellitus. *Arch. Dermatol.* 115:324, 1979.
Cantrell, A. R., and Martz, W. Idiopathic bullae in diabetics. Bullous diabeticorum. *Arch. Dermatol.* 96:42, 1967.
Paltzik, R. L. Bullous eruption of diabetes mellitus. Bullosis diabeticorum. *Arch. Dermatol.* 116:475–476, 1980.

Coma Bulla
Arndt, K. A., Mihm, M. C., Jr., and Parrish, J. A. Bullae: A cutaneous sign of a variety of neurologic diseases. *J. Invest. Dermatol.* 60:312, 1973.

IgA Pustular Dermatosis
Huff, J. C., Golitz, L. E., and Kunke, K. S. Intraepidermal neutrophilic IgA dermatosis. *N. Engl. J. Med.* 31:1643–1645, 1985.

Pemphigus Vulgaris
Emmerson, R. W., and Wilson-Jones, E. Eosinophilic spongiosis in pemphigus: A report of an unusual histological change in pemphigus. *Arch. Dermatol.* 97:252, 1968.
Hashimoto, T., Sugiura, M., Kurihara, S., et al. Atypical pemphigus showing eosinophilic spongiosis. *Clin. Exp. Dermatol.* 8:37, 1983.
Knight, A. G., Black, M. M., and Delaney, J. J. Eosinophilic spongiosis: Clinical, histologic and immunofluorescent correlation. *Clin. Exp. Dermatol.* 1:141, 1976.
Mutasim, D. F., Pelc, N. J., Anhalt, G. J. Paraneoplastic pemphigus, pemphigus vulgaris, and pemphigus foliaceus. *Clin. Dermatol.* 11:113–117, 1993.
Pisani, M., and Ruocco, V. Drug-induced pemphigus in M. J. Fellner and D. A. Zeide (Eds.), Unexpected drug reactions. *Clin. Dermatol.* 4:118, 1986.

Pemphigus Vegetans
Ahmed, A. R., and Blose, D. A. Pemphigus vegetans: Neumann type and Hallopeau type. *Int. Dermatol.* 23:135, 1984.
Director, W. Pemphigus vegetans: A clinicopathological correlation. *Arch. Dermatol. Syphilol.* 66:343, 1952.
Guerra-Rodrigo, F., and Morais-Cardoso, J. P. Pemphigus vegetans. *Arch. Dermatol.* 104:412, 1971.

Benign Familial Pemphigus
Gottlieb, S. K., and Lutzner, M. A. Hailey-Hailey disease—An electron microscopic study. *J. Invest. Dermatol.* 54:368, 1970.
Hernandez-Perez, E. Familial benign chronic pemphigus. *Cutis* 39:75, 1987.
Michel, B. "Familial benign chronic pemphigus" by Hailey and Hailey, April 1939. Commentary: Hailey–Hailey disease, familial benign chronic pemphigus. *Arch. Dermatol.* 118:774, 1982.
Palmer, D. D., and Perry, H. O. Benign familial chronic pemphigus. *Arch. Dermatol.* 86:493, 1962.
Steffen, C. G. Familial benign chronic pemphigus. *Am. J. Dermatopathol.* 9:58, 1987.

Keratosis Follicularis (Darier's Disease)
Getzler, N. A., and Flint, A. Keratosis follicularis: A study of one family. *Arch. Dermatol.* 93:545, 1966.
Gottlieb, S. K., and Lutzner, M. A. Darier's disease: An electron microscopic study. *Arch. Dermatol.* 107:225, 1973.

Suprabasilar

Ishibashi, Y., Kajiwara, Y., Andoh, I., et al. The nature and pathogenesis of dyskeratosis in Hailey–Hailey and Darier's disease. *J. Dermatol.* 11:335, 1984.

Transient Acantholytic Dermatosis
Ackerman, A. B. Focal acantholytic dyskeratosis. *Arch. Dermatol.* 106:702, 1972.
Bystryn, J. C. Immunofluorescence studies in transient acantholytic dermatosis (Grover's disease). *Am. J. Dermatopathol.* 1:325, 1979.
Chalet, M., Grover, R., and Ackerman, A. B. Transient acantholytic dermatosis. A reevaluation. *Arch. Dermatol.* 113:431, 1977.
Grover, R. W. Transient acantholytic dermatosis. *Arch. Dermatol.* 101:426, 1970.
Heaphy, M. R., Tucker, S. B., and Winkelmann, R. K. Benign papular acantholytic dermatosis. *Arch. Dermatol.* 112:814, 1976.
Horn, T. D., and Gruleau, G. E. Transient acantholytic dermatosis in immunocompromised febrile patients with cancer. *Arch. Dermatol.* 123:238, 1987.

Chapter 7

Neoplastic Patterns of
the Epidermis

I. Benign hyperplastic disorders
   A. Seborrheic keratosis
     1. Hyperkeratotic and papillary
     2. Acanthotic
     3. Adenoidal
     4. Irritated keratosis
     5. Inverted follicular keratosis
     6. Clonal seborrheic keratosis
   B. Linear epidermal nevus
   C. Acanthosis nigricans
   D. Verruca vulgaris
   E. Verruca plantaris
   F. Condyloma acuminatum
   G. Verruca plana
   H. Bowenoid papulosis
   I. Molluscum contagiosum
   J. Fibroepithelial polyp
   K. Warty dyskeratoma
   L. Clear cell acanthoma (Degos' tumor)
   M. Confluent and reticulated papillomatosis of Gougerot and Carteaud
   N. Large cell acanthoma
II. Hyperplastic disorders, unclassified
   A. Keratoacanthoma
   B. Pseudoepitheliomatous hyperplasia
III. Atypical keratinocytic proliferation
   A. Actinic keratosis
     1. Hypertrophic
     2. Atrophic
     3. Acantholytic
     4. Lichenoid
IV. Malignancy
   A. Squamous cell carcinoma
     1. Intraepidermal neoplasia (IEN) III
     2. Invasive
   B. Basal cell carcinoma
     1. Superficial (multifocal)
     2. Sclerosing (morpheaform)
     3. Basosquamous carcinoma
     4. Micronodular basal cell carcinoma
   C. Fibroepithelioma of Pinkus
   D. Paget's disease: breast and extramammary

Although epidermal hyperplasia can be quite irregular, three common patterns are recognized. A papillary pattern is generally present in benign neoplastic lesions such as verruca vulgaris. A psoriasiform pattern may reflect squamous cell carcinoma *in situ*. Platelike hyperplasia may occur in benign or malignant lesions such as eccrine poroma or squamous cell carcinoma in situ.

The Reactive Process and the Disease	Histopathology	Comments
I. Benign hyperplastic disorders		
A. Seborrheic keratosis (Fig. 7-1)		
1. Hyperkeratotic and papillary (Fig. 7-2)	1. Marked laminated hyperkeratosis	

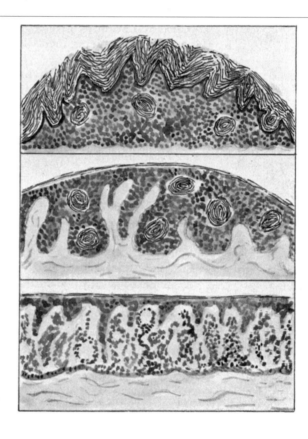

Fig. **7-1.** *Seborrheic keratosis. Three histologic patterns are illustrated here: the hyperkeratotic* (top), *acanthotic* (middle), *and adenoidal* (lower) *types.*

Fig. **7-2.** *Seborrheic keratosis, hyperkeratotic pattern. Epidermal nevi may also exhibit this histology. (Reprinted with permission from T. H. Kwan and M. C. Mihm. The Skin. In S. L. Robbins and R. S. Cotran (Eds.), Pathologic Basis of Disease (2nd ed.). Philadelphia: Saunders, 1979.)*

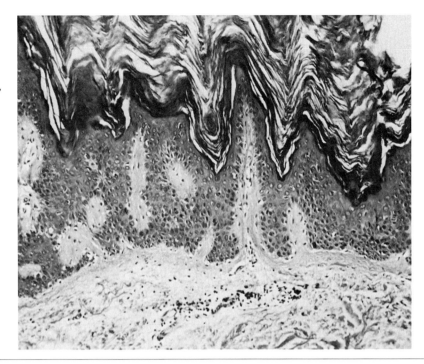

Cutaneous horn:

The cutaneous horn is a clinical entity describing a markedly hyperkeratotic, excrescent lesion that juts out from the normal skin. This lesion can exhibit a variety of histologic features beneath it, including a seborrheic keratosis, an actinic keratosis, a basal cell carcinoma, a squamous cell carcinoma, a trichilemmoma, a verruca vulgaris, and even, as rarely reported in the literature, a malignant melanoma or Kaposi's sarcoma. Thus, cutaneous horn is a clinical diagnosis the true nature of which can be determined only by histologic examination.

2. Papillary epidermal hyperplasia (papillomatosis)
3. Proliferation of basaloid cells
4. Horn pseudocysts may or may not be present

Papillary epidermal hyperplasia (papillomatosis) often seen in:

Seborrheic keratosis
Actinic keratosis
Epidermal nevus
Verruca vulgaris
Acanthosis nigricans
Acrokeratosis verruciformis (Hopf)
Fibroepithelial polyp
Reticulated and confluent papillomatosis

Seborrheic keratoses are usually elevated above the normal skin surface

Dermatosis papulosa nigra is a term used to describe a small, pigmented seborrheic keratosis occurring in people of color

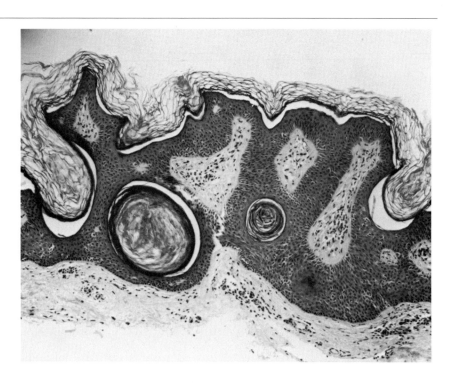

Fig. **7-3.** *Seborrheic keratosis of acanthotic type.*

2. Acanthotic (Fig. 7-3)

1. Hyperkeratosis
2. Sheets of basaloid cells
3. Keratin-filled horn pseudocysts

The basaloid cells of a seborrheic keratosis are small and cuboidal, with a low nuclear–cytoplasmic ratio. The basaloid cells in a basal cell carcinoma are larger and rounder, with a higher nuclear/cytoplasmic ratio

3. Adenoidal (see Fig. 7-4)

1. Hyperkeratosis
2. Lacelike strands of basaloid cells
3. Pseudocysts may be absent

Pseudocysts, invaginations of epidermal surface, give the appearance of cysts when cut in cross section

Fig. **7-4.** *Seborrheic keratosis. A mixture of adenoidal and acanthotic patterns is present.*

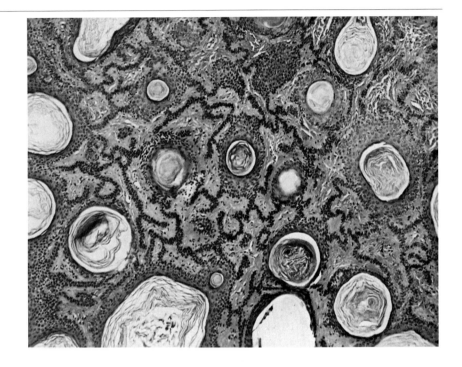

4. Irritated keratosis
   (Fig. 7-5)

1. Hyperkeratosis
2. Proliferation of basaloid cells often arising from a hair follicle
3. Exophytic growth
4. Squamous eddies (whorled focus of glassy eosinophilic keratinocytes)

Any seborrheic keratosis may have an associated inflammatory infiltrate. This may be referred to as an *inflamed seborrheic keratosis*

Fig. **7-5.** *Irritated seborrheic keratosis.*
A. *Papillary epidermal hyperplasia with areas of squamous change, squamous eddies, and chronic inflammation are typical.*
B. *Squamous eddies.*

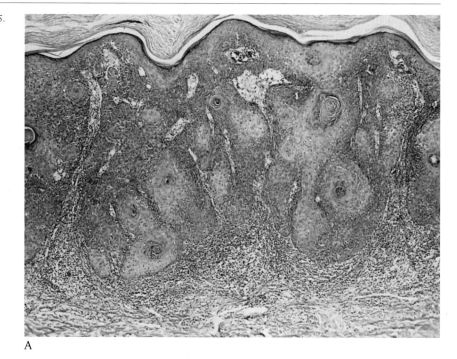

A

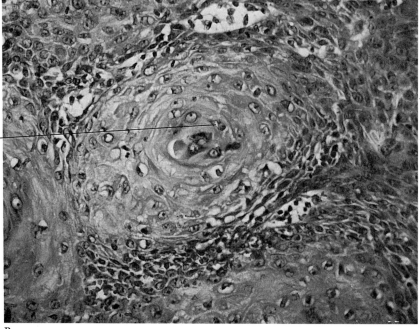

Squamous eddy

B

5. Inverted follicular keratosis

1. Hyperkeratosis
2. Proliferation of basaloid cells
3. Endophytic growth associated with hair follicles
4. Squamous eddies

6. Clonal seborrheic keratosis (Fig. 7-6)

1. Hyperkeratosis
2. Variable papillomatosis and epidermal hyperplasia
3. **Discrete nests of basaloid keratinocytes within the epidermis**
4. Intact basal cell layer and basement membrane

The concept of a clonal pattern within a tumor was originally described as an intraepidermal epithelioma

Other tumors that may exhibit a *clonal pattern* include:

Squamous cell carcinoma
Basal cell carcinoma
Malignant melanoma
Paget's disease
Eccrine poroma
Hidroacanthoma simplex
Pale cell acanthoma

B. Linear epidermal nevus

1. Hyperkeratosis
2. Focal parakeratosis
3. Papillomatosis and acanthosis, sometimes irregular or corrugated
4. Associated dermal abnormalities include abnormal placement of arrector pili muscle and/or irregular organization of reticular dermal collagen

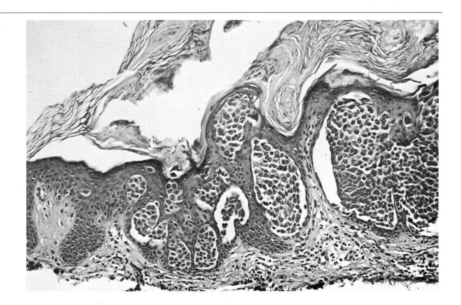

Fig. **7-6.** *Clonal seborrheic keratosis. The nests of basaloid cells exhibit intercellular bridges, indicating keratinocytic origin.*

C. Acanthosis nigricans

1. Marked hyperkeratosis
2. Irregular papillomatosis
3. Fusion of elongated rete ridges
4. Melanin deposition in basal layer, especially at the tips of the rete

D. Verruca vulgaris (Fig. 7-7A,B,C)

1. Marked hyperkeratosis
2. Marked focal **parakeratosis over papillary projections**
3. Papillomatosis
4. Exophytic growth pattern with elongated hyperplastic rete ridges
5. Large, vacuolated keratinocytes **(ballooning degeneration)** with deeply **basophilic inclusion bodies** present in the nucleus or in the cytoplasm, located in the granular and upper spinous layers
6. **Large keratohyaline granules** in vacuolated (infected) and nonvacuolated (noninfected) cells
7. Intracytoplasmic, irregularly shaped eosinophilic bodies within clear spaces
8. **Dilated, elongated vessels in papillary dermis**

Ballooning degeneration is a term used to describe the cytoplasmic swelling and vacuolization in keratinocytes that occur in some viral infections (see also Ch. 6, II.E)

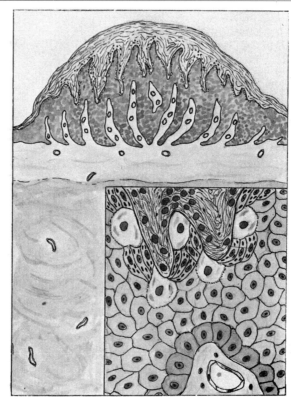

Fig. **7-7.** *Verruca vulgaris, condyloma acuminatum, verruca plantaris, and verruca plana. Epidermal hyperplasia, papillomatosis, hyperkeratosis, parakeratosis, densely basophilic nuclear inclusions, and disturbed keratohyaline granule formation are seen in varying degrees in lesions caused by the wart virus(es).*
A. *Verruca vulgaris. Inset: nuclear inclusions, large keratohyaline granules, and ballooning cytoplasmic changes.*

A

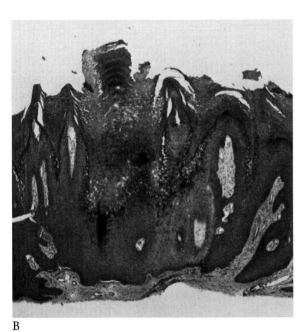

B

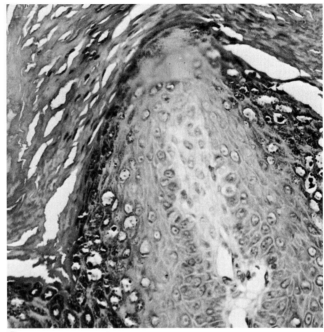

C

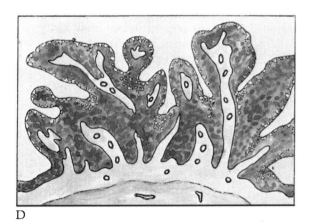

D

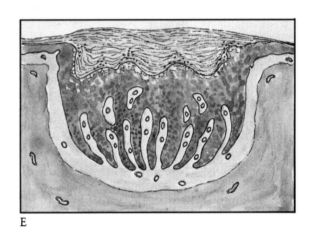

E

B. *Verruca vulgaris. Photomicrograph for comparison.*
C. *Higher magnification showing cytopathic effect of cells in the expanded granular layer.*
D. *Condyloma acuminatum.*
E. *Verruca plantaris.*
F. *Verruca plana.*

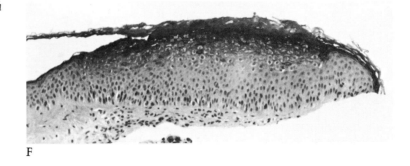

F

E. Verruca plantaris
(see Fig. 7-7E)

1. Marked hyperkeratosis
2. Marked focal **parakeratosis over papillary projections**
3. Blunted papillomatosis
4. **Endophytic growth pattern** with hyperplasia of elongated rete ridges curving inward toward the center of the lesion
5. Virally induced cytopathic changes are similar to those of verruca vulgaris. (see D.5, p. 108)
6. Some verruca plantaris lesions show prominent intracytoplasmic eosinophilic bodies (myrmecia)
7. Dilated elongated vessels in papillary dermis

F. Condyloma acuminatum
(see Fig. 7-7D)

1. Diffuse **parakeratosis**
2. Filiform papillary epidermal hyperplasia with thickening and elongation of the rete ridges
3. Inverted wedges of cells with perinuclear vacuolization (koilocytosis)
4. Eccentrically located, hyperchromatic irregularly shaped nuclei
5. Edematous dermis with dilated capillaries and moderately dense mononuclear cell infiltrate

Lesions usually occur on mucosal surfaces; pseudoepitheliomatous hyperplasia occurs rarely (giant condylomata of Buschke and Lowenstein)
Koilocytes, characteristic of human papillomavirus infections, are enlarged cells with a distinct perinuclear zone of cytoplasmic clearing surrounded by a peripheral zone of dense cytoplasm

G. Verruca plana
(see Fig. 7-7F)

1. Basketweave hyperkeratosis
2. Epidermal hyperplasia
3. Numerous vacuolated cells in the upper third of the epidermis—so-called **bird's-eye cells**
4. Nucleus has dense chromatin and prominent nucleolus
5. Dense basophilic inclusion bodies not observed

H. Bowenoid papulosis
(Fig. 7-8)

1. Variable hyperkeratosis
2. Mild acanthosis
3. Disarray and proliferation of keratinocytes with loss of normal polarity
4. Atypical mitotic figures throughout epidermis
5. Alteration or loss of granular cell layer

I. Molluscum contagiosum
(Fig. 7-9)

1. Epithelial hyperplasia extending downward in a lobulated fashion to form a cup-shaped lesion

Fig. **7-8.** Bowenoid papulosis. Acanthosis with full-thickness keratinocytic atypia and numerous mitotic figures are seen.

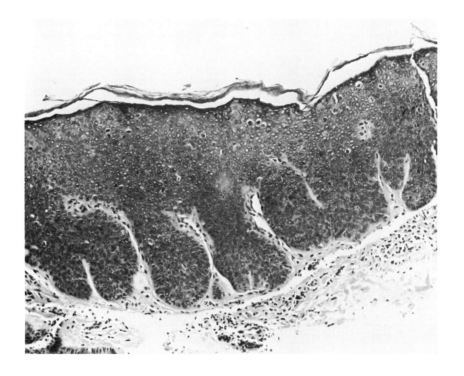

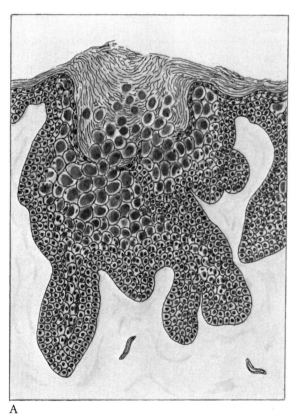

A

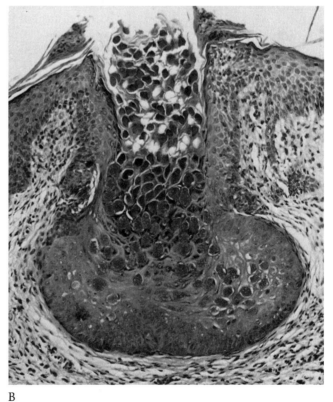

B

Fig. **7-9.** (A, B) Molluscum contagiosum. Hyperplasia and invagination of the epidermis and the characteristic eosinophilic cytoplasmic inclusions are diagnostic.

	2. Hyperkeratosis	
	3. **"Molluscum bodies"**	Molluscum bodies are homogeneous, eosinophilic intracytoplasmic inclusions that enlarge to compress and flatten the nucleus; these molluscum bodies become basophilic at the level of granular layer

J. Fibroepithelial polyp	1. Hyperkeratosis
	2. Papillomatosis
	3. Variable epidermal hyperplasia, sometimes resembling a seborrheic keratosis
	4. Dermal connective-tissue stalk composed of loose collagen fibers and capillaries
	5. Absence of epidermal appendages
		Differential diagnosis:
		  Supernumerary digit
		  Acquired digital fibrokeratoma
		  Accessory tragus

K. Warty dyskeratoma (Fig. 7-10)	1. Central cup-shaped invagination filled with hyperkeratotic and parakeratotic debris 2. Acanthosis of lining epithelium 3. Acantholytic and dyskeratotic cells at base of the lesion 4. Prominent papillary projections, called **villi,** are lined by basal cells	The histology of warty dyskeratoma may be identical to that of Darier's disease (keratosis follicularis)
L. Clear cell acanthoma (Degos' tumor)	1. Sharply demarcated area of epidermal hyperplasia with elongated, fused rete ridges 2. Parakeratosis 3. Surface commonly eroded 4. **Large, pale or "clear" keratinocytes** 5. Slight spongiosis 6. **Neutrophilic invasion** of epidermis and formation of neutrophilic microabscesses 7. Prominent vascular dilatation 8. Mixed infiltrate in dermis	Clear cells contain abundant glycogen, which is PAS-positive and diastase-labile. Glycogen accumulates in the pale cells due to absent phosphorylase. Thus, the glycogen cannot be metabolized
M. Confluent and reticulated papillomatosis of Gougerot and Carteaud	1. Hyperkeratosis 2. Papillomatous and slightly acanthotic epidermis 3. Increased basilar hyperpigmentation 4. Minimal inflammation	This may be a response pattern to tinea versicolor. Many cases will demonstrate yeast and hyphal forms with PAS stains
N. Large cell acanthoma	1. Hyperkeratosis without parakeratosis 2. Slight elongation of rete ridges but epidermis usually of normal thickness	The existence of this entity is controversial. Some believe these to represent variants of other keratinocytic proliferations

Fig. **7-10.** Warty dyskeratoma.
A. An epidermal invagination filled
   with keratinaceous material exhibits
   suprabasal cleft formation and
   villous papillary epidermal
   hyperplasia.
B. This higher magnification exhibits
   corps ronds (arrows) and
   papillomatosis.

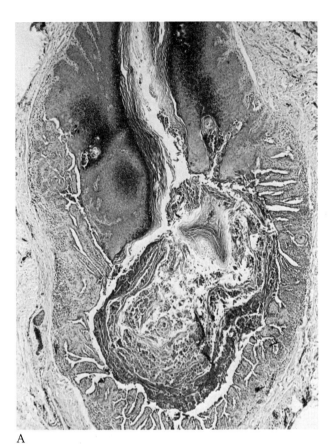

A

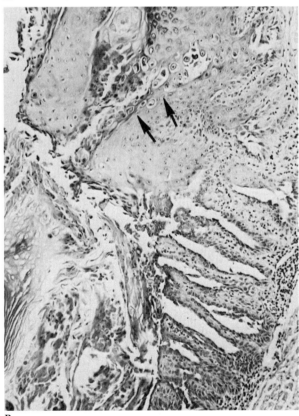

B

3. Enlarged keratinocytes with slightly altered maturation sequence
4. Absence of significant solar elastosis

Differential diagnosis:

Actinic keratosis
Lentigo simplex
Seborrheic keratosis
Solar lentigo

II. Hyperplastic disorders, unclassified
   A. Keratoacanthoma (Fig. 7-11)

1. **Cup-shaped** invagination of epidermis with keratin-filled central crater and lateral "lip-like" extensions over the sides of the crater
2. Most cells are **large, with pale, eosinophilic "glassy" cytoplasm**
3. The advancing lower margin of the lesion is characteristically infiltrating in spiky, irregular tongues of smaller keratinocytes, which entrap connective-tissue elements
4. Cells of the advancing border and peripheral margin may exhibit variable nuclear atypism. Centrally located cells do not show nuclear atypia
5. Mitoses common
6. **Intraepidermal neutrophilic abscesses** containing collagen, elastic fibers, and occasional dyskeratotic cell
7. Inflammatory infiltrate beneath proliferating epidermis common in later lesions

Keratoacanthomas may be difficult to distinguish from squamous cell carcinoma. Complete excision of the lesion is desirable for definitive classification

Resolving keratoacanthomas exhibit a hyperkeratotic mass above an epidermis that is flattened and rests on a bandlike zone of inflamed fibrous tissue

Unilocular intraepidermal neutrophilic abscesses with marked epidermal hyperplasia may be seen in:

Keratoacanthoma
Deep fungal infection
Iododerma and bromoderma
Pale cell acanthoma

   B. Pseudoepitheliomatous hyperplasia

1. Variable hyperkeratosis and parakeratosis
2. Extensive epidermal hyperplasia with elongated rete ridges
3. Normal maturation from basal layer to stratum corneum
4. Mitoses occasionally present

Extensive, irregular epidermal proliferation with cytologic atypia favors a diagnosis of squamous cell carcinoma

Fig. **7-11.** *Keratoacanthoma*
A. *Low magnification reveals the cup shape or crateriform architecture and well-demarcated borders.*
B. *Higher magnification shows the characteristic glassy, cytologic change in keratinocytes.*

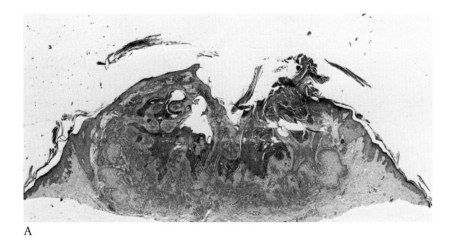

A

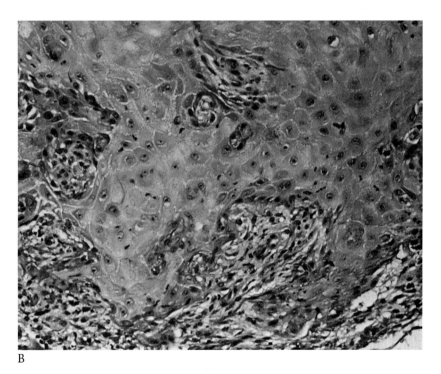

B

III. Atypical keratinocytic proliferation

A. Actinic keratosis (Fig. 7-12); intraepidermal neoplasia (IEN) I (see IV A. 1)	1. Hyperkeratosis common 2. Parakeratosis common 3. Epidermal atrophy alternating with hyperplasia 4. **Pleomorphism** of large, irregular hyperchromatic nuclei in the lower layers of the epidermis 5. **Loss of cellular polarity,** especially in lower epidermis 6. Teardroplike proliferation of cells in basal layer may be seen 7. Solar elastosis 8. Sparing of appendageal epithelium frequently observed	See Table 7-1 *Solar elastotic changes,* as well as a mononuclear cell infiltrate, are frequently found beneath an actinic keratosis Arsenical keratoses and other nonactinically induced premalignant keratoses exhibit similar cytologic atypia without underlying dermal elastosis
1. Hypertrophic	Changes described above, with emphasis on hyperkeratosis and acanthosis	It is not necessary to subclassify actinic keratoses for clinical reasons, but subtypes present distinctive histologic patterns and so are mentioned here
2. Atrophic	Changes described above, with emphasis on epidermal atrophy	Actinic keratoses may exhibit marked hyperpigmentation of keratinocytes; these lesions are sometimes called *pigmented* actinic keratosis
3. Acantholytic	Changes described above with acantholysis	
4. Lichenoid (see Fig. 10-4)	Changes described above, with dense, bandlike mononuclear cell infiltrate in the upper dermis and occasional keratinocytic dyskeratosis	Lichenoid actinic keratosis may be similar histologically to lichen planus (see also Ch. 12, XI)

Fig. **7-12.** (A, B) Actinic keratosis. The hallmark of this disorder is proliferation of atypical keratinocytes associated with solar elastosis. Parakeratosis and chronic inflammation frequently are present. In actinic keratosis, the atypical keratinocytes are not transepidermal, unlike squamous cell carcinoma in situ in which the atypical keratinocytes are present at all levels of the epidermis.

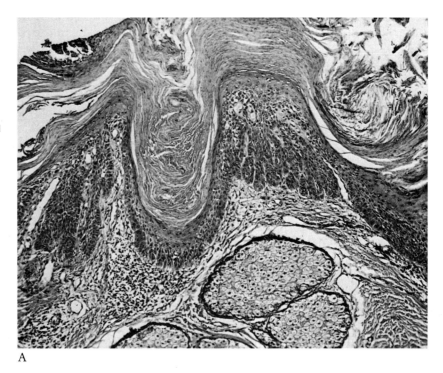

A

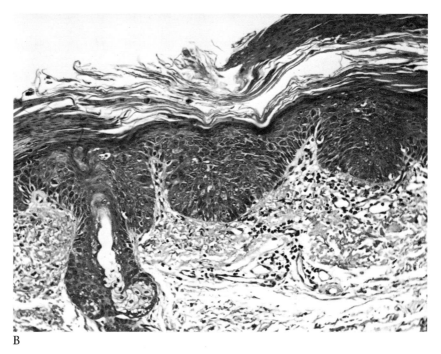

B

In dermatopathology, terms such as *Bowen's disease* and *erythroplasia of Queyrat* have been used in the past to describe squamous cell carcinoma *in situ* (Fig. 7-13) occurring in different areas of the body. Bowen's disease traditionally has referred to squamous cell carcinoma that appears in normal appearing skin in contrast to squamous cell carcinoma *in situ* that appears in association with an actinic keratosis. We believe it is more

Fig. **7-13.** *Squamous cell carcinoma in situ.*
A. *Transepidermal cytologic atypia is diagnostic.*
B. *Dyskeratosis, atypical mitotic figures, and cellular pleomorphism are present.*

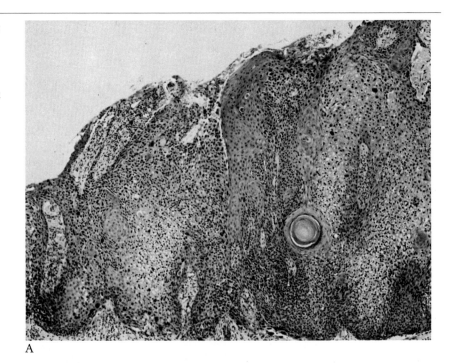

A

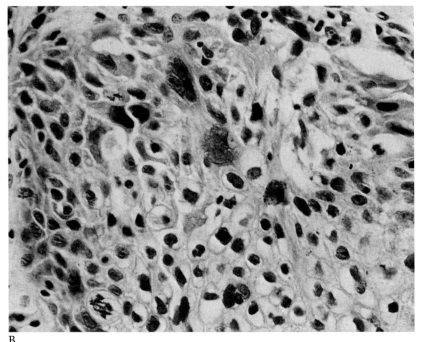

B

Table **7-1.** *Carcinoma In Situ or Intraepidermal Neoplasia (IEN)*

Grade	Histologic Features	Examples
I.	Basilar atypia/cellular pleomorphism	Actinic keratosis
II.	Atypism of lower two-thirds of epidermis	Arsenical keratosis, hypertrophic actinic keratosis
III.	Two-thirds to full-thickness atypia 1. Appendageal involvement 2. Loss of granular cell layer 3. Full thickness/loss of maturation	Squamous cell carcinoma *in situ*, Bowen's disease, erythroplasia of Queyrat, bowenoid papulosis

desirable to classify *in situ* carcinoma in a similar fashion to gynecologic pathology:

Vulvar intraepithelial neoplasia (VIN), grades I–III.

Cervical intraepithelial neoplasia (CIN), grades I–III.

Grade I is mild cytologic atypia, grade II is partial atypia, and grade III is full-thickness atypia. In the analogy to the skin, grades I and III are defined, but to date the concept of grade II (partial atypia) has no practical application regarding treatment or prognosis. For purposes of this text we define squamous cell carcinoma *in situ* in Table 7-1 as in IEN III.

IV. Malignancy

    A. Squamous cell carcinoma

        1. Intraepidermal neoplasia (IEN) III; squamous cell carcinoma *in situ*

1. Marked parakeratosis
2. Acanthosis common, but atrophy occasionally seen
3. Erosion may be present
4. **Loss of normal progression** from basal cell to granular keratinocyte
5. Atypia and pleomorphism of keratinocytes extending **throughout the entire epidermis**
6. Dyskeratosis
7. Mitotic figures may be numerous; atypical mitotic figures may be seen
8. Multinucleated epidermal cells

2. Invasive (Fig. 7-14)

1. Irregular masses of atypical cells proliferating downward in discontiguous islands detached from overlying epidermis
2. Variable keratinization with squamous pearls
3. Acantholysis may be present
4. Marked inflammatory dermal infiltrate composed predominantly of mononuclear cells

Atypism is minimal in well-differentiated squamous cell carcinoma and absent in verrucous carcinoma

Occasionally cells may be predominantly spindle-shaped (Fig. 7-15)

Morbidity and mortality are said to be greater in squamous cell carcinoma arising from non–sun-exposed skin, i.e., in chronic radiodermatitis, in sinus tracts, in ulcers, and on mucosal surfaces. An exception is squamous cell carcinoma arising in actinic cheilitis

A **squamous pearl** is a focus of keratinization or a dyskeratotic cell with a pyknotic nucleus surrounded by whorls of variably keratinized cells

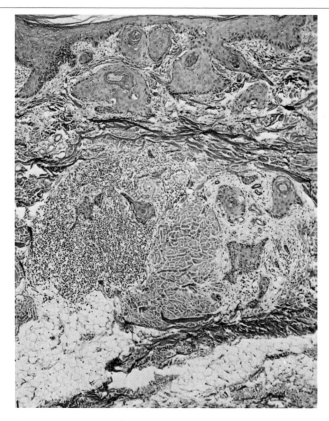

Fig. **7-14.** *Invasive squamous cell carcinoma. Irregular tongues of moderately well-differentiated squamous cell carcinoma invade the dermis. A lymphocytic infiltrate surrounds some tumor nests at left.*

Fig. **7-15.** *Spindle cell squamous cell carcinoma. The differential diagnosis of this spindle cell tumor (A) includes atypical fibroxanthoma and spindle cell or desmoplastic melanoma. Squamous cell carcinoma can be diagnosed if origin from epidermis is observed, if areas of squamous differentiation such as bridges and squamous pearls are present, or by appropriate immunoperoxidase profile, including positive stains for keratin (B). (Immunoperoxidase preparation courtesy of Geraldine Pinkus, M.D.)*

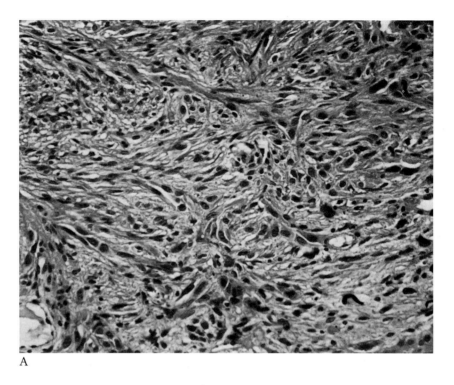

A

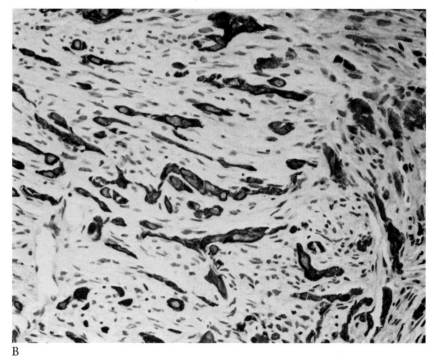

B

B. Basal cell carcinoma (nodular pattern) (Fig. 7-16)

1. Patterned proliferation of small cuboidal to round cells with a large nuclear–cytoplasmic ratio, basophilic cytoplasm, and hyperchromatic nuclei; nucleoli usually absent
2. Intercellular bridges are decreased to absent
3. **Peripheral palisading** of tumor cells
4. Tumor often surrounded by a fibrous and inflammatory stroma
5. **Separation (retraction) artifact** between tumor cells and stroma is frequently observed
6. Tumor lobules frequently connect to overlying epidermis or adjacent hair follicles

The histologic appearance of basal cell carcinoma varies considerably with regard to the presence or absence of surface ulceration, adnexal involvement, pigmentation, keratinization, acid mucopolysaccharide (mucin) deposition, or cystic spaces. Consequently descriptive adjectives such as *ulceronodular, cystic, pigmented,* and so forth, are often used in diagnosing basal cell carcinoma. For practical, prognostic, and therapeutic purposes, however, it is most important to qualify the diagnosis in three instances:
Superficial (multifocal) basal cell carcinoma
Sclerosing (morpheaform) basal cell carcinoma
Basosquamous carcinoma

An infiltrative (spiky border) pattern seems to be associated with an increased incidence of recurrence

1. Superficial (multifocal) (see Fig. 7-16C)

1. Small **buds** of deeply basophilic cells extend from the epidermis into superficial dermis
2. Separation artifact may be prominent

Superficial and sclerosing basal cell carcinomas may have microscopic extension far beyond clinically apparent borders

2. Sclerosing (morpheaform) (see Fig. 7-16B)

1. Small, often **linear and branching** aggregates of tumor cells embedded in a **fibrotic dermis**
2. Overlying epidermal attachment may be minimal to absent

Fibrous stroma may be the predominant feature since the total number of tumor cells present in sclerosing basal cell carcinoma may be quite small
Differential diagnosis:
Metastatic carcinoma, especially adenocarcinoma of the breast (helpful distinguishing feature: metastatic carcinoma grows in nonbranching lines)
Microcystic adnexal carcinoma

3. Basosquamous carcinoma (see Fig. 7-16D)

1. Areas of typical basal cell carcinoma with adjacent areas of invasive squamous cell carcinoma

Basosquamous carcinomas may be locally aggressive and may metastasize

4. Miconodular basal cell carcinoma

1. Well-circumscribed, small nests of basal keratinocytes
2. Separation of individual nests by abundant intervening collagen
3. Deep and lateral extension of nests throughout dermis

Fig. **7-16.** *Basal cell carcinoma.*
A. *Solid and pseudocystic patterns.*
B. *Basal cell carcinoma with an infiltrative pattern. Nests of tumor cells, some quite small, extend from the epidermis into the dermis.*

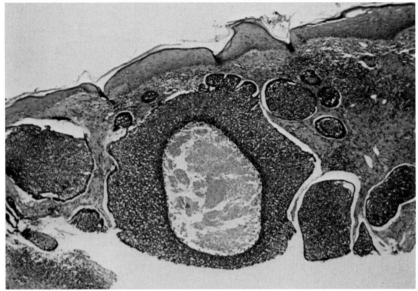

A

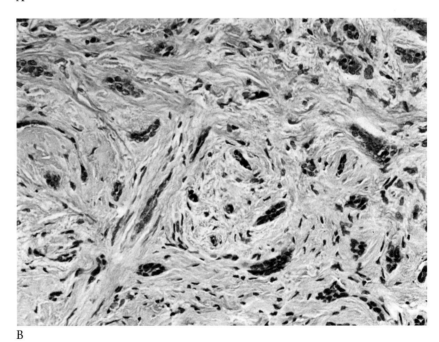

B

Fig. **7-16.** (continued)
C. *Superficial type.*
D. *Basosquamous carcinoma type.*

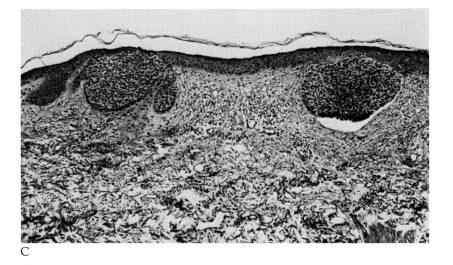

C

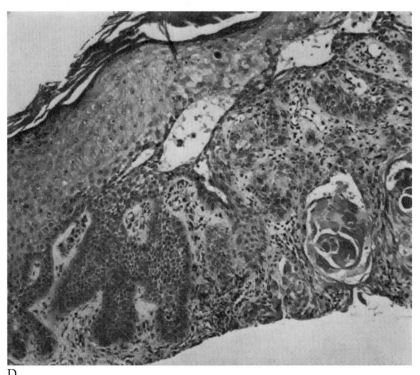

D

C. Fibroepithelioma of Pinkus (Fig. 7-17)

1. Narrow anastomosing strands of basophilic tumor cells extend from epidermis deep into dermis
2. Fibrotic stroma surrounds tumor

Controversy exists regarding the precise classification of this tumor—whether it is a premalignant tumor, a variant of a basal cell carcinoma, or a separate entity that may evolve into a basal cell carcinoma

Fig. **7-17.** *Fibroepithelioma of Pinkus. Basaloid cells within a fibrous stroma extend in an anastomosing trabecular pattern deep into the dermis.*

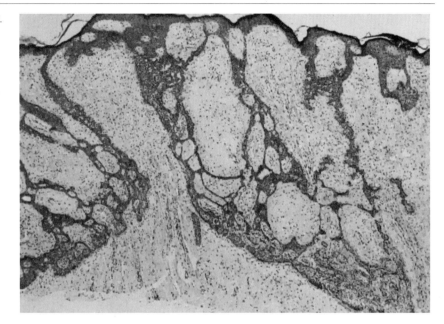

D. Paget's disease: breast and extramammary (Fig. 7-18)

1. Epidermal hyperplasia is frequent
2. Epidermal infiltration by single cells or groups of cells
3. **Paget's cells** are variably pleomorphic, with pale, often vacuolated cytoplasm, large nuclei, and no intercellular bridges
4. In the lower epidermis, tumor cells often compress or flatten the underlying basal cells
5. Mitoses common

Paget's cells are PAS-positive, diastase-resistant, and stain with alcian blue at pH 2.5

Differential diagnosis:
Malignant melanoma
Squamous cell carcinoma *in situ*

Compression of the basal cells is a finding that helps differentiate Paget's disease from malignant melanoma

Immunoperoxidase staining pattern:

Positive	Negative
Keratin	S-100
EMA	Vimentin
CEA	

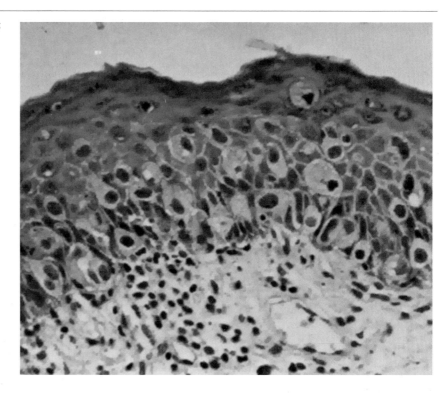

Fig. **7-18.** *Paget's disease. Large cells with pale, vacuolated cytoplasms and variably hyperchromatic nuclei pepper the epidermis.*

Suggested Reading

Seborrheic Keratosis

Bedi, T. R. Familial congenital multiple seborrheic verrucae. *Arch. Dermatol.* 113:1441, 1977.

Berman, A., and Winkelmann, R. K. Seborrheic keratoses: Appearance in course of exfoliative erythroderma and regression associated with histologic mononuclear cell infiltration. *Arch. Dermatol.* 118:615, 1982.

Braun-Falco, O., and Kint, A. Zur histogenese der verruca seborrhoica. I. Mittelung. *Arch. Klin. Exp. Dermatol.* 216:615, 1963.

Friedman-Birnbaum, R., and Haim, S. Seborrheic keratosis and papillomatosis: markers of breast adenocarcinoma. *Cutis* 32:161–162, 1983.

Lindelof, B., Sigurgeirsson, B., and Melander, S. Seborrheic keratosis and cancer. *J. Am. Acad. Dermatol.* 26:947–950, 1992.

Mevorah, B., and Mishima, Y. Cellular response of seborrheic keratosis following croton oil irritation and surgical trauma. *Dermatologica* 131:452, 1965.

Sanderson, K. V. The structure of seborrhoeic keratoses. *Br. J. Dermatol.* 80:588, 1968.

Sperry, K., and Wall, J. Adenocarcinoma of the stomach with eruptive seborrheic keratoses: The sign of Leser-Trelat. *Cancer* 45:2434, 1980.

Linear Epidermal Nevus

Altman, J., and Mehregan, A. H. Inflammatory linear verrucose epidermal nevus. *Arch. Dermatol.* 104:385, 1971.

Dupre, A., and Christol, B. Inflammatory linear verrucose epidermal nevus. A pathologic study. *Arch. Dermatol.* 113:767, 1977.

Kennedy, C. Inflammatory linear verrucous epidermal nevus (eczematous linear naevus). *Clin. Exp. Dermatol.* 5:471, 1980.

Solomon, L. M., Fretzin, D. F., and Dewald, R. L. The epidermal nevus syndrome. *Arch. Dermatol.* 97:273, 1968.

Acanthosis Nigricans

Brown, J., and Winkelmann, R. K. Acanthosis nigricans: A study of 90 cases. *Medicine* (Baltimore) 47:33–51, 1986.

Schwartz, R. A. Acanthosis nigricans. *J. Am. Acad. Dermatol.* 31:1–19, 1994.

Verruca

Gross, G., Pfister, H., Hagedorn, M., and Gissmann, L. Correlation between human papillomavirus (HPV) type and histology of warts. *J. Invest. Dermatol.* 78:160, 1982.

Molluscum Contagiosum

Lombardo, P. C. Molluscum contagiosum and acquired immunodeficiency syndrome. *Arch. Dermatol.* 121:834–835, 1985.

Lutzner, M. A. Molluscum contagiosum, verruca and zoster viruses: Electron microscopic studies in the skin. *Arch. Dermatol.* 87:436, 1963.

Mihara, M. Three-dimensional ultrastructural study of molluscum contagiosum in the skin using scanning-electron microscopy. *Br. J. Dermatol.* 125:557–560, 1991.

Warty Dyskeratoma

Szymanski, F. J. Warty dyskeratoma: A benign cutaneous tumor resembling Darier's disease microscopically. *Arch. Dermatol.* 75:567, 1957.

Tanay, A., and Mehregan, A. H. Warty dyskeratoma. (Review) *Dermatologica* 138:155, 1969.

Clear Cell Acanthoma

Brownstein, M., Fernando, S., and Shapiro, L. Clear cell acanthoma: Clinicopathologic analysis of 37 new cases. *Am. J. Clin. Pathol.* 59:306, 1973.

Trau, H., Fisher, B. K., and Schewach-Millet, M. Multiple clear cell acanthomas. *Arch. Dermatol.* 116:433, 1980.

Keratoacanthoma

Fathizadeh, A., Medenica, M. M., Soltani, K., et al. Aggressive keratoacanthoma and internal malignant neoplasm. *Arch. Dermatol.* 118:112, 1982.

Fisher, E. R., McCoy, M. M., and Wechsler, H. L. Analysis of histopathologic and electron microscopic determinants of keratoacanthoma and squamous cell carcinoma. *Cancer* 29:1387, 1972.

Hodak, E., Jones, R. E., and Ackerman, A. B. Solitary keratoacanthoma is a squamous cell carcinoma: three examples with metastases. *Am. J. Dermatopathol.* 15:332–342, 1993.

Kern, W. H., and McCray, M. K. The histopathologic differentiation of keratoacanthoma and squamous cell carcinoma of the skin. *J. Cutan. Pathol.* 7:318, 1980.

King, D. F., and Barr, R. J. Intraepithelial elastic fibers and intracytoplasmic glycogen: Diagnostic aids in differentiating keratoacanthoma from squamous cell carcinoma. *J. Cutan. Pathol.* 7:140, 1980.

Lapins, N. A., and Helwig, E. G. Perineural invasion by KA. *Arch. Dermatol.* 37:791, 1980.

Reed, R. J. Keratoacanthoma: Entity or syndrome? *Bull. Tulane Univ. Med. Fac.* 26:117, 1967.

Reid, B. J., and Cheesbrough, M. J. Multiple KA: A unique case and review of current classification. *Acta Dermatol. Venereol.* (*Stockh.*) 58:169, 1978.

Takaki, Y., Masutani, M., and Kawada, A. Electron microscopic study of keratoacanthoma. *Acta Derm. Venereol.* 51:21, 1971.

Wade, T. R., and Ackerman, A. S. The many faces of KA. *J. Dermatol. Surg. Oncol.* 4:498, 1978.

Actinic Keratosis

Ackerman, A. B., and Reed, R. J. Epidermolytic variant of solar keratosis. *Arch. Dermatol.* 107:104, 1973.

Shapiro, L., and Ackerman, A. Solitary lichen planus-like keratosis. *Dermatologica* 132:386, 1966.

Subert, P., Jorizzo, J. L., and Apisarnthanarax, P. Spreading pigmented actinic keratosis. *J. Am. Acad. Dermatol.* 8:63, 1983.

Wade, T. R., and Ackerman, A. B. The many faces of solar keratoses. *J. Dermatol. Surg. Oncol.* 4:730, 1978.

Squamous Cell Carcinoma

Johnson, W. C., and Helwig, E. B. Adenoid squamous cell carcinoma (adenoacanthoma): A clinicopathologic study of 155 patients. *Cancer* 19:1639, 1966.

Lichtiger, B., Mackay, B., and Tessmer, C. F. Spindle-cell variant of squamous carcinoma. *Cancer* 26:1311, 1970.

Schlegel, R., Banks-Schlegel, S., McLeod, J. A., and Pinkus, G. S. Immunoperoxidase localization of keratin in human neoplasms. *Am. J. Pathol.* 101:41, 1980.

Stern, R. S., Thibodeau, L. A., Kleinerman, R. A., et al. Risk of cutaneous carcinoma in patients treated with oral methoxsalen photochemotherapy for psoriasis. *N. Engl. J. Med.* 300:809, 1979.

Strayer, D. S., and Santa Cruz, D. J. Carcinoma *in situ* of the skin: A review of histopathology. *J. Cutan. Pathol.* 7:244, 1980.

Taylor, D. R., Jr., and South, D. A. Bowenoid papulosis: A review. *Cutis* 27:92, 1981.

Ulbright, T. M., Stehman, F. B., Roth, L. M., et al. Bowenoid dysplasia of the vulva. *Cancer* 50:2910, 1982.

Wade, T. R., Kopf, A. W., and Ackerman, A. B. Bowenoid papulosis of the penis. *Cancer* 42:1890, 1978.

Basal Cell Carcinoma

Borel, D. M. Cutaneous basosquamous carcinoma. Review of the literature and report of 35 cases. *Arch. Pathol.* 95:293, 1973.

DeFaria, J. L. Basal cell carcinoma of the skin with areas of squamous cell carcinoma: A basosquamous cell carcinoma? *J. Clin. Pathol.* 38:1273, 1985.

Farmer, E. R., and Helwig, E. B. Metastatic basal cell carcinoma: A clinicopathologic study of seventeen cases. *Cancer* 46:748, 1980.

Jacobs, G. H., Rippey, J. J., and Altini, M. Prediction of aggressive behavior in basal cell carcinoma. *Cancer* 49:533, 1982.

Lang, P. G., Jr., and Maize, J. C. Histologic evolution of recurrent basal cell carcinoma and treatment implications. *J. Am. Acad. Dermatol.* 14:186, 1986.

McGibbon, D. H. Malignant epidermal tumors. *J. Cutan. Pathol.* 12:224, 1985.

Mehregan, A. H. Acantholysis in basal cell epithelioma. *J. Cutan. Pathol.* 6:280, 1979.

Okun, M. R., and Blumethal, G. Basal cell epithelioma with giant cells and nuclear atypicality. *Arch. Dermatol.* 89:598, 1964.

Siegle, R. J., MacMillan, J., and Pollack, S. V. Infiltrative basal cell carcinoma: A nonsclerosing subtype. *J. Dermatol. Surg. Oncol.* 12:830, 1986.

Sloane, J. P. The value of typing basal cell carcinomas in predicting recurrence after surgical excision. *Br. J. Dermatol.* 96:127, 1977.

Wade, T. R., and Ackerman, A. B. The many faces of basal cell carcinoma. *J. Dermatol. Surg. Oncol.* 4:23, 1978.

Extramammary Paget's Disease   Helwig, E. B., and Graham, J. H. Anogenital extramammary Paget's disease: A clinicopathologic review. *Cancer* 16:387, 1963.

Jones, R. E., Austin, C., and Ackerman, A. B. Extramammary Paget's disease: A critical reexamination. *Am. J. Dermatopathol.* 1:101, 1979.

Merot, Y., Mazoujian, G., Pinkus, G., et al. Extramammary Paget's disease of the perianal and perineal regions. *Arch. Dermatol.* 121:750, 1985.

Chapter 8

*Atrophic Processes of
the Epidermis*

Atrophy of the epidermis may occur as a result of aging or various disease processes. Other than in a congenital setting, it is rarely a primary feature; however, epidermal atrophy is a prominent feature in the diseases enumerated in this chapter.

The nosology of parapsoriasis is uncertain. Among the entities that have been given the term parapsoriasis are parapsoriasis en plaques (large and small plaque types), *parapsoriasis* guttata, parapsoriasis lichenoides, and parapsoriasis variegata. Many of these entities will be mentioned in other chapters. Some of the entities, such as parapsoriasis en plaques and parapsoriasis variegata, may exhibit atrophy of the epidermis. It is important to recognize that the use of the term *parapsoriasis* does not imply a common etiology.

The Reactive Process and the Disease	Histopathology	Comments
I. Lichen sclerosus et atrophicus (Figs. 8-1, 12-2)		
A. Early	1. Variable hyperkeratosis 2. Epidermal atrophy	

> *Epidermal atrophy* may be a prominent feature in:
>
> Atrophic actinic keratosis
> Atrophic lichen planus
> Scleroderma
> Lentigo maligna
> Chronic graft-versus-host reaction
> Aged or actinically damaged skin
> Following chronic use of topical corticosteroid preparations
> Acrodermatitis chronica atrophicans
> Radiodermatitis
> Necrobiosis lipoidica
> Lupus erythematosus
> Dermatomyositis
> Aplasia cutis congenita
> Epidermis overlying tumors

	Histopathology	Comments
	3. Vacuolization of dermo-epidermal junction	See also Ch. 11, II.L
	4. Markedly edematous and **homogenized, broadened papillary dermis**	
	5. Vascular ectasia and extravasation of erythrocytes	
	6. Bandlike mononuclear cell infiltrate beneath the edematous papillary dermis extending about and between venules and into the upper reticular dermis	See also Ch. 12, II

Fig. **8-1.** *Lichen sclerosus et atrophicus. Massive upper dermal edema is present with atrophy of the epidermis and a bandlike lymphocytic infiltrate.*

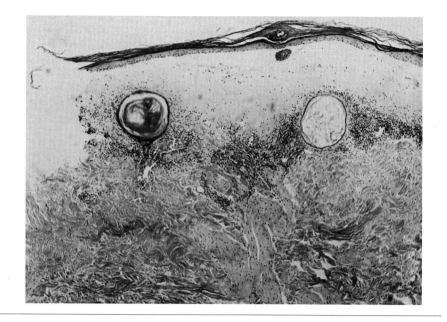

B. Late

1. Marked hyperkeratosis
2. **Hyperkeratotic invagination of the epidermis (follicular plugging)**
3. Marked epidermal **atrophy** alternating with epidermal hyperplasia
4. **Vacuolization** along the dermoepidermal interface
5. **Squamatization** of basal cell layer
6. **Homogenization of upper dermis** with **sclerosis** of collagen
7. Variable patchy mononuclear cell infiltrate in upper dermis

Subepidermal hemorrhagic bulla occasionally present
Differential diagnosis:
  Morphea
  Lupus erythematosus
  Chronic radiodermatitis

See also Ch. 11, II.L

Epidermal atypism may occur in vulvar lichen sclerosus et atrophicus
Lichen sclerosus et atrophicus may occur in association with morphea

II. Parapsoriasis

Parapsoriasis variegata and parapsoriasis en plaques at times may exhibit variable atrophy of the epidermis

See also Ch. 5, I.E; Ch. 12, IX

III. Porokeratosis

1. **Cornoid lamella:** A column of parakeratotic stratum corneum arising within a keratin-filled invagination of epidermis
2. **Absence of granular layer at the base of the coronoid lamella;** cells may be vacuolated or dyskeratotic

There are various clinical forms of porokeratosis that may be histologically indistinguishable. The four types of porokeratosis are classic porokeratosis (Mibelli), disseminated superficial actinic porokeratosis, porokeratosis palmaris et plantaris disseminata, and linear porokeratosis

3. Epidermis overlying the central portion of the lesion may be normal, atrophic, or even hyperplastic
4. Mild lymphocytic perivascular infiltrate in dermis

The cornoid lamella and associated changes often are less well formed in disseminated superficial actinic porokeratosis, which is often associated with solar elastosis

Cornoid lamella has been reported in:

Seborrheic keratosis
Scar
Verruca vulgaris
Milia
Actinic keratosis
Squamous cell carcinoma *in situ*
Basal cell carcinoma

IV. Acrodermatitis chronica atrophicans

    A. Inflammatory phase

1. Hyperkeratosis
2. Parakeratosis
3. Epidermal atrophy with spongiosis
4. Grenz zone
5. Bandlike lymphocytic infiltrate in upper dermis
6. Atrophic sebaceous glands and hair follicles; eccrine glands preserved

Spirochetes may be found using silver stains

    B. Atrophic phase

1. Profound **atrophy of epidermis, dermis, and subcutaneous fat**
2. Inflammatory infiltrate scant to absent

See also Ch. 12, VII; Ch. 20, XI

V. Poikiloderma vasculare atrophicans (Fig. 8-2)

1. Hyperkeratosis
2. Focal parakeratosis
3. **Epidermal atrophy** with flattening of rete ridges
4. Dyskeratosis

Poikiloderma may be:

Congenital
Idiopathic
Associated with dermatomyositis
Associated with mycosis fungoides
Associated with chronic radiation dermatitis

5. **Vacuolization** along dermoepidermal interface

See also Ch. 10, VI; Ch. 12, VIII

Fig. **8-2.** *Poikiloderma vasculare atrophicans. Thinning of the epidermis, vacuolization of the dermoepidermal junction, lymphocytes lined up in the basal layer, and bandlike chronic inflammation of the dermis are characteristic.*

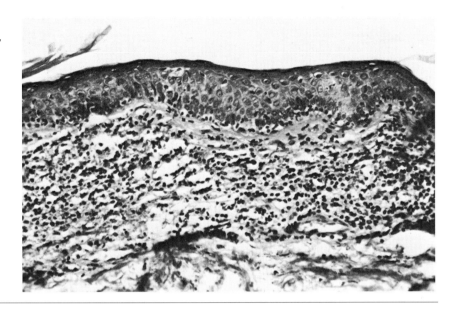

	6. **Bandlike lymphocytic dermal infiltrate**	See also Ch. 12, VIII
	7. Vascular ectasia	
	8. Pigment incontinence may be prominent	
VI. Lupus erythematosus (see Fig. 12-3)	1. Hyperkeratosis	Direct immunofluorescence studies are often helpful in diagnosis
	2. Hyperkeratotic invagination of epidermis (follicular lugging)	
	3. Epidermal atrophy may be prominent	
	4. Squamatization of basal cell layer may be present	
	5. Thickened basement membrane zone in older lesion	Demonstration of thickened basement membrane with PAS stain is helpful in diagnosis of lupus erythematosus
	6. **Vacuolization** along dermal epidermal junction, both **above and below basement membrane zone**	Based on histology alone, it is not possible to differentiate the various subsets of lupus erythematosus
	7. Edema of papillary dermis	
	8. Vascular ectasia	
	9. Extravasation of erythrocytes in early lesions	
	10. Lymphohistiocytic dermal infiltrate may be:	
	a. Bandlike, occasionally obscuring the dermal interface	See also Ch. 12, III
	b. Patchy and disposed about vessels and appendages in reticular dermis, occasionally extending into subcutaneous fat	See also Ch. 16, I.B.1; Ch. 26, I.B.1

11. Neutrophils and nuclear debris may be present in early lesions
12. Pigment incontinence common
13. Increased deposition of acid mucopolysaccharide in reticular dermis

VII. Thermal burn

First degree:
1. Death of keratinocytes through coagulative necrosis;
2. Basal epidermis generally spared
3. Little or no inflammation

Second degree:
4. Variable depth of dermal necrosis
5. Deep portions of adnexal structures spared
6. Subepidermal bulla may arise

Third degree:
7. All of dermis and possibly deeper tissues necrotic

Only first-degree burns are limited to the epidermis

Second- and third-degree burns are discussed here for the sake of convenience

---

Ulceration may be due to:

Thermal burn
Chondrodermatitis nodularis helicis
Neoplasm
Mechanical trauma
Vasculitis
Infection, especially herpes viruses

See also Ch. 11, I

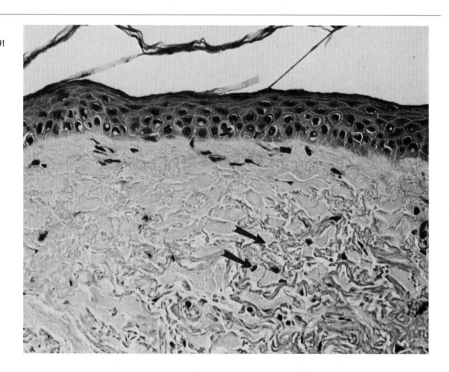

Fig. **8-3.** *Aged skin. The epidermis is thinned, with loss of the normal pattern of rete ridges. Solar elastosis is present (arrows).*

VIII. Aged skin (Fig. 8-3)

1. Thinning of the epidermis with attenuation of rete ridge pattern
2. Decreased numbers of melanocytes
3. Altered elastotic material (solar elastosis) in basophilic clumps or thickened, wavy fibers
4. Dermal hemorrhage without significant inflammation characterizes purpuric patches

Suggested Reading

Lichen Sclerosus et Atrophicus

Aberer, E., and Stanek, G. Histological evidence for spirochetal origin of morphea and lichen sclerosus et atrophicus. *Am. J. Dermatopathol.* 9(5):374–379, 1987.

Bergfeld, W. F., and Lesowitz, S. A. Lichen sclerosus et atrophicus. *Arch. Dermatol.* 101:247, 1970.

Steigleder, G. K., and Raab, W. P. Lichen sclerosus et atrophicus. *Arch. Dermatol.* 84:219, 1961.

Parapsoriasis

Bonvalet, D. The different forms of parapsoriasis en plaques. A report of 90 cases. *Acta Derm. Venereol. (Stockh.)* 104:18, 1977.

Hu, C. H., and Winklemann, R. K. Digitate dermatosis. A new look at symmetrical, small plaque parapsoriasis. *Arch. Dermatol.* 107:65, 1973.

Samman, P. D. The natural history of parapsoriasis en plaques (chronic superficial dermatitis) and prereticulotic poikiloderma. *Br. J. Dermatol.* 87:405, 1972.

Sanchez, J. F., and Ackerman, A. B. The patch stage of mycosis fungoides. Criteria for histologic diagnosis. *Am. J. Dermatopathol.* 1:5, 1979.

Porokeratosis

Lederman, J. S., Sober, A. J., and Lederman, G. S. Immunosuppression: A cause of porokeratosis? *J. Am. Acad. Dermatol.* 13:75–79, 1985.

Mikhail, G. R., and Wertheimer, F. W. Clinical variants of porokeratosis (Mibelli). *Arch. Dermatol.* 98:124, 1968.

Reed, R. J., and Leone, P. Porokeratosis—A mutant clonal keratosis of the epidermis. I. Histogenesis. *Arch. Dermatol.* 101:340, 1970.

Wade, T. R., and Ackerman, A. B. Cornoid lamellation: A histologic reaction pattern. *Am. J. Dermatopathol.* 2:5–15, 1980.

Acrodermatitis Chronica Atrophicans

Åsbrink, E., Brehmer-Anderson, E., and Hovmark, A. Acrodermatitis chronica atrophicans—a spirochetosis. *Am. J. Dermatopathol.* 8:209–219, 1986.

Burgdorf, W. H. C., Worret, W. I., and Schultka, O. Acrodermatitis chronica atrophicans. *Int. J. Dermatol.* 18:595, 1979.

de Koning, J., Tazelaar, D. J., Hoogkamp-Korstanje, J. A., and Elema, J. D. Acrodermatitis chronica atrophicans: A light and electron microscopic study. *J. Cutan. Pathol.* 22:23–32, 1995.

Montgomery, H., and Sullivan, R. R. Acrodermatitis atrophicans chronica. *Arch. Dermatol. Syphilol.* 51:32, 1945.

Patmas, M. A. Lyme disease: The evolution of erythema chronicum migrans into acrodermatitis chronica migrans. *Cutis* 52:169–170, 1993.

Poikiloderma Vasculare Atrophicans

McMillan, E. M., Wasik, R., and Everett, M. A. In situ demonstration of T cell subsets in atrophic parapsoriasis. *J. Am. Acad. Dermatol.* 6:32–39, 1982.

Watsky, M. S., and Lynfield, Y. L. Poikiloderma vasculare atrophicans. *Cutis* 17:938, 1976.

Wolf, D. J., and Selmanowitz, V. J. Poikiloderma vasculare atrophicans. *Cancer* 25:682, 1970.

Lupus Erythematosus

Bangert, J., Freeman, R., Sontheimer, R. D., and Gilliam, J. N. Subacute cutaneous lupus erythematosus and discoid lupus erythematosus. Comparative histologic findings. *Arch. Dermatol.* 120:332–337, 1984.

Bielsam, I., Herrero, C., Collado, A., Cobos, A., Palou, J., and Mascaro, J. M. Histopathologic findings in cutaneous lupus erythematosus. *Arch. Dermatol.* 130:54–58, 1994.

Biesecker, G., Lavin, L., Ziskind, M., and Koffler, D. Cutaneous localization of the membrane attack complex in discoid and systemic lupus erythematosus. *N. Engl. J. Med.* 306:264, 1982.

Brown, M. M., and Yount, W. J. Skin immunopathology in systemic lupus erythematosus. *JAMA* 243:38, 1980.

Callen, J. P., and Klein, J. Subacute cutaneous lupus erythematosus. Clinical, serologic, immunogenetic, and therapeutic considerations in 72 patients. *Arthritis Rheum.* 31:1007–1013, 1988.

Clark, W. H., Reed, R. J., and Mihm, M. C., Jr. Lupus erythematosus: Histopathology of cutaneous lesions. *Hum. Pathol.* 4:157, 1973.

Dubois, E. L. *Lupus Erythematosus: A Review of the Current Status of Discoid and Systemic Lupus Erythematosus and Their Variants* (2nd ed.). Los Angeles: University of Southern California Press, 1974.

Jerdan, M. S., Hood, A. F., Moore, G. W., and Calleu, J. P. Histopathologic comparison of subsets of lupus erythematosus. *Arch. Dermatol.* 126:52–55, 1990.

McCreight, W. G., and Montgomery, H. Cutaneous changes in lupus erythematosus. *Arch. Dermatol. Syphilol.* 61:1, 1950.

Provost, T. T., Zone, J. J., Synkowski, D., et al. Unusual cutaneous manifestations of systemic lupus erythematosus. I. Urticaria-like lesions. Correlation with clinical and serological abnormalities. *J. Invest. Dermatol.* 75:495, 1980.

Prunieras, M., and Montgomery, H. Histopathology of cutaneous lesions in systemic lupus erythematosus. *Arch. Dermatol.* 74:177, 1956.

Prystowsky, S. D., and Gilliam, J. N. Discoid lupus erythematosus as part of a larger disease spectrum. *Arch. Dermatol.* 111:1448, 1975.

Synkowski, D. R., Reichlin, M., and Provost, T. T. Serum autoantibodies in systemic lupus erythematosus and correlation with cutaneous features. *J. Rheumatol.* 9:380, 1982.

Tuffanelli, D. L., Kay, D., and Fukuyama, K. Dermal-epidermal junction in lupus erythematosus. *Arch. Dermatol.* 99:652, 1969.

Winkelmann, R. K. Spectrum of lupus erythematosus. *J. Cutan. Pathol.* 6:457, 1979.

Chapter 9

Disorders of the Melanocyte

I. Hypermelanosis
   A. Circumscribed
      1. Ephelis (freckle)
      2. Café-au-lait spot
      3. Postinflammatory hyperpigmentation
      4. Melasma
   B. Diffuse
II. Hyperplasia
   A. Lentigo simplex
   B. Solar lentigo
III. Neoplasia
   A. Benign
      1. Nevocellular nevus
         a. Junctional nevus
         b. Dermal nevus
         c. Compound nevus
         d. Congenital nevocellular nevus
         e. Halo nevus
      2. Blue nevus
         a. Common
         b. Cellular
         c. Blue nevus with focal hypercellularity
      3. Mongolian spot
      4. Nevus of Ota (nevus fuscoceruleus ophthalmomaxillaris), nevus of Ito (nevus fuscoceruleus acromiodeltoideus)
      5. Spindle and epithelioid cell nevus (compound nevus of Spitz)
      6. Pigmented spindle cell nevus
      7. Combined nevus
      8. Recurrent nevus
      9. Genital nevus
      10. Acral nevus
      11. Deep penetrating nevus
      12. Desmoplastic nevus
   B. Atypical (dysplastic) nevus
   C. Malignant
      1. *In situ*
         a. Melanoma in situ
         b. Lentigo maligna
      2. Invasive
         a. Lentigo maligna melanoma
         b. Superficial spreading melanoma
         c. Acral lentiginous melanoma
         d. Nodular melanoma
         e. Melanoma with desmoplasia and neurotropism
         f. Nevoid melanoma
         g. Nevoid melanoma arising in a congenital nevus
         h. Malignant blue nevus
         i. Pigment synthesizing (animal/equine) melanoma

IV. Hypomelanosis
  A. Circumscribed
    1. Vitiligo and piebaldism
    2. Halo nevus
    3. Postinflammatory hypopigmentation
  B. Generalized
    1. Albinism, oculocutaneous
    2. Vitiligo
    3. Chediak–Higashi syndrome

Certain entities described in this chapter are the focus of spirited debate. The terminology employed by dermatopathologists to classify nevocellular nevi occurring in the familial atypical mole syndrome (dysplastic nevi), and to classify melanomas, is changing and will continue to change. We prefer to be inclusive rather than selectively exclusive of terms, concepts, and diagnoses that might not be universally accepted. Thus, for example, atypical (dysplastic) nevus and subtypes of melanoma are described. As the scholarly dialogue continues on these topics, we hope that the reader will follow along with critical thought and an open mind.

The Reactive Process and the Disease	Histopathology	Comments
I. Hypermelanosis		
A. Circumscribed		
1. Ephelis (freckle) (Figs. 9-1, 9-2)	Increased melanin in basal cell layer; normal number of melanocytes	
2. Café-au-lait spot	Increased melanin in basal cell layer; variable increased number of melanocytes	Solitary café-au-lait spots are seen in the general population, but when multiple they may be associated with neurofibromatosis or Albright's syndrome
3. Postinflammatory hyperpigmentation	1. Increased melanin in basal cell layer; occasional increased number of melanocytes 2. Free and/or phagocytized melanin in dermis	Postinflammatory hyperpigmentation is seen in association with or following disorders that involve the dermoepidermal junction, such as lichen planus, lupus erythematosus, and drug eruptions

Fig. **9-1.** *Some disorders of intraepidermal melanocytes.*
A. *Normal: one melanocyte for every four to nine basal cells is usual.*
B. *Freckle: increased pigmentation of basal cells but normal numbers of melanocytes are seen.*
C. *Lentigo simplex: increased pigmentation of basal cells with increased numbers of melanocytes and elongation of rete ridges is typical.*
D. *Lentigo senilis: similar to lentigo simplex but elongation of rete ridges is pronounced.*
E. *Lentigo maligna: increased numbers of atypical melanocytes on a background of sun-damaged skin with epidermal atrophy and solar elastosis.*

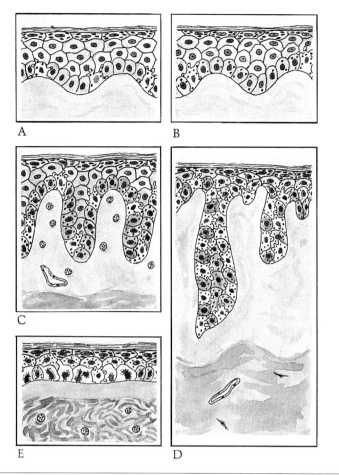

4. Melasma

1. Increased melanin in basal cell layer
2. Free and/or phagocytized melanin in dermis

B. Diffuse

1. Increased melanin in basal cell layer; apparently normal number of melanocytes
2. Free and/or phagocytized melanin in dermis in variable quantities

Diffuse hypermelanosis may be seen in a wide variety of diseases including:

Addison's disease
Argyria
Hemochromatosis
Porphyria cutanea tarda
Arsenic intoxication
Busulfan administration
Progressive systemic sclerosis
Chronic hepatic insufficiency
Whipple's disease
Malignant melanoma
Radiation exposure
Ultraviolet light exposure
Graft-versus-host disease

Fig. **9-2.** *Ephelis; Lentigo.*
A. *Ephelis. Basilar hyperpigmentation is evident.*
B. *Lentigo. Melanocytic hyperplasia, hyperpigmented elongated rete ridges, and dermal melanophages are characteristic.*

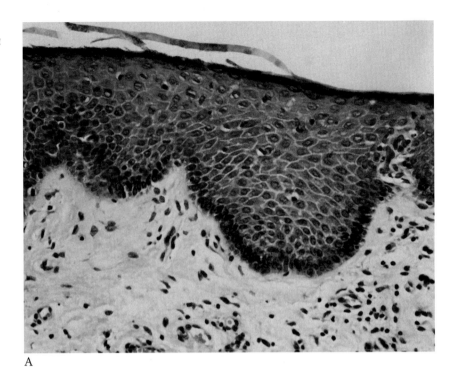

A

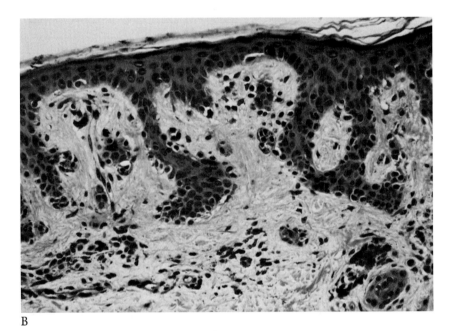

B

II. Hyperplasia

A. Lentigo simplex (see Figs. 9-1, 9-2)

1. **Elongation of rete ridges**
2. **Increased number of melanocytes**
3. **Increased melanin** in melanocytes, basal cells, and keratinocytes
4. Occasionally, small nests of nevus cells at the dermoepidermal junction
5. Melanophages in upper dermis
6. Occasionally, mild superficial mononuclear cell infiltrate

These histologic features also may be observed in:
Nevus spilus
Peutz-Jeghers syndrome
Becker's nevus
Centrofacial lentiginosis
Eruptive lentiginosis
Moynahan's syndrome
LEOPARD syndrome
LAMB syndrome

A pigmented actinic keratosis may show proliferative "buds" and hyperpigmentation somewhat resembling a lentigo. Such a keratosis may contain atypical keratinocytes. See also Ch. 7, III.A

B. Solar lentigo

1. **Elongated, club-shaped rete ridges**
2. Increased number of melanocytes
3. Increased melanin in basal cells
4. Melanophages in upper dermis

Lentigines induced by psoralen and ultraviolet light (PUVA) therapy may show similar histology but may show melanocytic atypia

III. Neoplasia

A. Benign

1. Nevocellular nevus

These lesions are composed of polygonal nevus cells (cells of neuroectodermal origin) and are subclassified into junctional, compound, and dermal types

a. Junctional nevus

1. Relatively symmetrical, round nests of cohesive cells within the lower part of the epidermis
2. Characteristics of junctional and subjacent dermal nevus cells (also referred to as type A nevus cells):

Shape: cuboidal, oval, or spindle
Cytoplasm: gray, often distinctly outlined; may exhibit short dendritic processes
Nucleus: large, round to oval
Nucleolus: small
Melanin: when present, disposed in variably large clumps

Fig. **9-3.** Neurotized nevus.
A. Dermal nevus with neurotization of
   deeper areas.
B. At higher magnification, the small,
   polygonal nevus cells (small arrow)
   can be contrasted with larger,
   neurotized cells (large arrow).

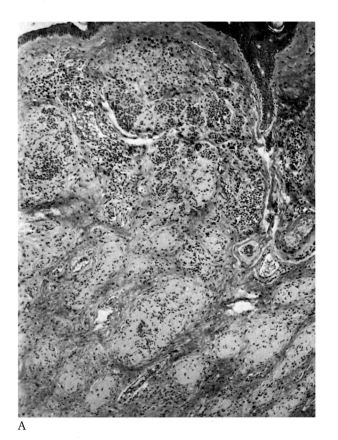

A

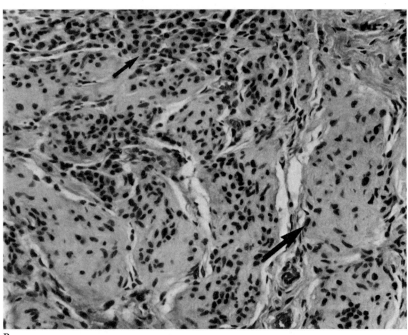

B

C. Fibrillar stroma of neurotized zones
   is illustrated.

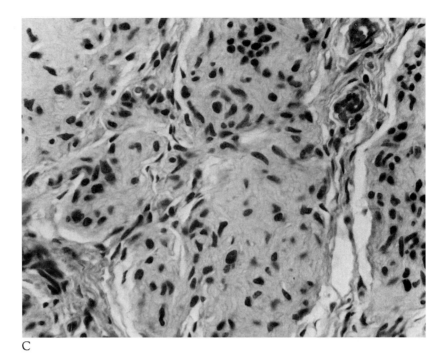

C

---

b. Dermal nevus

1. Nevus cells in nests and cords
   and singly arrayed in the dermis
2. Nevus cell characteristics vary
   according to location within the
   nevus

Upper dermis (type B nevus cells):

Shape: cuboidal or oval
Cytoplasm: distinctly outlined,
   homogeneous
Nucleus: large, round or oval, pale
   or vesicular; may show
   eosinophilic cytoplasmic
   inclusions; usually
   multinucleate giant forms noted
Melanin: when present, finely
   granular

Lower dermis (type C nevus cells):

Shape: elongate or spindle
Cytoplasm: pale blue-gray,
   homogeneous without distinct
   cellular outline (syncytial)
Nucleus: spindle-shaped
Melanin: usually absent; melanin
   may be present in adjacent
   melanophages

Lower dermal portions of nevi
sometimes exhibit a neuroid
appearance composed of wavy
spindle cells, fine, collagenous
stroma, and increased numbers
of mast cells; these changes are
referred to as neurotization
(Fig 9-3)

In contrast, collections of dendritic melanin-producing melanocytes in the dermis are characteristic of blue nevi

The progression in these nevi from type A to type C nevus cells is generally referred to as *maturation*

c. Compound nevus (Fig. 9-4)

These nevi show combined characteristics of junctional and dermal nevi; no striking stromal proliferation observed

Nevus cells in common acquired nevi are predominantly situated in the epidermis, the papillary, and the upper reticular dermis

d. Congenital nevocellular nevus

The lesions may have the pattern of any nevocellular nevus. Typical histologic features that suggest congenital onset include:

1. Nevus cells in the middle to **lower dermis** and subcutis
2. Nests of nevus cells within appendages, vessels, and/or nerves
3. Nevus cells in single-cell array between collagen bundles of deep reticular dermis

Fig. **9-4.** (A, B) Compound nevus. Nests of nevus cells are present within both the epidermis and dermis.

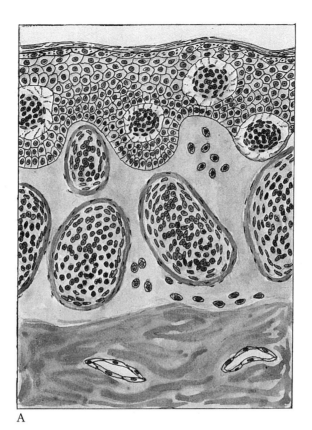

A

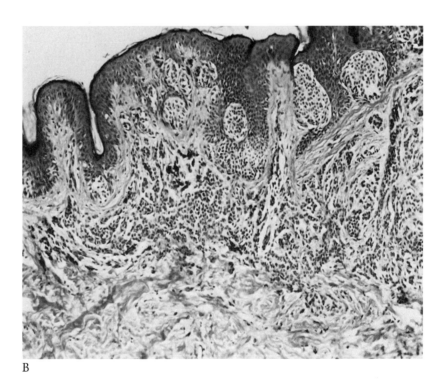

B

e. Halo nevus
(Fig. 9-5)

1. **Nevus cells associated with an intense infiltrate of lymphocytes and histiocytes**
2. Infiltrate may obscure nevus architecture
3. Some nevus cells show large nuclei with prominent nucleoli and ample eosinophilic cytoplasm
4. Dermal fibrosis may be prominent
5. **Absence of epidermal melanocytes within the depigmented halo**
6. Lymphocytes tagging along the basal layer, with vacuolopathy, and focal lymphocyte-melanocytic satellitosis, beyond the dermal nevic component

Halo nevus is a term used clinically to describe a nevus with a peripheral rim of hypopigmentation. Histologically the term most commonly describes a nevus with the features enumerated to the left. Clinical and histologic halo phenomena may occur in association with any melanocytic proliferative process—benign, atypical, or malignant

Although most halo nevi have benign cellular characteristics, some halo nevi are difficult to distinguish from melanomas with a prominent inflammatory infiltrate

Identification of nevus cells may be facilitated by the use of immunohistochemistry for S-100 protein

Older lesions may exhibit fibrosis without inflammation

Fig. **9-5.** Halo nevus. At the right and lower portions of the field, nevus cells are admixed with lymphocytes and histiocytes. Nevus cells without much inflammation are present in the upper portions of the micrograph. Older lesions of halo nevus may exhibit less inflammation and more fibrosis.

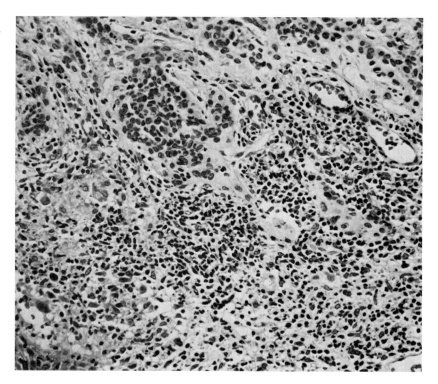

2. Blue nevus

a. Common
(Fig. 9-6)

1. Epidermis normal
2. Elongated, slender **dendritic melanocytes** are filled with fine melanin granules and are irregularly dispersed in the reticular dermis
3. **Melanophages** filled with coarse melanin granules
4. Dermal fibrosis

Dermal melanocytes in blue nevi similar to but more numerous than those seen in Mongolian spot

Differential diagnosis:
  Mongolian spot
  Nevus of Ota
  Nevus of Ito
  Tattoo

b. Cellular

Biphasic pattern with:
1. Zones of **pigmented dendritic melanocytes,** melanophages, and fibrosis
2. Intersecting bundles of aggregated, large, **spindle-shaped and epithelioid cells** with ovoid nuclei, and abundant pale cytoplasms, containing **little or no melanin**
3. Spindle-shaped cells may exhibit nuclear pleomorphism
4. Mitoses may be numerous but not atypical

Differential diagnosis:
  Malignant melanoma
  Dermatofibrosarcoma protuberans (Bednar variant)
  Dermatofibroma, pigmented variant
  Plexiform neurofibroma
  Pigmented schwannoma

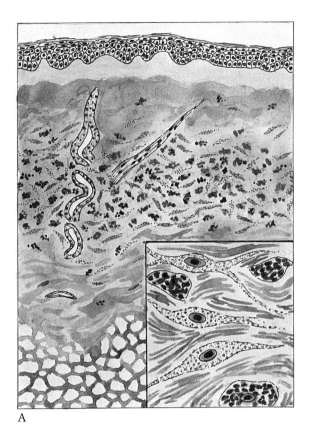

A

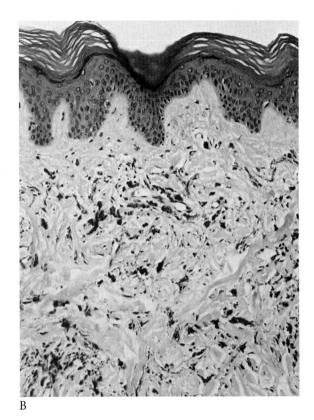

B

Fig. **9-6.** Blue nevus.

A. The low-power impression is that of numerous pigmented cells in the dermis. Inset: At higher power two populations can be distinguished; dendritic melanocytes with rather delicate pigment (blue nevus cells) and numerous polygonal melanophages with abundant coarse cytoplasmic pigment.

B. Micrograph for comparison with A. Fibrosis, here delicate, frequently accompanies blue nevi.

C. A spindled cell with melanin-containing dendrocyte (arrows) is typical of the blue nevus.

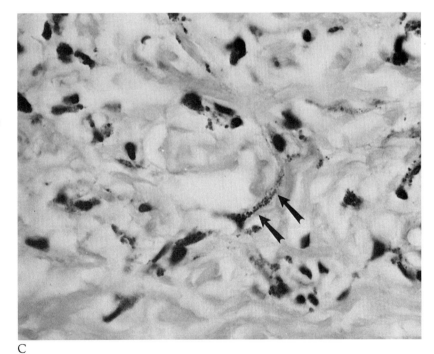

C

c. Blue nevus, with focal hyper-cellularity	1. **Focal areas of increased cellularity,** intermingled with areas of common blue nevus at low power 2. Cellular zones, limited to the reticular dermis and occasionally to the superficial areas of the subcutaneous fat 3. Cellular areas at high power examination exhibit hyperchromatic spindle cells 4. Mitoses rare or absent 5. Necrosis absent	

3. Mongolian spot	1. Ribbonlike, **wavy dendritic cells** containing evenly dispersed melanin granules are scattered in the reticular dermis and at times the subcutis
	2. Melanophages absent
		Differential diagnosis:
		   Blue nevus
		   Nevus of Ota
		   Nevus of Ito
		   Tattoo

4. Nevus of Ota (nevus fuscoceruleus oph-thalmomaxillaris), nevus of Ito (nevus fuscoceruleus acromiodeltoideus)	1. Ribbonlike, **wavy dendritic cells** with evenly dispersed melanin granules are distributed in the superficial reticular dermis, often lying parallel to the epidermis 2. Numerous melanophages	
5. Spindle and epithelioid cell nevus (compound nevus of Spitz) (Figs. 9-7, 9-8)	1. Symmetrical, often dome-shaped lesion composed of prominent nests of nevus cells, nests may be variable in size and shape 2. **Epidermal hyperplasia** common 3. Compound pattern most common, but purely junctional or dermal proliferation may occur	This lesion may be extremely difficult to distinguish from malignant melanoma Kamino bodies, brightly eosinophilic globular structures, are commonly present in superficial nests. These represent apoptotic keratinocytes

Fig. **9-7.** *Spindle and epithelioid cell nevus.*

A. Plump spindle cells with variable amounts of amphophilic cytoplasm and melanin pigment are organized into nests at the dermoepidermal junction and into fascicles within the dermis. Inset: Nucleoli may appear very prominent.

B. Photomicrograph for comparison. Numerous junctional nests here are composed of spindle cells. A mitotic figure is present in the center of the field.

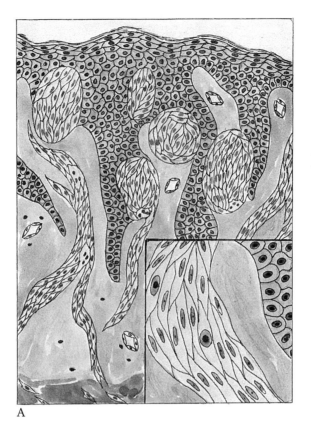

A

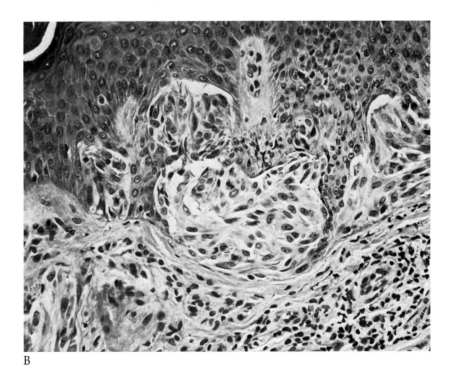

B

Fig. **9-8.** *Halo spindle cell nevus.*
A. *Note the typical pattern of spindle cell nevus (compare with Fig. 9-7).*
B. *Superimposed upon this nevus is an inflammatory process composed of numerous lymphocytes in close association with nevus cells. See also Ch. 9, III.A.1.e.*

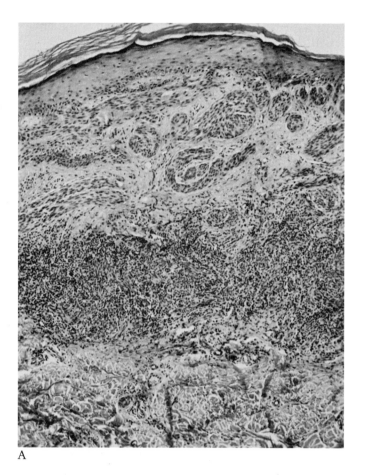

A

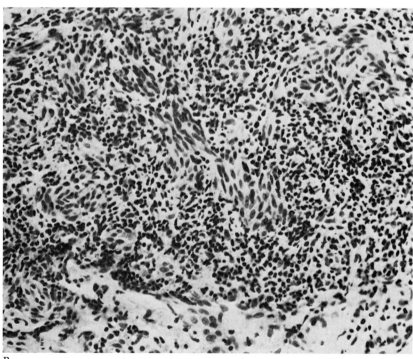

B

4. Cell type characteristics
   a. **Spindle-shaped:** characteristically arranged in fascicles, which may lie parallel or perpendicular ("raining down") to the epidermis
   b. **Epithelioid:** large, polygonal, well-dermarcated cells with pale, variably staining cytoplasm; sometimes multinucleate
   c. Cells decrease in size ("mature") from superficial to deep but maintain same nuclear/cytoplasmic features
5. Chromatin finely disposed around the nuclear membrane; cytoplasm often "wispy" and variably pigmented
6. Edema of upper dermis with ectatic capillary venules
7. **Mitotic figures may be present superficially,** but atypical mitoses are not observed
8. Nevus cells at lower border infiltrate between collagen bundles
9. Chronic inflammatory infiltrate may be present

Tumor cells may be predominantly spindle shaped, epithelioid, or a mixture of both

Scattered epithelioid cells may possess bizarre nuclei with large nucleoli; nevoid giant cells often present

Pagetoid Spitz nevus, an unusual variant, may exhibit numerous single epithelioid cells throughout the epidermis and simulate melanoma *in situ*; clues to the correct diagnosis include confinement of cells throughout to the area of junctional nesting, and benign characteristics of the cells

6. Pigmented spindle cell nevus

1. **Circumscribed symmetrical nested proliferation of intraepidermal pigmented spindle cells**
2. Papillary dermal nodule of similar cells
3. Cell characteristics
   a. Elongate, fusiform (not dendritic)
   b. Nucleus: ovoid with delicate chromatin and tiny nucleoli
   c. Variable cytoplasmic pigmentation
   d. Normal mitotic figures, especially in nodule
   e. Cellular morphology uniform in both epidermal and dermal components
4. Inflammatory infiltrate usually absent
5. Melanophages present, often numerous
6. Stromal fibrosis slight

Lesions most common on dorsal surfaces, especially legs of young women

Purely intraepidermal proliferations can be observed

Differential diagnosis:
Atypical (dysplastic) nevus
Superficial spreading melanoma

This lesion is distinguished from a dysplastic nevus by the relative uniformity of cells characteristically present in the pigmented spindle cell nevus

Variants of spindle cell nevus occur, such as desmoplastic Spitz nevus and agminated Spitz nevus. See the Suggested Reading at the end of the chapter

7. Combined nevus (Fig. 9-9)

Occasionally nevi may occur in combination. A common pattern is the **acquired nevocellular nevus and blue nevus** in which clearly identifiable zones of dermal nevus cell nests are opposed or commingled with cells of blue nevus

Fig. **9-9.** *Combined nevus.*
A. *Intradermal proliferation of melanocytic cells*
B. *The higher magnification shows the dendritic melanin-laden blue nevus cells admixed with plump bland nevocellular nevus cells.*

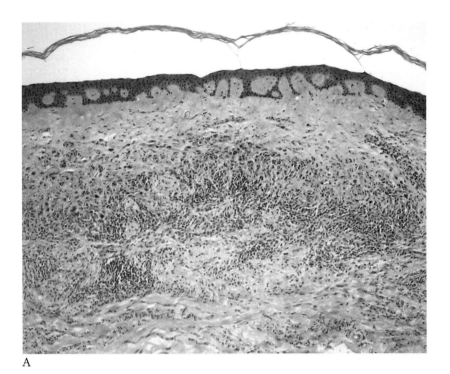

A

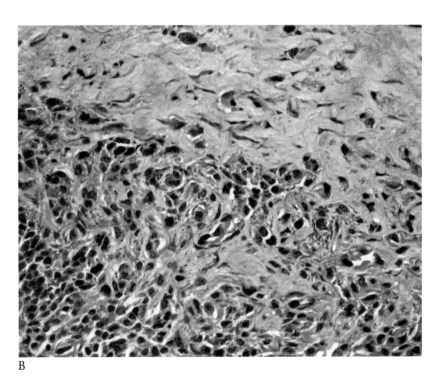

B

8. Recurrent nevus
   (Fig. 9-10)

1. Low-power observation reveals **dermal scar** with epidermis exhibiting effacement of rete ridges
2. **Lentiginous melanocytic hyperplasia** usually of round to oval melanocytes with prominent nuclei present overlying scar
3. In periphery of scarred area residual intraepidermal and/or dermal nests present
4. Sometimes residual dermal nests are found beneath scar
5. Intraepidermal component high-power shows uniformity of cells without remarkable atypia
6. Sometimes focal pagetoid spread evident

Differential diagnosis includes regressed melanoma which shows extensive melanophages, coarse fibrosis, and increased vascularity with markedly atypical cells in epidermis overlying the regressed area when present; clinical history often helpful; recurrent nevi occur rapidly within the first year or so after removal; recurrent melanomas occur usually later several years after removal

9. Genital nevus

1. Lentiginous junctional or compound nevus with focal bridging or extension along the adnexae
2. Junctional component often with **large irregular nests of variable shape**
3. Nests comprised of epithelioid and spindle-shaped cells with small nucleoli; atypia, when present, is mild
4. Mitoses sparse or absent
5. Migration, not extensive, of cells in the lower part of the epidermis; no true pagetoid spread noticed
6. Foci of inflammatory reaction may occur in the dermis
7. Melanophages apparent and often in great number
8. Scarring of superficial dermis often observed
9. Fibroplasia of the papillary dermis is reminiscent of dysplastic nevus
10. Genital nevi with severe atypia most common in children and young adults

Differential diagnosis is dysplastic nevus which exhibits more pattern fibroplasia and a more diffuse rte hyperplasia with proliferation of melanocytes; two atypical variants of melanoma of the lentiginous type which show more cytologically atypical features

10. Acral nevus

1. Prominent uniform intraepithelial nesting of type A nevus cells
2. Dermal component may or may not be present
3. Prominent pagetoid spread of benign nevomelanocytes confined to the areas above and between the intraepidermal nests (60% of cases)

The histologic differential diagnosis is acral melanoma in situ, which exhibits nests of irregular sizes and extensive pagetoid spread of atypical melanocytic cells

Fig. **9-10.** *Recurrent nevus.*
A. *Low-power view with melanocytic proliferation overlying a scar in the reticular dermis.*
B. *Nests of melanocytic cells are irregular in size and distribution; scattered single cells also seen within the epidermis. Melanophages are present between the epidermis and scar.*

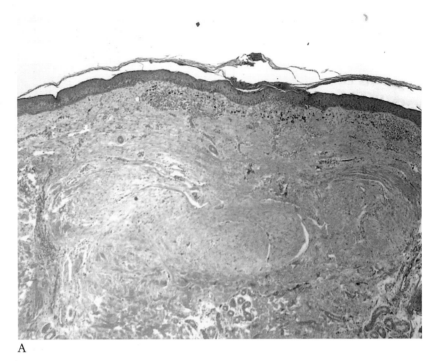

A

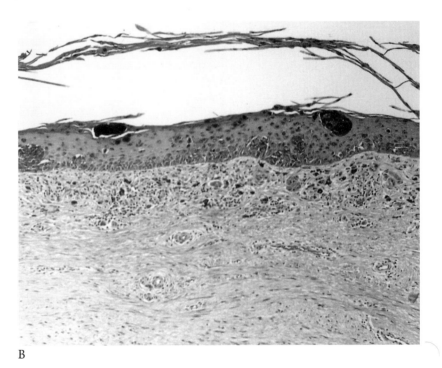

B

4. Pagetoid spread does not extend beyond the lateral nested confines of the lesion

11. Deep penetrating nevus

1. Cells extend from the superficial dermis into deep dermis, usually **along the follicle and/or along neurovascular bundles**
2. Nests of spindle or epithelioid cells usually surrounded by melanophages
3. Characteristic epithelioid or dermal type A cells have small sometimes hyperchromatic nuclei and ample cytoplasm with scattered pigment granules
4. Usually no mitoses
5. Deep expansile aggregates, especially when associated with mitoses, are a sign of atypia and possible recurrence
6. Usually combined with commonly acquired nevi and sometimes blue nevi

12. Desmoplastic nevus

1. Low-power appreciation of cellular areas defined by collagenous stroma often in pattern of inverted triangle
2. Epidermal hyperplasia, or atrophy, with or without nesting may overly the dermal component
3. High-power observation of dermal cells reveals within the collagenous stroma, typical epithelioid or spindle cell nevus types
4. The collagenous stroma defines the lesion and is usually of a brightly eosinophilic dense nature

Differential diagnosis, desmoplastic melanoma easily differentiated by the presence of prominent epithelioid cells in the desmoplastic nevus, abscess of inflammation, and absence of mucinosis

B. Atypical (dysplastic) nevus (Fig. 9-11)

1. Types of cells
   a. Cells with variably hyperchromatic, angular nuclei surrounded by dark-staining narrow rim of cytoplasm separated from adjacent keratinocytes by an obvious clear space; cells in nests are not cohesive

The atypical (dysplastic) nevus is a recently described entity with clincopathologic correlation; it is still evolving as a concept

Fig. **9-11.** *Atypical (dysplastic) nevus. The illustration shows several features that characterize nevi from persons with the dysplastic nevus syndrome: horizontally disposed nests, lamellar fibroplasia* (arrows), *melanocytic hyperplasia, and lentiginous epidermal change.*

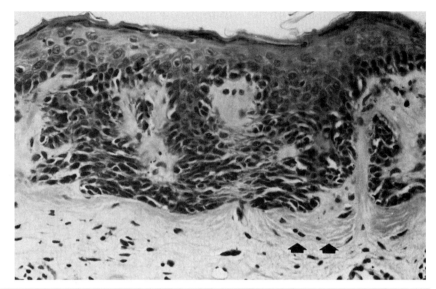

b. Cells with round, variably hyperchromatic nuclei surrounded by ample melanin-laden cytoplasm clearly abutting adjacent keratinocytes; nested cells are variably cohesive and have small nuclear to cytoplasmic ratios
c. Mixtures of a and b
2. Architectural features
    a. Asymmetry: intraepidermal population of atypical cells extend asymmetrically lateral to the dermal component
    b. Epidermal findings
        1. Hyperplasia with elongation of rete ridges (most common change); elongated rete ridges connected by horizontally disposed nests of nevus cells
        2. Normal epidermis
        3. Atrophy of epidermis uncommon
        4. Nevus cells and nevus cell nests are irregularly disposed in the epidermis
        5. Single-cell spread upward into epidermis observed

Lesions showing these architectural changes but lacking cytologic atypia are called *compound nevi with architectural features of the dysplastic nevus*

3. Stromal changes
   a. Inflammatory infiltrate: lymphocytes scattered and in patchy array
   b. Collagenous eosinophilic concentric or lamellar fibrosis
   c. Vascular capillary venules variably prominent and ectatic

C. Malignant

   1. In situ

Melanoma in situ may occur *de novo* or in association with preexisting nevi

   a. Melanoma in situ

   1. Irregular spread of tumor throughout epidermis and/or adnexal epithelium
   2. Replacement of lower epidermis by tumor cells
   3. Tumor cells in the most common presentation are usually **large, round cells containing fine, dispersed melanin granules**
   4. Nuclei are usually large and round but variable in size and shape, with irregularly dispersed chromatin patterns
   5. Large, pink nucleoli
   6. Large nuclear/cytoplasmic ratios
   7. Mitoses frequent, occasionally atypical
   8. Dermal invasion absent

Differential diagnosis:
   Paget's disease
   Intraepidermal epithelioid cell nevus

Melanoma in situ occurring in acral areas has a distinct histologic appearance (see C.2.c)

   b. Lentigo maligna (Fig. 9-12)

   1. Increased number of intraepidermal pleomorphic melanocytes with variable nuclear hyperchromatism, vacuolated cytoplasm, and melanin granules
   2. **Melanocytes haphazardly** or **contiguously dispersed along basal cell layer** with occasional extension into the upper epidermis and downward extension into basilar region of hair follicles and, sometimes, eccrine ducts
   3. **Epidermal atrophy common**
   4. **Solar elastosis** of upper dermis
   5. Bandlike mononuclear-cell infiltrate may be present
   6. Melanophages

The differential diagnosis of lentigo maligna includes lentigines, pigmented actinic keratoses, and dysplastic nevi

Fig. **9-12.** *Lentigo maligna.*
A. Nests of tumor cells are most
   prominent at the dermoepidermal
   junction of both the epidermis and
   the hair follicles. Prominent solar
   elastosis and epidermal atrophy
   accompany this tumor frequently.
B. Flattening of the epidermis is
   apparent with upward migration of
   atypical melanocytes.

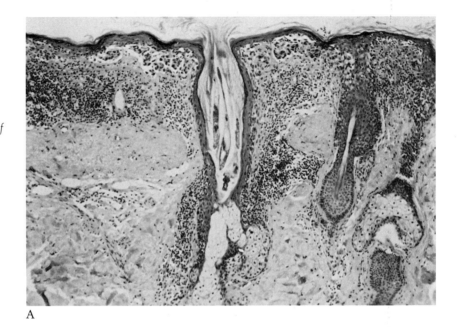

A

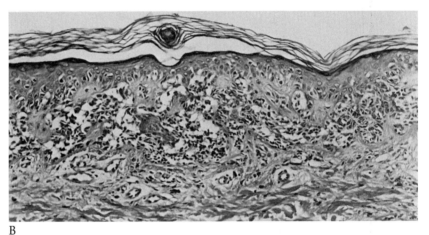

B

2. Invasive

<table>
<tr><td>

a. Lentigo maligna melanoma
</td><td>

1. For intraepidermal component, see C.1.b
2. Invasion of dermis by spindle-shaped or, less commonly, epithelioid tumor cells with large nuclear-cytoplasmic ratios
3. Malignant spindle cells have hyperchromatic nuclei and tend to be disposed in fascicles and large aggregates within the dermis
4. Epithelioid cells have irregularly hyperchromatic nuclei and ample pigment-laden cytoplasm
5. Mitoses present, varying from rare to abundant; atypical forms may be observed
6. Variable inflammatory infiltrate
7. Melanophages are common and may be abundant
</td><td>

Desmoplastic response and neurotropism may be noted
</td></tr>
<tr><td>

b. Superficial spreading melanoma (Fig. 9-13)
</td><td>

1. For intraepidermal component see C.1.a
2. Invasion of papillary dermis by single cells or small nests of cells with similar morphology to those found in the epidermis in early lesion (level II)
3. Aggregates of cells in papillary dermis and extending more deeply, composed of cells with often differing morphologies from the intraepidermal cells (levels III, IV, V)
4. Invasive cells are commonly round, with large nuclei and prominent nucleoli
5. Nuclear chromatin is often coarse and irregularly disposed
6. Cytoplasm dusky-pink and filled with fine melanin granules
7. Dermal mitoses often present and may be atypical
8. Inflammatory host response common beneath intraepidermal component but variable beneath dermal tumor
</td><td>

Fibrosis and focal absence of tumor are considered evidence of spontaneous regression
</td></tr>
</table>

Fig. **9-13.** Malignant melanoma, superficial spreading type.
A. Horizontal and vertical growth phases are evident at lower magnification.
B. Fibrosis and chronic inflammation within the dermis are frequently associated with tumor cells.

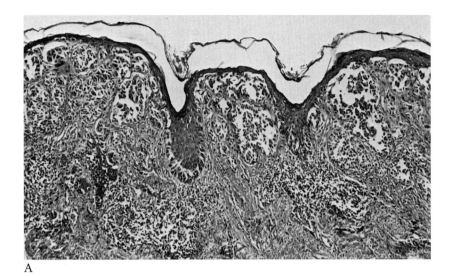

A

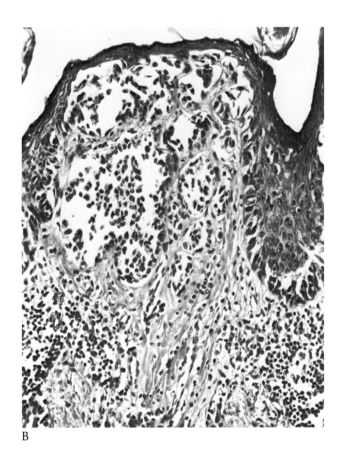

B

Melanoma, which is intraepidermal (level I) or superficially invasive to papillary dermis (level II), has been designated *radial growth phase disease*. Melanoma that forms a discrete nodule in the papillary dermis (level III) and infiltrates into the reticular dermis (level IV) or subcutaneous fat (level V) has been designated *vertical growth phase disease*. Cells of the vertical growth phase may be cytologically different from those of the radial growth phase. This classification has prognostic significance in that radial growth phase disease is virtually curable by surgery; vertical growth disease has an increasing potential for metastasis with increasing depth of invasion. *The most useful prognostic indicator is the measured depth of the tumor expressed in millimeters.* Measurement is taken with an ocular micrometer from the top of the granular layer to the deepest tumor cell. The best prognosis is found in lesions less than 1.0 mm in thickness. Risk for recurrence and metastasis increases with thickness. Individuals with tumors greater than 4.0 mm in thickness are considered at very high risk for recurrence and metastasis.

In vertical growth phase, tumor cells at the base of the lesion often (but not always) appear to "push" or compress the collagen, rather than infiltrate between collagen bundles; the presence of a "pushing border" may be helpful in distinguishing between melanoma and spindle and epithelial cell nevus.

Melanomas with problems in Breslow microstratification include polypoid melanoma, due to its abnormal orientation, and melanoma arising in a congenital nevus in a multifocal pattern and without connection with the overlying epidermis.

Thin melanomas with risk of metastasis: The concept of the early vertical growth phase includes the presence of an expansile nodule composed of a countable number of melanoma cells, usually 25 to 50, of different cytomorphology, than the intraepidermal horizontal growth phase cells. Mitoses are often noted. Furthermore, thin melanomas with Level IV, and/or extensive regression, may also metastasize.

c. Acral lentiginous melanoma

1. Cells with large cytoplasm, large nuclei, and prominent nucleoli contiguously dispersed in the basilar epidermis
2. Cytoplasm contains melanin granules, often highlighting dendritic processes
3. Single-cell spread present but most common in invasive areas
4. Epidermis hyperplastic with retention of rete pattern
5. Infiltration of papillary dermis by single cells associated with inflammatory infiltrate and melanophages
6. Nodule or invasion of deep dermis associated with round or spindle-shaped tumor cells
7. Perineural invasion common in spindle cell or desmoplastic tumors
8. Infiltration of dermal eccrine ducts often noted
9. Stromal fibrosis with lymphocytic infiltrate may be observed

Mucosal melanomas with radial growth phase often exhibit a lentiginous melanoma

d. Nodular mela-
noma (Fig. 9-14)

1. Pleomorphic tumor cells invade dermis in aggregates, fascicles, and sheets, with little or no lateral intraepidermal present
2. Lateral spread (atypical melanocytic cells within the epidermis) is usually confined to three or fewer rete ridges
3. Nuclei exhibit irregular clumping of chromatin
4. Nucleoli large and sometimes multiple
5. Cells may be spindle or round (epithelioid) in shape
6. Mitoses commonly observed

Fig. **9-14.** *Malignant melanoma, nodular type.*
A. *Lack of lateral spread within the epidermis and nodular downward growth characterize this tumor.*
B. *Cytologic features of this tumor can vary widely. Large vesicular nuclei with prominent nucleoli and amphophilic cytoplasm with dusty pigment are illustrated here.*

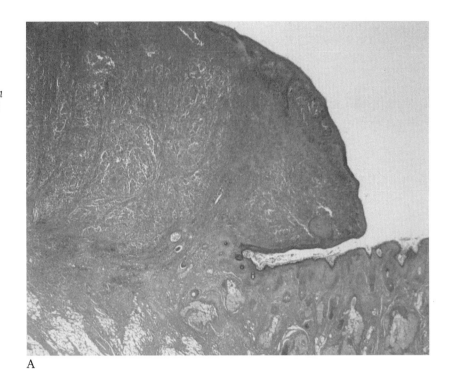

A

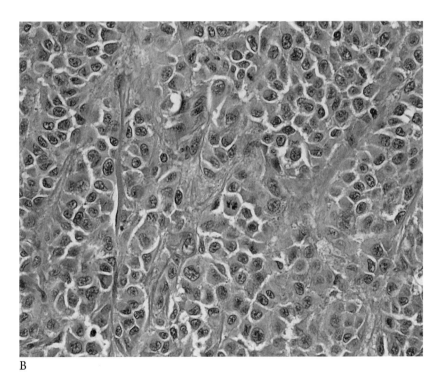

B

e. Melanoma with desmoplasia and neurotropism

1. Intraepidermal component, if identifiable, is usually characterized by single-cell spread of tumor cells along basal layer
2. Pleomorphic spindle cells form an expansile nodule and infiltrating tongues
3. Cells may be **nested,** in a tightly **fascicular pattern,** or in **single-cell array dispersed in a dense fibrosis**
4. Variable pigmentation with melanophages common
5. Areas of dense fibrosis distant from obvious tumor mass
6. **Foci of chronic inflammation** commonly present in tumor nodules
7. **Perineural infiltration,** sometimes at significant distance from main tumor mass
8. Mast cell hyperplasia and associated mucin deposition common

Desmoplasia and neurotropism in melanoma are most commonly associated with lentigo maligna melanoma but may also occur in acral lentiginous melanoma and melanomas of mucocutaneous sites

f. Nevoid melanoma

1. Lesion resembles dermal or spitz nevus on low power observation but with obvious hyperchromated cells
2. Lesional cells form an **expansile nodule** with effacement of ridges in the epidermis; nodular expansion widens the papillary dermis and/or infiltrates the reticular dermis
3. Intraepidermal component may be lentiginous, nested or in some cases may be absent
4. Comprising cells are either type B, spindle, epithelioid or, a mixture of these cells
5. These cells are hyperchromatic with large nuclear–cytoplasmic ratios and prominent nucleoli often focally obscured by the marked hyperchromasia
6. **Mitotic figures** are frequently easily observed
7. **Pseudomaturation** with cells appearing to diminish in size but actually retaining markedly atypical histologic features

Nevoid melanomas are often confused with atypical nevi but the presence of mitotic figures and absence of maturation allow for differentiation; most lesions appear to recur locally before metastasis occurs

g. Nevoid melanoma arising in a congenital nevus

1. Distinctly separate expansile nodules present in dermal component of the nevus
2. Intraepidermal or dermal origin sites may be present
3. Intraepidermal component may resemble superficial spreading or acrolentiginous melanoma
4. Expansile dermal nodules composed of uniformly atypical cells with increased mitoses and individual cell necrosis

h. Malignant blue nevus

1. Large expansile nodules, infiltrating dermis and subcutaneous fat on low power and deforming the architecture of the skin
2. Epidermis usually intact unless ulcerated
3. Nodules composed predominantly of pleomorphic spindle cells, with focal epithelioid cell areas
4. Mitoses often observed and easily visualized
5. Zones of necrosis common
6. Characteristic infiltration of subcutaneous fat by individual malignant cells or by cellular fascicles
7. Scattered lymphocytic infiltrates, often noted
8. Remnants of blue nevus usually identifiable in the periphery or admixed with the malignant cellular areas

i. Pigment synthesizing (animal/equine) melanoma

1. Large nodules of heavily pigmented cells, filling dermis, and usually extending into subcutaneous fat
2. The great majority of cells are malignant, with few melanophages
3. The cytomorphology of the cells varies from atypical to highly malignant
4. Prominent nucleoli, easily observed
5. Mitoses variable, but often numerous
6. Central mass, characterized by fascicles of spindle and epithelioid cells

Differential diagnosis includes cellular blue nevus, spindle and epithelioid cell nevus with hyperpigmentation, and malignant blue nevus

7. Peripheral infiltrating cells are spindle-shaped, with dendrites engorged with plump pigment granules
8. Lymphocytic infiltration common
9. Some tumors exhibit perifollicular prominence
10. Epidermis usually uninvolved, but occasionally dendritic cells are present in the basilar layer

IV. Hypomelanosis

A. Circumscribed

1. Vitiligo and piebaldism — Absence of melanocytes
2. Halo nevus — Melanocytes are absent in areas of hypopigmentation
3. Postinflammatory
   1. Decreased melanin in basal cells but melanocytes are present
   2. Pigment incontinence hypopigmentation

Melanocyte populations are difficult to define on H&E-stained sections; electron microscopy will define cells with melanosomes (the ultrastructural hallmark of the melanocyte); DOPA oxidase preparations define enzymatic functional activity in these cells; immunohistochemical stains that identify melanocytes (such as S-100) can be very helpful.

B. Generalized

1. Albinism, oculocutaneous — Absence of melanin in basal cells; melanocytes present
2. Vitiligo — Absence of melanocytes
3. Chédiak–Higashi syndrome — Irregularly shaped, large melanin granules in basal cells, upper dermis, and within melanophages

Suggested Reading

Hypermelanosis and Hypomelanosis

Halder, R. M., Walters, C. S., Johnson, B. A., et al. Aberrations in T lymphocytes and natural killer cells in vitiligo: A flow cytometric study. J. Am. Acad. Dermatol. 14:733–737, 1986.

Hori, Y., et al. Acquired bilateral nevus of Ota-like macules. J. Am. Acad. Dermatol. 10:961, 1984.

Jimbow, K., Fitzpatrick, T. B., Szabo, T., et al. Congenital circumscribed hypomelanosis: A characterization based on electron microscopic study of tuberous sclerosis, nevus depigmentosus, and piebaldism. J. Invest. Dermatol. 64:50, 1975.

Lever, W. F., and Schaumburg-Lever, G. *Histopathology of the Skin* (7th ed.). Philadelphia: J. B. Lippincott Co., 1990.

Miller, R. A. Psoralens and UV-A–induced stellate hyperpigmented freckling. Arch. Dermatol. 118:619, 1982.

Mishima, Y. Histopathology of functional pigmentary disorders. *Cutis* 21:225, 1978.

Morris, T. J., Johnson, W. G., and Silvers, D. N. Giant pigment granules in biopsy specimens from café au lait spots in neurofibromatosis. Arch. Dermatol. 118:385, 1982.

Mosher, D. B., Fitzpatrick, T. B., and Ortone, J. P. Abnormalities of Pigmentation. In T. B. Fitzpatrick et al. (Eds.), *Dermatology in General Medicine* (2nd ed.). New York: McGraw-Hill, 1979.

Nevocellular Nevus

Bhawan, J. Melanocytic nevi. A review. J. Cutan. Pathol. 6:153, 1979.

Clark, W. H., Reimer, R. R., Greene, M., et al. Origin of familial malignant melanomas from heritable melanocytic lesions, "the B-K mole syndrome." Arch. Dermatol. 114:732, 1978.

Clark, W. H., Jr. The dysplastic nevus syndrome. Arch. Dermatol. 124:1207–1210, 1988.

Clemente, C., et al. Histopathologic diagnosis of dysplastic nevi: Concordance among pathologists. Hum. Pathol. 22:313–319, 1991.

Elder, D. E., Goldman, L. I., Goldman, S. C., et al. Dysplastic nevus syndrome: A phenotypic association of sporadic cutaneous melanoma. *Cancer* 46:1787, 1980.

Halaban, R., Ghosh, S., Duray, P., et al. Human melanocytes cultured from nevi and melanomas. J. Invest. Dermatol. 87:95–101, 1986.

Rhodes, A. R., Neoplasms: Benign Neoplasias, Hyperplasias, and Dysplasias of Melanocytes. In T. B. Fitzpatrick et al. (Eds.), *Dermatology in General Medicine* (3rd ed.). New York: McGraw-Hill, 1987.

Shaffer, B. Pigmented nevi. Arch. Dermatol. 72:120, 1955.

Congenital Nevus

Barnhill, R. L., and Busam, K. J. Congenital Melanocytic Neoplasms, Congenital and Childhood Melanoma. In *Pathology of Melanocytic Nevi and Malignant Melanoma*. Boston: Butterworth-Heinemann, 1995, p. 79.

Barnhill, R. L., and Fleischli, M. Histologic features of congenital melanocytic nevi in infants 1 year of age or younger. J. Am. Acad. Dermatol. 33:780–785, 1995.

Hendrickson, M. R., and Ross, J. C. Neoplasms arising in congenital giant nevi: Morphologic study of seven cases and a review of the literature. Am. J. Surg. Pathol. 5:109, 1981.

Jauniaux, E., de Meeeus, M. C., Verellen, G., Lachapelle, J. M., and Hustin, J. Giant congenital melanocytic nevus with placental involvement: Long-term follow-up of a case and review of the literature. Pediatr. Pathol. 13:717–721, 1993.

Mark, G. J., Mihm, M. C., and Liteplo, M. G. Congenital melanocytic nevi of the small and garment type. Clinical, histologic and ultrastructural studies. Hum. Pathol. 4:395, 1973.

Rhodes, A. R., Weinstock, M. A., Fitzpatrick, T. B., et al. Risk factors for cutaneous melanoma. A practical method for recognizing predisposed individuals. J.A.M.A. 258:3147–3154, 1987.

Halo Nevus

Mihm, M. C., and Googe, P. B. *Problematic Pigmented Lesions*. Philadelphia: Lea & Febger, 1990.

Wayte, D. M., and Helwig, E. B. Halo nevi. *Cancer* 22:69, 1968.

Blue Nevus

Ainsworth, A. M., Folberg, R., Reed, R. J., et al. Melanocytic Nevi, Melanocytomas, Melanocytic Dysplasias, and Uncommon Forms of Melanoma. In W. H. Clark, L. I. Goldman, and M. J. Mastrangelo (Eds.), *Human Malignant Melanoma*. Orlando, FL: Grune & Stratton, 1979.

Dorsey, C. S., and Montgomery, H. Blue nevus and its distinction from Mongolian spot and the nevus of Ota. J. Invest. Dermatol. 22:225, 1954.

Leopold, J. G., and Richards, D. B. Cellular blue naevi. J. Pathol. Bact. 94:247, 1967.

Rodriguez, H. A., and Ackerman, L. V. Cellular blue nevus. Cancer, 21:393, 1968.

Spindle and Epithelioid Cell Nevus

Ainsworth, A. M., Folberg, R., Reed, R. J., et al. Pigmented Spindle Cell Tumor. In W. H. Clark, L. I. Goldman, and M. J. Mastrangelo (Eds.), *Human Malignant Melanoma*. Orlando, FL: Grune & Stratton, 1979.

Barnhill, R. L., and Mihm, M. C., Jr. Pigmented spindle cell nevus and its variants: Distinction from melanoma. Br. J. Dermatol. 121:717, 1989.

McWhorter, H. E., and Woolner, L. B. Treatment of juvenile melanomas and malignant melanomas in children. J.A.M.A. 156:695, 1954.

Mihm, M. C., Jr., and Murphy, G. F. *Pathobiology and Recognition of Malignant Melanoma*. Baltimore: Williams & Wilkins, 1988.

Paniago-Pereira, C., Maize, J. C., and Ackerman, A. B. Nevus of large spindle and/or epithelioid cells (Spitz's nevus). Arch. Dermatol. 114:1811, 1978.

Reed, R. J., Ichinose, H., Clark, W. H., Jr., and Mihm, M. C., Jr. Common and uncommon melanocytic nevi and borderline melanomas. Semin. Oncol. 2:119, 1975.

Weedon, D. Unusual features of nevocellular nevi. J. Cutan. Pathol. 9:284–292, 1982.

Genital Nevus

Clark, W. H., Hood, A. F., Tucker, M. A., and Jampel, R. M. Atypical melanocytic nevi of the genital type with a discussion of reciprocal parenchymal–stromal interactions in the biology of neoplasia. Hum. Pathol. 29:S1–S24, 1998.

Melanoma

Balch, C., Murad, T. M., Soong, S.-J., et al. A multifactorial analysis of melanoma: Prognostic histopathological features comparing Clark's and Breslow's staging methods. Ann. Surg. 188:732, 1978.

Balch, C. M., Milton, G. W., Shaw, H. M., et al. *Cutaneous Melanoma: Clinical Management and Treatment Results Worldwide*. Philadelphia: J. B. Lippincott, 1985.

Barnhill, R. L., and Busam, K. J. Congenital melanocytic neoplasms, congenital and childhood melanoma. In: *Pathology of Melanocytic Nevi and Malignant Melanoma*. Boston: Butterworth-Heinemann, 1995, p. 79.

Clark, W. H., Elder, D. E., Guerry, D. G., et al. A model predicting survival in stage I melanoma based upon tumor progression. J. Natl. Cancer Inst. 81:1893–1904, 1989.

Clark, W. H., Jr., Elder, D. E., and van Horn, M. The biologic forms of malignant melanoma. Hum. Pathol. 17:443–450, 1986.

Crowson, A. N., Magro, C. M., Mihm, M. C. The Melanocytic Proliferations. A *comprehensive Texbook of Pigmented Lesions*. New York: Wiley-Liss, 2001.

Day, C. L., Mihm, M. C., Sober, A. J., et al. Narrower margins for clinical stage I malignant melanoma. N. Engl. J. Med. 306:479, 1982.

Elder, D. E. (Ed.). *Pathobiology of Malignant Melanoma*. New York: Karger, 1987.

Elder, D. E., and Clark, W. H., Jr. Tumor Progression and Prognosis in Malignant Melanoma. In D. E. Elder (Ed.), *Pathobiology of Malignant Melanoma*. New York: Karger, 1987.

Elwood, J. M. (Ed.). *Melanoma and Nevi: Incidence, Interrelationships and Implications*. New York: Karger, 1988.

Feibleman, C. E., Stoll, H., and Maize, J. C. Melanomas of the palm, sole and nailbed; a clinicopathologic study. Cancer 46:2492, 1980.

Gromet, M. A., Epstein, W. L., and Blois, M. S. The regressing thin malignant melanoma, a distinctive lesion with metastatic potential. Cancer 42:2282, 1978.

Kopf, A. W., Bart, R. S., Rodriguez-Sains, R. S., et al. *Malignant Melanoma*. New York: Masson, 1979.

McGovern, V. J., Shaw, H. M., Milton, G. W., et al. Prognostic significance of the histological features of malignant melanoma. Histopathology 3:385, 1979.

Sober, A. J., Fitzpatrick, T. B., and Mihm, M. C. Primary melanoma of the skin: Recognition and management. J. Am. Acad. Dermatol. 2:179, 1980.

Sober, A. J., Rhodes, A. R., Mihm, M. C., Jr., and Fitzpatrick, T. B. Neoplasms: Malignant melanoma. In T. B. Fitzpatrick et al. (Eds.), *Dermatology in General Medicine* (3rd ed.). New York: McGraw-Hill, 1987.

Part III

Basement Membrane Zone, Papillary Dermis, and Superficial Vascular Plexus

Chapter **10**

*Vacuolization of the
Basement Membrane
Zone*

    I. Erythema multiforme
   II. Graft-versus-host reaction (GVHR), acute
  III. Morbilliform viral exanthem
  IV. Fixed drug eruption, chronic
   V. Dermatomyositis
  VI. Poikiloderma vasculare atrophicans (idiopathic)
 VII. Erythema dyschromium perstans
VIII. Phototoxic drug eruption
  IX. Postinflammatory hyperpigmentation
   X. Pinta, tertiary stage

Many inflammatory and vesiculobullous cutaneous diseases are characterized histologically by the presence of vacuoles along the dermoepidermal junction. These vacuoles may be located above the basement membrane, below the basement membrane, or both above and below, as in lupus erythematosus. Coalescence of the vacuoles may result in subepidermal cleft formation or clinical blisters. Vacuolization along the dermoepidermal junction may or may not be accompanied by inflammation. Disease with inflammation may be subdivided further into those with or without squamatization of the basal layer, a situation in which the normally cuboidal or columnar basal cells are replaced by polygonal or even flattened keratinocytes (see Fig. 2-12). The term *interface dermatitis* refers to the combination of basal vacuolization, dyskeratosis, and a variably intense superficial perivascular or interstitial mononuclear cell infiltrate. Diseases other than those discussed in this chapter display vacuolization of the basement membrane zone (e.g., lichen planus and lichen sclerosus et atrophicus), yet are placed elsewhere in the text because they possess other distinctive features.

The Reactive Process and the Disease

I. Erythema multiforme (Fig. 10-1)

Histopathology

1. Focal dyskeratosis
2. Focal intercellular edema
3. **Vacuolization** of basal layer with **lymphocytes along the dermoepidermal junction**
4. Perivascular lymphocytic infiltrate
5. Endothelial cell hypertrophy of affected cutaneous vessels
6. Melanin incontinence may be present
7. Subepidermal bulla formation may be noted

Comments

The histopathology of fixed drug eruption may be indistinguishable from erythema multiforme

See also Ch. 6 II.L; Ch. 11, II.I

Fig. **10-1.** *Erythema multiforme. A mild lymphocytic infiltrate with exocytosis, basal layer vacuolization, and dyskeratotic keratinocytes* (arrow) *are present.*

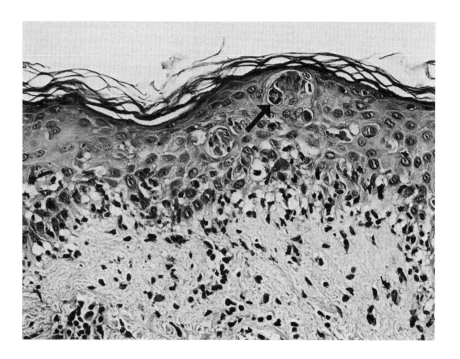

II. Graft-versus-host reaction (GVHR), acute (Fig. 10-2)

1. **Loss of polarity of epidermal cells** (due to pretreatment regimens)
2. **Dyskeratotic epidermal cells** rarely associated with a lymphocyte (satellite necrosis)
3. **Vacuolization** at dermoepidermal junction
4. Mild perivascular infiltrate with extension into epidermis
5. Melanin incontinence
6. Clefting and subepidermal bullae characteristic of more severe forms of GVHR

Early lesions may be confused with erythema multiforme; the prominent loss of polarity of epidermal cells and sparse infiltrate in GVHR help differentiate the entities

See Ch. 11, I.D; Ch. 12, XVI; Ch. 20, IV

III. Morbilliform viral exanthem

1. Focal dyskeratosis
2. Multinucleated keratinocytes may be present depending on the causative agent
3. Vacuolization along dermo-epidermal junction
4. Focal, scant lymphohistiocytic perivascular infiltrate
5. Focal extravasation of erythrocytes may be present

Except for multinucleate keratinocytes, this pattern is nonspecific

In the absence of multinucleate giant cells, a morbilliform drug eruption should be considered

Fig. **10-2.** *Acute graft-versus-host reaction.*
A. *Basal layer vacuolization is prominent in this photomicrograph. Other findings include exocytosis and dyskeratotic keratinocytes (arrow).*
B. *The more prominent keratinocytic dysmaturation in this photomicrograph is due to chemotherapy effect.*

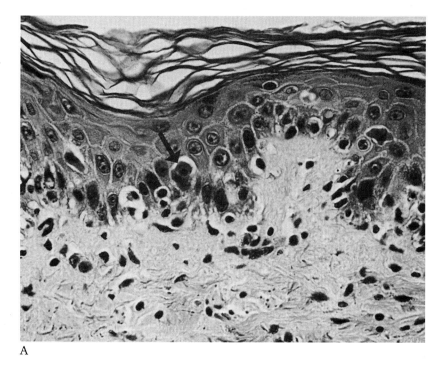

A

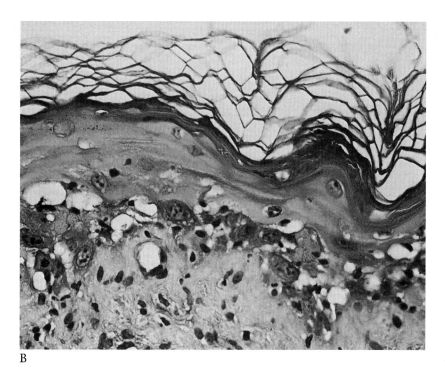

B

IV. Fixed drug eruption, chronic (Fig. 10-3)

1. Variable, slight parakeratosis
2. Focal slight intercellular edema
3. Rare dyskeratotic cells
4. **Vacuolization** along dermoepidermal junction
5. Slight papillary dermal fibrosis
6. Scattered melanophages, especially between venules

Ch. 11, II.J

V. Dermatomyositis (Fig. 10-4)

1. Normal to atrophic epidermis
2. Marked dermal edema with deposition of acid mucopolysaccharides
3. Scanty lymphocytic infiltrate present about venules in superficial dermis
4. Older lesions may have extensive dermal calcification, especially in children

Edematous, erythematous lesions may be indistinguishable histologically from lupus erythematosus

Older lesions clinically and histologically may resemble poikiloderma (See also Ch. 10, V)

VI. Poikiloderma vasculare atrophicans (idiopathic) (see Fig. 8-2)

1. Hyperkeratosis
2. Focal parakeratosis
3. Epidermal atrophy
4. Dyskeratosis in lower epidermal cells
5. Vacuolization at the dermoepidermal interface
6. Bandlike lymphocytic dermal infiltrate with exocytosis
7. Dilated dermal capillaries common
8. Melanophages

See also Ch. 8, V; Ch. 12, VIII

VII. Erythema dyschromium perstans

1. Vacuolization along the dermal-epidermal junction
2. Variable lymphocytic infiltrate in upper dermis
3. Melanophages in upper dermis

VIII. Phototoxic drug eruption

1. Dyskeratosis may be prominent
2. Squamatization of the basal layer
3. Vacuolization along dermoepidermal junction
4. Papillary dermal edema
5. Vessel ectasia
6. Variable superficial perivascular mononuclear cell infiltrate

IX. Postinflammatory hyperpigmentation

1. Epidermis normal to slightly atrophic (depending on etiologic agent)
2. Prominent vacuolization along dermoepidermal junction

This entity represents an end stage caused by various factors; for example, late lesions of lichen planus may show only postinflammatory pigmentation

Fig. **10-3.** Fixed drug eruption. Basal layer vacuolization with dyskeratotic keratinocytes and dermal melanophages (arrow) are seen.

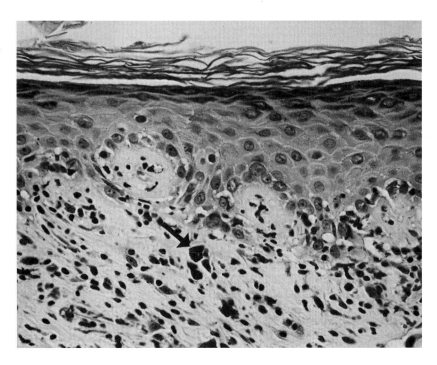

Fig. **10-4.** Dermatomyositis. Frequently, the histologic changes are minimal. Here there are vacuolization and a slight perivascular lymphocytic infiltrate with exocytosis. Increased mucin in the dermis (not seen here) is also common.

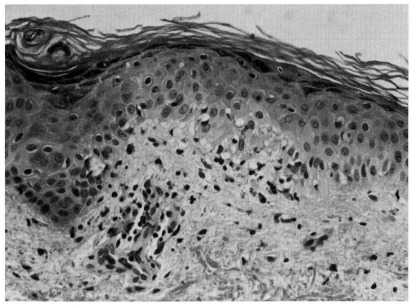

	3. Scattered melanophages in perivascular and intervascular array in papillary dermis	
	4. Occasional lymphocyte present	
X. Pinta, tertiary stage	1. Variable epidermal atrophy	Vacuolization appears in inflammatory first stage
	2. Marked vacuolization along dermoepidermal junction	
	3. Numerous melanophages in upper dermis	

Suggested Reading

Erythema Multiforme

Ackerman, A. B., Penneys, N. S., and Clark, W. H. Erythema multiforme exudativum: Distinctive pathological process. Br. J. Dermatol. 84:554–566, 1971.

Bastuji-Garin, S., Rzany, B., Stern, R. S., Shear, N. H., Naldi, L., and Roujeau, J. C. Clinical classification of cases of toxic epidermal necrolysis, Stevens–Johnson syndrome and erythema multiforme. Arch. Dermatol. 129:92–96, 1993.

Fabbri, P., and Panconesi, E. Erythema multiforme ("minus" and "maius") and drug intake. Clin. Dermatol. 11:479–489, 1993.

Howland, W. W., Golitz, L. E., Weston, W. E., et al. Erythema multiforme: Clinical, histopathologic, and immunologic study. J. Am. Acad. Dermatol. 10:438–446, 1984.

Huff, J. C., Weston, W. L., and Tonnesen, M. G. Erythema multiforme: A critical review of characteristics, diagnostic criteria, and causes. J. Am. Acad. Dermatol. 8:763–775, 1983.

Lever, W. F. My concept of erythema multiforme. Am. J. Dermatopathol. 7:141–142, 1985.

Orfanos, C. E., Schaumberg-Lever, G., and Lever, W. F. Dermal and epidermal types of erythema multiforme: A histologic study of 24 cases. Arch. Dermatol. 109:682–688, 1974.

Roujeau, J. C. What is going on in erythema multiforme? Dermatology 188: 249–250, 1994.

Graft-versus-host Reaction (GVHR), Acute

Bauer, D. J., Hood, A. F., and Horn, T. D. Histologic comparison of autologous graft-vs-host reaction and cutaneous eruption of lymphocyte recovery. Arch. Dermatol. 129:855–858, 1993.

Brubaker, D. B. Transfusion-associated graft-versus-host disease. Hum. Pathol. 17:1085–1088, 1986.

Einsele, H., Ehninger, G., Schneider, E. M., et al. High frequency of graft-versus-host-like syndromes following syngeneic bone marrow transplantation. Transplantation 45:579–585, 1988.

Elliot, C. J., Sloane, J. P., Sanderson, K. V., et al. The histological diagnosis of cutaneous graft versus host disease: Relationship of skin changes to marrow purging and other clinical variables. Histopathology 11:145–155, 1987.

Farmer, E. R. The histopathology of graft-versus-host disease. Adv. Dermatol. 1:173–188, 1986.

Hood, A. F., Black, L. P., Vogelsang, G. B., et al. Acute graft-versus-host disease following autologous and syngeneic bone marrow transplantation. Arch. Dermatol. 123:745–750, 1987.

Hood, A. F., Soter, N. A., Rappeport, J., and Gigli, I. Graft-versus-host reaction: Cutaneous manifestations following bone marrow transplantation. Arch. Dermatol. 113:1087–1091, 1977.

Hymes, S. R., Farmer, E. R., Lewis, P. G., et al. Cutaneous graft-versus-host reaction. Prognosis features seen by light microscopy. J. Am. Acad. Dermatol. 12:468–474, 1985.

Lerner, K. G. Histopathology of graft-versus-host reaction (GVHR) in human recipients of marrow from HLA-matched sibling donors. Transplant Proc. 6:367–371, 1974.

Sale, G. E., Lerner, K. G., Berker, E. A., et al. The skin biopsy in the diagnosis of acute graft-versus-host disease in man. Am. J. Pathol. 89:621–636, 1977.

Santos, G. W., Hess, A. D., and Vogelsang, G. B. Graft-versus-host reactions and disease. Immunol. Rev. 88:169–192, 1985.

Fixed Drug Eruption

Korkij, W. K., and Soltani, K. Fixed drug eruption. A brief review. Arch. Dermatol. 120:520–524, 1984.

Mahboob, A., and Haroon, T. S. Drugs causing fixed eruptions: A study of 450 cases. Int. J. Dermatol. 37:833–838, 1998.

Sharma, V. K., Dhar, S., and Gill, A. N. Drug related involvement of specific sites in fixed eruptions: A statistical evaluation. J. Dermatol. 23:530–534, 1996.

Dermatomyositis

Bowyer, S. L., Clark, R. A., Ragsdale, C. G., Hollister, J. R., and Sullivan, D. B. Juvenile dermatomyositis: Histologic findings and pathogenetic hypothesis for the associated skin changes. J. Rheumatol. 13:753–759, 1986.

Callen, J. P. Dermatomyositis and malignancy. Clin. Dermatol. 11:61–65, 1993.

Hanno, R., and Callen, J. P. Histopathology of Gottrom's papules. *J. Cutan. Pathol.* 12:389–394, 1985.

Janis, J. F., and Winkelmann, R. K. Histopathology of the skin in dermatomyositis: A histopathologic study of 55 cases. *Arch. Dermatol.* 97:640–650, 1968.

Mascaro, J. M., Jr., Hausmann, G., Herrero, C., Grau, J. M., Cid M. C., Palou, J., and Mascaro, J. M. Membrane attack complex deposits in cutaneous lesions of dermatomyositis. *Arch. Dermatol.* 131:1386–1392, 1995.

Magro, C. M., and Crowson, A. N. The immunofluorescent profile of dermatomyositis: A comparative study with lupus erythematosus. *J. Cutan. Pathol.* 24: 543–552, 1997.

Phototoxic Reactions

Epstein, J. H. Adverse Cutaneous reactions to the Sun. In: Malkinson, F. D., and Pearson, R. W. (Eds.). *Year Book of Dermatology.* Chicago: Year Book Medical Publishers; 1971, pp. 5–43.

Epstein, J. H. Photosensitivity: I. Mechanisms. *Clin. Dermatol.* 4:81–87, 1986.

Epstein, J. H. Phototoxicity and photoallergy in man. *J. Am. Acad. Dermatol.* 8:141–147, 1983.

Pinta

Hasselmann, C. M. Comparative studies on the histopathology of syphilis, yaws and pinta. *Br. J. Vener. Dis.* 33:5–23, 1957.

Pardo-Castello, V., and Ferrer, I. Pinta. *Arch. Dermatol. Syph.* 45:843–864, 1942.

Rodriguez, H. A., Albores-Saavedra, J., Lozano, M. M., et al. Langerhans' cells in late pinta. *Arch. Pathol.* 91:302–306, 1971.

Williams, H. U. Pathology of yaws. *Arch. Pathol.* 20:596–630, 1935.

Chapter 11

Subepidermal Clefting, Blister, or Pustule Formation

I. Cell poor
  A. Porphyria cutanea tarda
  B. Epidermolysis bullosa
  C. Toxic epidermal necrolysis
  D. Graft-versus-host reaction (GVHR), acute
  E. Acute radiodermatitis
  F. Bullous dermatosis of diabetes mellitus
  G. Bullous dermatosis of renal failure
  H. Electrical burn
  I. Thermal burn
II. With inflammation
  A. Bullous pemphigoid
  B. Herpes gestationis
  C. Dermatitis herpetiformis
  D. Bullous lupus erythematosus
  E. Linear IgA dermatosis
  F. Chronic bullous disease of childhood
  G. Focal embolic lesions in gonococcemia and acute meningococcemia
  H. Epidermolysis bullosa acquisita
  I. Erythema multiforme
  J. Fixed drug eruption
  K. Bullous lichen planus
  L. Lichen sclerosus et atrophicus
  M. Bullous drug eruption
  N. Light eruption
  O. Mastocytosis
  P. Perniosis

Subepidermal clefts and blisters arise due to a wide variety of causes. The clefts may be focal along the dermoepidermal junction or may coalesce to form vesicles or bullae. The age of the lesion sampled is critical in determining the extent of blister formation. Older lesions may exhibit reepithelialization of the blister floor from adnexal epithelium, giving the impression of an intraepidermal plane of separation. This chapter examines immunologically mediated bullous disorders (e.g., pemphigoid), mechanobullous disorders (e.g., epidermolysis bullosa simplex), bullous disorders due to physical agents (e.g., radiodermatitis), and metabolically mediated bullous disorders (e.g., bullous dermatosis of renal failure).

In evaluating a suspected bullous disorder, it is crucial to identify the level of clefting within the skin, the predominant type of infiltrating inflammatory cell, and the presence or absence of dyskeratotic keratinocytes. Where possible and appropriate, histologic diagnoses should be correlated with the results of direct and indirect immunofluorescence testing. In the case of hereditary forms of epidermolysis bullosa, definitive diagnosis will rest upon electron microscopy. Nonetheless, light microscopy is very useful to determine the level of cleavage in epidermolysis bullosa, especially when combined with immunohistochemical analysis of basement membrane components in relation to the split in the skin (Fig. 11-1).

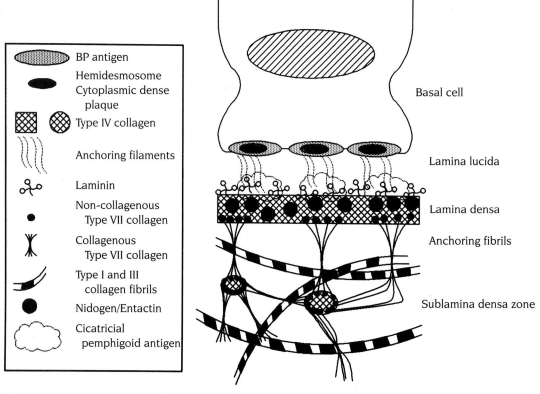

BP antigen

Hemidesmosome
Cytoplasmic dense
plaque

Type IV collagen

Anchoring filaments

Laminin

Non-collagenous
Type VII collagen

Collagenous
Type VII collagen

Type I and III
collagen fibrils

Nidogen/Entactin

Cicatricial
pemphigoid antigen

Basal cell

Lamina lucida

Lamina densa

Anchoring fibrils

Sublamina densa zone

Fig. **11-1.** *Basement membrane zone. Schematic diagram of the basement membrane zone. (From Anhalt, G. A. In D. J. Demis (Ed.), Clinical Dermatology. Philadelphia: J. B. Lippincott, 1992.)*

The Reactive Process and the Disease	Histopathology	Comments
I. Cell poor		
A. Porphyria cutanea tarda (Fig. 11-2)	1. **Subepidermal bulla** with intact epidermal roof 2. Dermal papillae protrude irregularly into bulla cavity, giving a ragged appearance to the base of the blister ("festooning") 3. **PAS-positive, diastase-resistant hyaline material deposited around dermal capillaries** in some lesions	Hyaline material is type IV collagen

Fig. **11-2.** *Porphyria cutanea tarda.*
A. *Subepidermal cleft formation with "festooning." The latter refers to the remarkably well-preserved shape of dermal papillae.*
B. *PAS-positive material encircles superficial capillary-venules.*

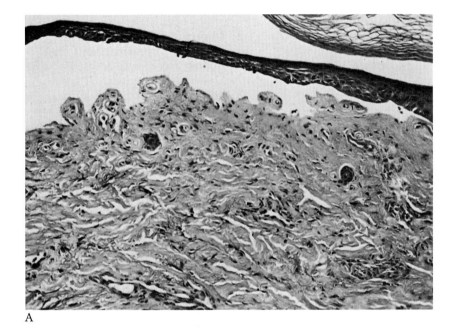

A

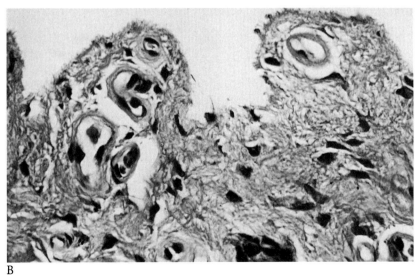

B

	4. Extravasation of erythrocytes into epidermis and bulla cavity 5. Older lesions may contain neutrophils	
B. Epidermolysis bullosa (Fig. 11-3)	1. Normal overlying epidermis 2. Subepidermal bulla 3. Paucicellular infiltrate	
C. Toxic epidermal necrolysis (Fig. 11-4)	1. **Partial or full-thickness epidermal necrosis with subepidermal bullae** 2. Vacuolization along dermoepidermal junction adjacent to necrotic epidermis 3. Dermal infiltrate characteristically sparse	Full-thickness necrosis occasionally may be observed in erythema multiforme (EM); some observers consider toxic epidermal necrolysis to be a type of noninflammatory EM
D. Graft-versus-host reaction (GVHR) (see Fig. 10-2), acute	1. **Loss of polarity** of epidermal cells due to pretreatment regimens 2. **Dyskeratotic epidermal cells** rarely associated with a lymphocyte 3. **Vacuolization** at dermoepidermal junction 4. Mild perivascular infiltrate with extension into epidermis 5. Melanin incontinence 6. Subepidermal clefting and bullae characterize more severe forms of a GVHR	Early lesions may be confused with erythema multiforme; the prominent loss of polarity of epidermal and sparse infiltrate in GVHR helps differentiate the entities See also Ch. 10, II; Ch. 12, XVI; Ch. 20, IV

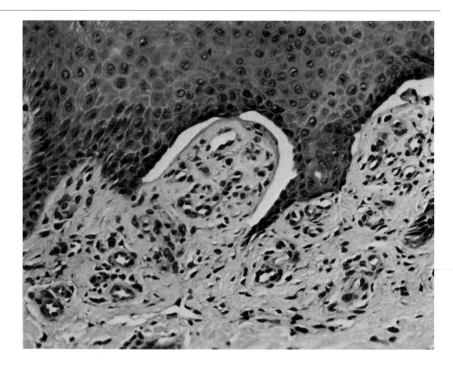

Fig. **11-3.** *Epidermolysis bullosa. A sharp subepidermal cleft is present in this tissue of junctional epidermolysis bullosa. Note that the underlying dermis lacks significant inflammatory cell infiltrate.*

Fig. **11-4.** (A,B) *Toxic epidermal necrolysis. Intact epidermis overlying a subepidermal blister without significant inflammation. There is widespread necrosis of keratinocytes in the epidermis.*

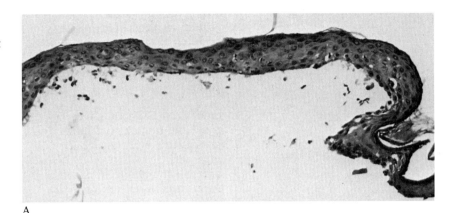

A

B

E. Acute radiodermatitis	1. Focal dyskeratosis 2. Epidermal necrosis may be present 3. Vacuolization along the dermoepidermal junction 4. Subepidermal bulla formation occasionally observed 5. Edema of papillary and upper reticular dermis 6. Variable pyknosis of fibroblasts and histiocytes 7. Vacuolization of endothelial cells	See also Ch. 20, VI.A
F. Bullous dermatosis of diabetes mellitus	1. Blister often subepidermal; may be midepidermal 2. Extensive epidermal necrosis in blister roof 3. Venules in upper dermis are **thick walled,** characteristic of vessel changes in diabetes mellitus	
G. Bullous dermatosis of renal failure	Findings similar or identical to porphyria cutanea tarda	This "pseudoporphyria" occurs in patients on hemodialysis who have normal porphyrin studies

H. Electrical burn

1. Subepidermal bulla
2. Nuclei of basal keratinocytes attenuated and vertically disposed, in parallel array
3. Coagulative necrosis of upper dermis

I. Thermal burn

1. Epidermal necrosis with **ghostlike nuclear remnants**
2. **Intrablister hemorrhage** common
3. Variable appendageal necrosis, depending on extent of injury
4. Pyknosis of fibroblasts, with loss of refractility of affected collagen
5. Neutrophilic infiltrate of subcutis variable, but characterizes third-degree burns

See also Ch. 8, VII

II. With inflammation

A. Bullous pemphigoid (Fig. 11-5).

1. **Subepidermal bulla** with roof composed of relatively normal epidermis
2. Vacuolization along dermo-epidermal junction adjacent to bulla.
3. Eosinophils may migrate into the epidermis in early lesions

> *Epidermal invasion by eosinophils* may be seen in:
>
> Bullous pemphigoid
> Pemphigus vulgaris and foliaceus
> Arthropod bite reaction
> Allergic contact dermatitis
> Incontinentia pigmenti

4. Bulbous edematous papillae may protrude into blister cavity
5. Early lesions characterized by eosinophils at dermoepidermal junction
6. Scattered superficial and deep dermal infiltrate of **eosinophils and lymphocytes** with some aggregation about venules

The number of eosinophils varies; when present in great numbers, they may extend through the dermis and into subcutaneous fat; immunofluorescence studies are usually diagnostic

B. Herpes gestationis (pemphigoides gestationis)

1. Changes may resemble bullous pemphigoid
2. Occasional dyskeratotic keratinocytes in blister roof

Immunofluorescence findings similar to bullous pemphigoid

Fig. **11-5.** Bullous pemphigoid.
A. Subepidermal cleft formation with lymphocytes and eosinophils is characteristic.
B. Subepidermal cleft formation with numerous eosinophils and lymphocytes within the bulla and dermis is characteristic.

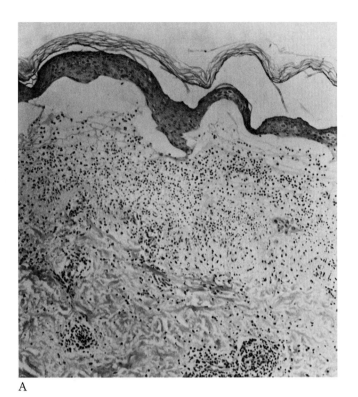

A

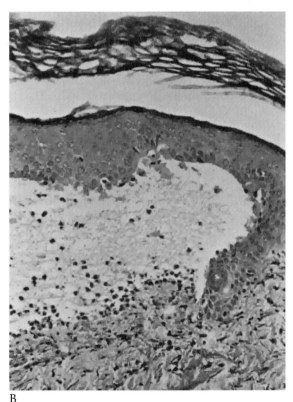

B

C. Dermatitis herpetiformis (Fig. 11-6)	1. Accumulation of neutrophils and basophilic debris below the basement membrane zone 2. Subsequent accumulation of **neutrophils in papillary dermal microabscesses** 3. Separation at the basement membrane zone above microabscesses to form subepidermal clefts 4. Eosinophils appear in the papillary dermis and bulla cavity as lesion evolves 5. Necrosis of epidermis in roof of bulla is not seen until late 6. Perivascular infiltrate of lymphocytes and polymorphonuclear leukocytes	The presence of neutrophils and nuclear dust below the basement membrane zone is observed in acute dermatitis herpetiformis, linear IgA dermatosis, and bullous lupus erythematosus; immuno-fluorescence studies are helpful in differentiating these disorders
D. Bullous lupus erythematosus	Bullous lesions occurring in systemic lupus erythematosus may be histologically indistinguishable from dermatitis herpetiformis except eosinophils are not present	
E. Linear IgA dermatosis (Fig. 11-7)	1. Accumulation of neutrophils and nuclear dust, especially at the tips of rete ridges 2. Separation at the basement membrane zone adjacent to scattered neutrophils in vacuoles 3. Eosinophils appear in the bulla and dermis as the lesion evolves 4. Perivascular infiltrate of lymphocytes and neutrophils	At times (e.g., drug-induced linear IgA dermatosis and chronic bullous disease of childhood), eosinophils may be admixed with neutrophils at the dermoepidermal junction. Direct immunofluorescence studies are required to confirm the diagnosis
F. Chronic bullous disease of childhood	Histologic (including direct immunofluorescence) findings are very similar to linear IgA dermatosis	
G. Focal embolic lesions in gonococcemia and acute meningococcemia	1. Necrotic epidermis 2. **Subepidermal pustules** 3. **Vasculitis** with variable fibrinoid necrosis of venules and striking inflammatory infiltrate of lymphocytes, histiocytic cells, neutrophils, and nuclear dust 4. **Fibrin thrombi in involved vessels** 5. Extravasation of erythrocytes	See also Ch. 16, II.B Gram-negative intracellular and extracellular organisms are easily demonstrated in acute meningococcemia; organisms are rarely demonstrated in gonococcemia
H. Epidermolysis bullosa acquisita	The histopathology of epidermolysis bullosa may be identical to bullous pemphigoid	

Fig. **11-6.** Dermatitis herpetiformis. Neutrophilic microabscesses and fibrin are present within dermal papillae. Vacuolization and early cleft formation are evident at right and centrally.

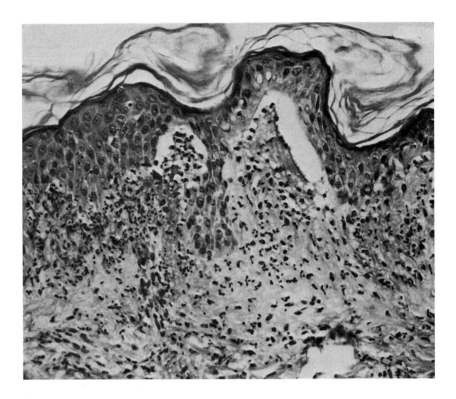

Fig. **11-7.** Linear IgA dermatosis. Subepidermal cleft with a moderate number of lymphocytes and granulocytes in the blister cavity. These features could also represent bullous pemphigoid; direct immunofluorescence is required.

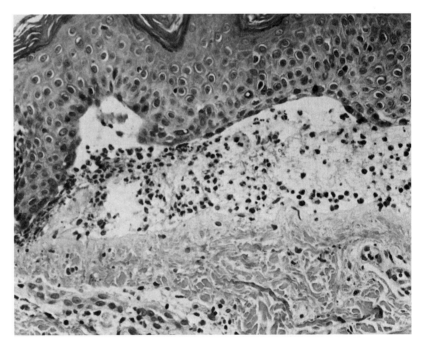

I. Erythema multiforme (Fig. 11-8)

1. Focal dyskeratosis
2. Focal intercellular edema
3. Vacuolization of basal cell layer with lymphocytes along the dermoepidermal junction
4. Subepidermal bulla formation may be noted
5. Perivascular lymphocytic infiltrate
6. Endothelial cell hypertrophy of affected cutaneous vessels
7. Melanin incontinence may be present

The histopathology of fixed drug eruption may be indistinguishable from erythema multiforme

See also Ch. 6, II.L; Ch. 10, I

J. Fixed drug eruption

1. Intercellular edema
2. Focal dyskeratosis most prominent along the basal layer; also present in clusters in mid-epidermis
3. Exocytosis of lymphocytes into lower epidermal region
4. **Vacuolization along dermoepidermal** junction
5. Perivascular lymphocytic infiltrate about superficial and deep vessels
6. Lymphocytic infiltrate along dermoepidermal junction sometimes bandlike
7. **Melanin incontinence**

In late stages, epidermal changes are minimal, but vacuolization persists, associated with numerous melanophages and sometimes a slight inflammatory infiltrate

Differential diagnosis:
Erythema multiforme
Lichenoid drug eruption
Graft-versus-host reaction

See also Ch. 10, IV

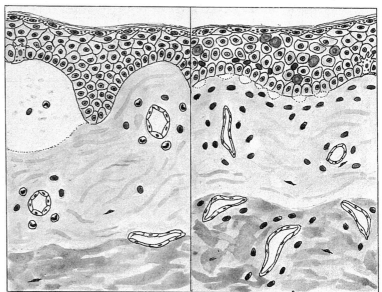

Fig. **11-8.** *Erythema multiforme, inflammatory type. Dermoepidermal junction changes include vacuolization and lymphocytic infiltration. The infiltrate is also disposed about superficial vessels and focally within the epidermis. Spongiosis and dyskeratosis are typical.*
A. *Comparison of the noninflammatory and inflammatory types of erythema multiforme. Left: Subepidermal cleft formation with edema of the papillary dermis and sparse mononuclear infiltrates is typical of the noninflammatory type of erythema multiforme, of which toxic epidermal necrolysis can be considered an example. Right: Dyskeratosis and spongiosis within the epidermis, vacuolization at the dermoepidermal interface, and lymphocytes lined up at the same location and around venules are characteristic of an early lesion of erythema multiforme, inflammatory type.*

A

B. *An early lesion with minimal dyskeratosis.*
C. *A later lesion with numerous dyskeratotic cells and separation at the dermoepidermal junction.*

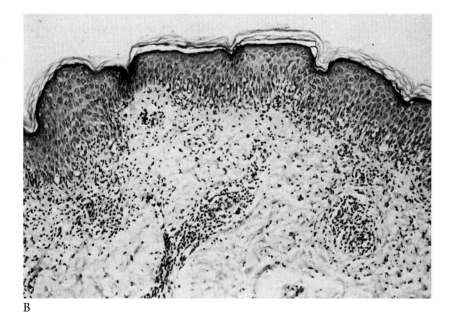

B

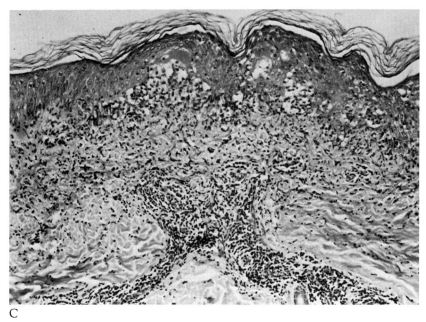

C

K. Bullous lichen planus

1. Hyperkeratosis
2. **Wedge-shape hypergranulosis**
3. Irregular hyperplasia of epidermis with characteristic **sawtooth** changes of the rete ridges
4. Homogeneous, eosinophilic hyaline bodies **(Civatte bodies)** in the epidermis and papillary dermis
5. Squamatization of basal cell layer
6. **Vacuolization of basal cell layer**
7. Vacuoles may coalesce to form clefts (Max-Joseph clefts) or subepidermal bulla — See Fig. 2-12
8. **Bandlike infiltrate** of lymphocytes, histiocytes, and macrophages, which may obscure the dermoepidermal interface — See also Ch. 12, I
9. Variable number of melanophages

L. Lichen sclerosus et atrophicus

1. Variable hyperkeratosis — See also Ch. 8, I; Ch. 12, II
2. Epidermal atrophy
3. Marked vacuolization at dermoepidermal junction
4. Subepidermal hemorrhagic bullae occasionally present
5. **Edematous, homogeneous, broadened upper dermis**
6. Sparse patchy or bandlike lymphocytic infiltrate may be present beneath edematous zone
7. Collagen may also assume a sclerotic or hyalinized appearance

M. Bullous drug eruption

1. Vacuolization along dermoepidermal junction
2. Edema of papillary dermis
3. **Subepidermal bullae**
4. Variable perivascular lymphocytic and eosinophilic infiltrate in superficial and deep dermis

Differential diagnosis:
  Bullous pemphigoid
  Epidermolysis bullosa
    acquisita
  Erythema multiforme

N. Light eruption (Fig. 11-9)
1. Focal dyskeratotic keratinocytes
2. Upper dermal edema, often marked
3. **Extravasation of erythrocytes**
4. Variably intense perivascular infiltrate, predominantly lymphocytes

O. Mastocytosis
1. Epidermis normal or attenuated
2. Extensive upper dermal edema causing subepidermal bulla
3. Variably intense infiltrate of mast cells in perivascular and interstitial array

Giemsa, Leder, and toluidine blue stains confirm presence of mast cells

See also Ch. 12, XIV; Ch. 13, IV; Ch. 18, IV.

P. Perniosis
1. Unremarkable epidermis
2. Papillary dermal edema, often extensive
3. Superficial and deep perivascular lymphocytic infiltrate
4. Peri-eccrine lymphocytic infiltrate
5. "Fluffy edema" and lymphocytic infiltration of vessel walls

Differential diagnosis of perniosis:

1. Dermatomyositis
2. Lupus erythematosus
3. Polymorphous light eruption

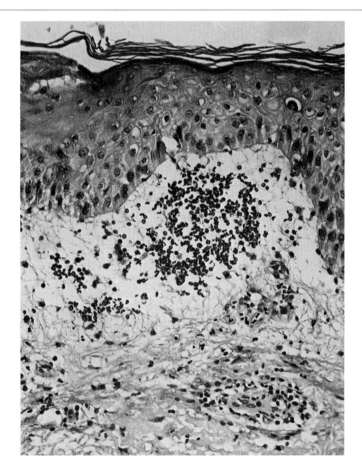

Fig. **11-9.** *Light eruption (polymorphous light eruption). Intense dermal edema is present with extravasation of erythrocytes. The dermis also contains a perivascular lymphocytic infiltrate. Scattered dyskeratotic cells are present in the overlying epidermis.*

Suggested Reading

Porphyria

Cormane, R. H., Szabo, E., and Hoo, T. T. Histopathology of the skin in acquired and hereditary porphyria cutanea tarda. *Br. J. Dermatol.* 85:531, 1972.

Epstein, J. H., Tuffanelli, D. L., and Epstein, W. L. Cutaneous changes in the porphyrias: A microscopic study. *Arch. Dermatol.* 107:689, 1973.

Feldaker, M., Montgomery, H., and Brunsting, L. A. Histopathology of porphyria cutanea tarda. *J. Invest. Dermatol.* 24:131, 1955.

Harber, L. C., and Bickers, D. R. Porphyria and pseudoporphyria. *J. Invest. Dermatol.* 82:207–209, 1984.

Hogan, D., Card, R. T., Ghadially, R., McSheffrey, J. B., and Lane, P. Human immunodeficiency virus infection and porphyria cutanea tarda. *J. Am. Acad. Dermatol.* 20:17–20, 1989.

LaCour, J. P., Bodokh, I., Castanet, J., Bekri, S., and Ortonne, J. P. Porphyria cutanea tarda and antibodies to hepatitis C. *Br. J. Dermatol.* 128:121–123, 1993.

Maynard, B., and Peters, M. S. Histologic and immunofluorescence study of cutaneous porphyrias. *J. Cutan. Pathol.* 19:40–47, 1991.

Young, J. W. and E. T. Conte, Porphyrias and porphyrins. *Int. J. Dermatol.* 30:399–406, 1991.

Epidermolysis Bullosa

Bergman, R. Immunohistopathologic diagnosis of epidermolysis bullosa. *Am. J. Dermatopathol.* 21:185–192, 1999.

Briggaman, R. A. Hereditary epidermolysis bullosa with special emphasis on newly recognized syndromes and complications. *Dermatol. Clin.* 1:263–280, 1983.

Briggaman, R. A., and Wheeler, C. E., Jr. Epidermolysis bullosa dystrophica recessive: A possible role of anchoring fibrils in the pathogenesis. *J. Invest. Dermatol.* 65:203, 1975.

Fine, J.-D. Epidermolysis bullosa: Clinical aspects, pathology, and recent advances in research. *Int. J. Dermatol.* 25:143–157, 1986.

Fine, J.-D., Bauer, E. A., Briggman, R. A., et al. Revised clinical and laboratory criteria for subtypes of inherited epidermolysis bullosa. *J. Am. Acad. Dermatol.* 24:119–135, 1991.

Haneke, E., and Anton-Lamprecht, I. Ultrastructure of blister formation in epidermolysis bullosa hereditaria: V. Epidermolysis bullosa simplex localisata type Weber-Cockayne. *J. Invest. Dermatol.* 78:219, 1982.

Katz, S. I. The epidermal basement membrane zone—Structure, ontogeny, and role in disease. *J. Am. Acad. Dermatol.* 11:1025–1037, 1984.

Pearson, R. W., Potter, B., and Strauss, F. Epidermolysis bullosa hereditaria letalis: Clinical and histological manifestations and course of the disease. *Arch. Dermatol.* 109:349, 1974.

Roenigk, H. H., Jr., Ryan, J. G., and Bergfeld, W. F. Epidermolysis bullosa acquisita. *Arch. Dermatol.* 103:1, 1971.

Yaoita, H., Briggaman, R. A., Lawley, T. J., et al. Epidermolysis bullosa acquisita: Ultrastructural and immunological studies. *J. Invest. Dermatol.* 76:288, 1981.

Toxic Epidermal Necrolysis

Lyell, A. Toxic epidermal necrolysis (the scalded skin syndrome): A reappraisal. *Br. J. Dermatol.* 100:69, 1979.

Rasmussen, J. E. Toxic epidermal necrolysis. *Med. Clin. North Am.* 64:901–920, 1980.

Roujeau, J.-C. The spectrum of Stevens–Johnson syndrome and toxic epidermal necrolysis: A clinical classification. *J. Invest. Dermatol.* 102:28S–30S, 1994.

Roujeau, J.-C., Chosidow, O., Saiaig, P., and Guillaume, J.-C. Toxic epidermal necrolysis (Lyell syndrome). *J. Am. Acad. Dermatol.* 23:1039–1058, 1990.

Graft-versus-host Reaction

Hood, A. F., Soter, N. A., Rappeport, J., and Gigli, I. Graft-versus-host reaction: Cutaneous manifestations following bone marrow transplantation. *Arch. Dermatol.* 113:1087, 1977.

Lerner, K. G. Histopathology of graft-versus-host reaction (GVHR) in human recipients of marrow from HLA-matched sibling donors. *Transplant. Proc.* 6:367, 1974.

Radiodermatitis

Hood, I. C., and Young, J. E. M. Late sequelae of superficial irradiation. *Head Neck Surg.* 7:65, 1984.

Rudolph, R., Gragahese, T., and Woodward, M. The ultrastructure and etiology of chronic radiotherapy damage in human skin. *Ann. Plast. Surg.* 9:282, 1982.

Bullous Dermatosis of Renal Failure   Gilchrest, B., Rowe, J., and Mihm, M. C., Jr. Bullous dermatosis of hemodialysis. *Ann. Intern. Med.* 83:480–483, 1975.

Poh-Fitzpatrick, M. B., Masullo, A. S., and Grossman, M. E. Porphyria cutanea tarda associated with chronic renal disease and hemodialysis. *Arch. Dermatol.* 116:191–195, 1980.

Burns   Foley, F. D. Pathology of cutaneous burns. *Surg. Clin. North Am.* 50:1200, 1970.

Bullous Pemphigoid   Bean, S. F., Michel, B., Furey, N., et al. Vesicular pemphigoid. *Arch. Dermatol.* 112:1402, 1976.

Eng, A. M., and Moncada, B. Bullous pemphigoid and dermatitis herpetiformis. *Arch. Dermatol.* 110:51, 1974.

Pearson, R. W. Advances in the Diagnosis and Treatment of Blistering Diseases: A Selective Review. In F. D. Malkinson and R. W. Pearson (Eds.), *Year Book of Dermatology*. Chicago: Year Book, 1977.

Mutasim, D. F., Takahashi, Y., Labib, R. S., et al. A pool of bullous pemphigoid antigen(s) is intracellular and associated with the basal cell cytoskeleton–hemidesmosome complex. *J. Invest. Dermatol.* 84:47, 1985.

Herpes Gestationis   Carruthers, J. A., Black, M. M., and Ramnarain, N. Immunopathological studies in herpes gestationis. *Br. J. Dermatol.* 96:35, 1977.

Hertz, K. C., Katz, S. I., Maize, J., and Ackerman, A. B. Herpes gestationis: A clinicopathologic study. *Arch. Dermatol.* 112:1543, 1976.

Schaumburg-Lever, G., Saffold, O. E., Orfanos, C. E., and Lever, W. F. Herpes gestationis: Histology and ultrastructure. *Arch. Dermatol.* 107:888, 1973.

Dermatitis Herpetiformis   Bose, S. K., Lacour, J. P., Bodokh, I., and Ortonne, J. P. Malignant lymphoma and dermatitis herpetiformis. *Dermatology*, 188:177–181, 1994.

Buckley, D. B., English, J., Molloy, W., Doyle, C. I., and Whelton, M. J. Dermatitis herpetiformis: A review of 119 cases. *Clin. Exp. Dermatol.* 8:477–487, 1983.

Connor, B. L., Marks, R., and Wilson-Jones, E. Dermatitis herpetiformis: Histological discriminants. *Trans. St. Johns Hosp. Dermatol. Soc.* 58:191, 1972.

Fry, L., and Seah, P. P. Dermatitis herpetiformis: An evaluation of diagnostic criteria. *Br. J. Dermatol.* 90:137, 1974.

Hall, R. P. Dermatitis herpetiformis. *J. Invest. Dermatol.* 99:873–881, 1992.

Katz, S. L., and Strober, W. The pathogenesis of dermatitis herpetiformis. *J. Invest. Dermatol.* 70:63, 1978.

Lawley, T. J., and Yancey, K. B. Dermatitis herpetiformis. *Dermatol. Clin.* 1:187, 1983.

Pazderka Smith, E., and Zone, J. J. Dermatitis herpetiformis and linear IgA bullous dermatosis. *Dermatol. Clin.* 11:511–526, 1993.

Seah, P. P., and Fry, L. Immunoglobulins in the skin in dermatitis herpetiformis and their relevance in diagnosis. *Br. J. Dermatol.* 92:157, 1975.

Bullous Lupus Erythematosus   Barton, D. D., Fine, J.-D., Gammon, W. R., and Sams, W. M., Jr. Bullous systemic lupus erythematosus: An unusual clinical course and detectable circulating autoantibodies to the epidermolysis bullosa acquisita antigen. *J. Am. Acad. Dermatol.* 15:369–373, 1986.

Burrows, N. P., Bhogal, B. S., Black, M. M., Rustin, M. H. A., Ishida-Yamamoto, A., Kirtschig, G., and Russell Jones, R., Bullous eruption of systemic lupus erythematosus: A clinicopathologic study of four cases. *Br. J. Dermatol.* 128:332–338, 1993.

Penneys, N. S., and Wiley, H. E. Herpetiform blisters in systemic lupus erythematosus. *Arch. Dermatol.* 115:1427, 1979.

Linear IgA Dermatosis and Chronic Bullous Disease of Childhood   Bhogal, B., Woinarowska, F., Marsden, R. A., et al. Linear IgA bullous dermatosis of adults and children: An immunoelectronmicroscopic study. *Br. J. Dermatol.* 117:289, 1987.

Smith, S. B., Harrist, T. J., Murphy, G. F., et al. Linear IgA bullous dermatosis v. dermatitis herpetiformis. *Arch. Dermatol.* 120:324, 1984.

Epidermolysis Bullosa Acquisita   Briggaman, R. A., Gammon, W. R., and Woodely, D. T. Epidermolysis bullosa acquisita of the immunopathologic type (dermolytic pemphigoid). *J. Invest. Dermatol.* 85(1, Suppl.): 79s–84s, 1985.

Woodley, D. T., Briggaman, R. A., O'Keefe, E. J., et al. Identification of the skin basement membrane autoantigen in epidermolysis bullosa acquisita. N. *Engl. J. Med.* 310:1007–1013, 1984.

Woodley, D. T., Burgeson, R. E., Lunstrum, G., et al. The epidermolysis bullosa acquisita antigen is the globular carboxyl terminus of type VII procollagen. J. *Clin. Invest.* 81:683–687, 1988.

Yaoita, H., Briggaman, R. A., Lawley, T. J., et al. Epidermolysis bullosa acquisita: Ultrastructural and immunological studies. J. *Invest. Dermatol.* 76:288–292, 1981.

Erythema Multiforme

Ackerman, A. B., Penneys, N. S., and Clark, W. H., Jr. Erythema multiforme exudativum: Distinctive pathological process. Br. J. *Dermatol.* 84:554, 1971.

Bedi, T. R., and Pinkus, H. Histopathological spectrum of erythema multiforme. Br. J. *Dermatol.* 95:243, 1976.

O'Loughlin, S., Schroeter, A. L., and Jordon, R. E. Chronic urticaria-like lesions in systemic lupus erythematosus. A review of 12 cases. *Arch. Dermatol.* 114:879, 1978.

Orfanos, C. E., Schaumburg-Lever, G., and Lever, W. F. Dermal and epidermal types of erythema multiforme. *Arch. Dermatol.* 109:682, 1974.

Fixed Drug Eruption

Korkij, W. K., and Soltani, K. Fixed drug eruption. A brief review. *Arch. Dermatol.* 120:520, 1984.

Lichen Planus

Altman, J., and Perry, H. O. The variations and course of lichen planus. *Arch. Dermatol.* 84:179, 1961.

Bellman, B., Reddy, R., and Falanga, V. Gereralized lichen planus associated with hepatitis C virus immunoreactivity. J. *Am. Acad. Dermatol.* 35:770–772, 1996.

Ellis, F. A. Histopathology of lichen planus based on analysis of one hundred biopsy specimens. J. *Invest. Dermatol.* 48:143, 1967.

Pereyo, N. G., Lesher, J. L., Jr., and Davis, L. S. Hepatitis C and its association with lichen planus and porphyria cutanea tarda. J. *Am. Acad. Dermatol.* 1995(32), 1995.

Ragaz, A., and Ackerman, A. B. Evolution, maturation and regression of lesions of lichen planus: New observations and correlations of clinical and histologic findings. *Am. J. Dermatopathol.* 3:5, 1981.

Shiohara, T., Moriya, N., Mochizuki, T., et al. Lichenoid tissue reactions (LTR) induced by local transfer of Ia-reactive T-cell clones. II. LTR by epidermal invasion of cytotoxic lymphokine-producing autoreactive T cells. J. *Invest. Dermatol.* 89:8, 1987.

Shklar, G. Erosive and bullous oral lesions of lichen planus. *Arch. Dermatol.* 97:411, 1968.

Van den Haute, V., Antoine, J. L., and Lachapelle, J. M. Histopathological discriminant criteria between lichenoid drug eruption and idiopathic lichen planus: retrospective study on selected samples. *Dermatologica* 179:10–13, 1989.

Lichen Sclerosus et Atrophicus

Bergfeld, W. F., and Lesowitz, S. A. Lichen sclerosus et atrophicus. *Arch. Dermatol.* 101:247, 1970.

Steigleder, G. K., and Raab, W. P. Lichen sclerosus et atrophicus. *Arch. Dermatol.* 84:219, 1961.

Mastocytosis

Johnson, W. C., and Helwig, E. B. Solitary mastocytosis. *Arch. Dermatol.* 84:148, 1961.

Chapter **12**

Bandlike Infiltrate
at the Dermoepidermal
Junction

I. Lichen planus and variants
  A. Hypertrophic lichen planus
  B. Atrophic lichen planus
  C. Bullous lichen planus
  D. Mucosal lichen planus
II. Lichen sclerosus et atrophicus
III. Lupus erythematosus
IV. Arthropod bite reaction
V. Lichen planus-like drug eruption
VI. Some persistent light eruptions, including actinic reticuloid
VII. Acrodermatitis chronica atrophicans
VIII. Poikiloderma vasculare atrophicans
IX. Parapsoriasis
X. Cutaneous T-cell lymphoma, mycosis fungoides variant, patch or plaque
XI. Lichenoid actinic keratosis
XII. Lichenoid keratosis
XIII. Secondary syphilis
XIV. Urticaria pigmentosa: papular lesion
XV. Progressive pigmented purpura
XVI. Graft-versus-host reaction, lichenoid stage
XVII. Lichen nitidus

Several inflammatory disorders of the skin exhibit a bandlike infiltrate that occupies the papillary dermis and may or may not be associated with epidermal changes. Some of those associated with epidermal alterations have been described in Chapters 5, 8, and 10 but are included again here for completeness and contrast.

The Reactive Process and the Disease	Histopathology	Comments
I. Lichen planus and variants (Fig. 12-1)	1. Hyperkeratosis 2. Rare parakeratosis 3. **Wedgelike hypergranulosis** 4. Irregular epidermal hyperplasia with **sawtooth** rete ridges 5. Eosinophilic hyaline cell remnants (**Civatte bodies**) in the epidermis and papillary dermis 6. Squamatization of basal cell layer 7. **Vacuolization** of basal cell layer	Parakeratosis more commonly observed in lichenoid drug eruptions and hypertrophic lichen planus Civatte bodies and dyskeratosis, terms that are used somewhat interchangeably, are the result of apoptosis

> *Lichenoid infiltrates* and *Civatte bodies* may be seen in many disorders, including:
>
> Lichen planus
> Lichen planopilaris
> Graft-versus-host reaction
> Lupus erythematosus
> Poikiloderma vasculare atrophicans
> Lichen planus-like drug eruption
> Lichenoid actinic keratosis
> Lichenoid keratosis

8. **Dense bandlike infiltrate** of lymphocytes, histiocytes, and macrophages that may obscure the dermoepidermal interface
9. Melanin incontinence common
10. Eosinophils uncommon

> Differential diagnosis of *bandlike infiltrate*:
>
> Lichen planus
> Lichen sclerosus et atrophicus
> Lupus erythematosus
> Arthropod bite reaction
> Lichen planus-like drug eruption
> Persistent light eruption
> Acrodermatitis chronica atrophicans
> Parapsoriasis
> Poikiloderma vasculare atrophicans
> Mycosis fungoides
> Actinic keratosis
> Secondary syphilis
> Histiocytosis X

Fig. **12-1.** (A,B) *Lichen planus.
Typical features include irregular
acanthosis ("sawtoothing"),
hyperkeratosis, hypergranulosis, a
lymphocytic infiltrate that "hugs" the
basal layer, vacuolization at the
dermoepidermal junction, Civatte bodies
(anucleate pink bodies near the
dermoepidermal junction), and a
squamatized basal layer.*

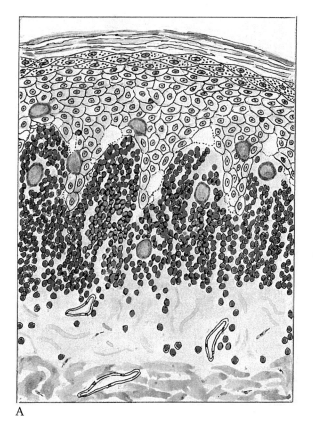

A

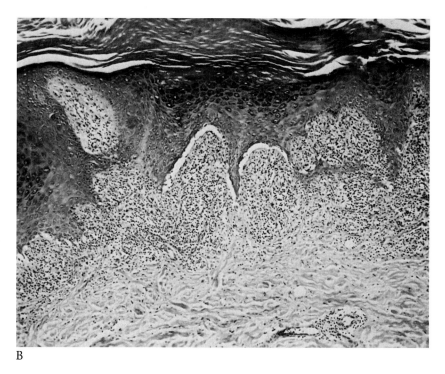

B

Vacuoles may coalesce to form subepidermal clefts (Max-Joseph spaces) (see Fig. 2-12)

The presence of numerous eosinophils raises the question of lichen planus-like drug eruption

Melanophages are often associated with inflammation in the area of the dermoepidermal junction

A. Hypertrophic lichen planus*

1. Hyperkeratosis and parakeratosis
2. Marked hypergranulosis
3. **Marked epidermal hyperplasia**
4. Hyperplastic papillary dermis often contains melanophages
5. Lymphocytic infiltrate focally along dermoepidermal junction and around superficial venules

When no bandlike infiltrate is present, consider lichen simplex chronicus or prurigo nodularis

B. Atrophic lichen planus*

1. Epidermal **atrophy**
2. Vacuolization of dermoepidermal junction

Atrophic lichen planus may be difficult to distinguish from lupus erythematosus or lichenoid actinic keratosis

C. Bullous lichen planus*

1. **Subepidermal bulla** with marked squamatization of basal cells in roof of bulla
2. Sawtooth papillae may protrude into base of bulla

See also Ch. 11, II.K

D. Mucosal lichen planus*

1. **Hypergranulosis with parakeratosis**
2. Squamatization and bandlike infiltrate

The presence of keratohyaline granules in most mucosal epithelium except for the hard palate represents hypergranulosis since the granular cell layer is normally absent

II. Lichen sclerosus et atrophicus (Fig. 12-2) (see Fig. 8-1)

1. Variable hyperkeratosis
2. Epidermal atrophy
3. **Edematous homogeneous, broadened upper dermis**
4. Vacuolization at the dermoepidermal junction
5. Vascular ectasia
6. Bandlike mononuclear cell infiltrate beneath edematous papillary dermis extending around and between venules and into the upper reticular dermis

See also Ch. 8, I, Ch. 11, II.L

* I.A through I.D are characterized by squamatization, vacuolization, and bandlike infiltrate.

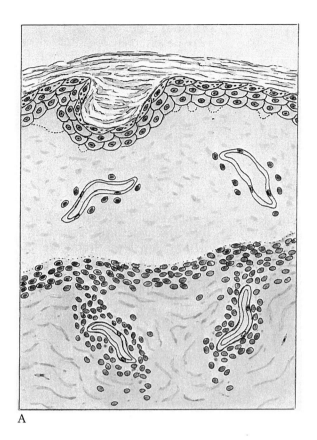

A

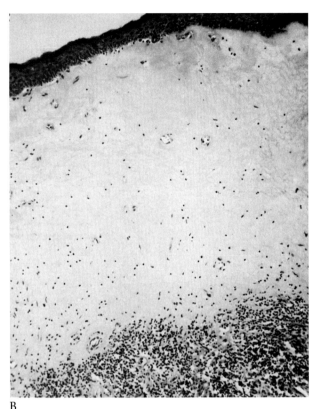

B

Fig. **12-2.** (A,B,C) *Lichen sclerosus et atrophicus.* Vacuolization at the dermoepidermal interface (A,C), homogenization of the upper dermis, and an underlying bandlike lymphocytic infiltrate are the hallmarks of this disorder. Follicular plugging and epidermal atrophy frequently accompany the features described above.

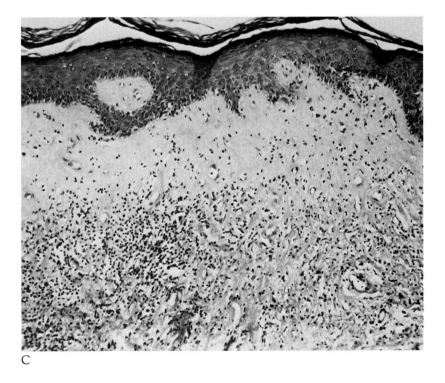

C

III. Lupus erythematosus
(Fig. 12-3)

1. Hyperkeratosis
2. Follicular plugging
3. Epidermal atrophy
4. Squamatization of basal cell layer
5. Thickened basement membrane zone
6. **Vacuolization along dermoepidermal junction both above and below basement membrane**
7. Edema of papillary dermis
8. Vascular ectasia
9. Bandlike and/or patchy **perivascular and periappendageal lymphocytic dermal infiltrate**
10. Extravasation of erythrocytes

Cutaneous lupus erythematosus may be associated with a cell-rich (bandlike) infiltrate or a cell-poor infiltrate *completely independent* from the deep periappendageal infiltrate

Special stains (see Ch. 3) are helpful in demonstrating increased acid mucopolysaccharide deposition in the dermis
See also Ch. 8, VI; Ch. 16, I.B.1.; Ch. 26, I.B.1

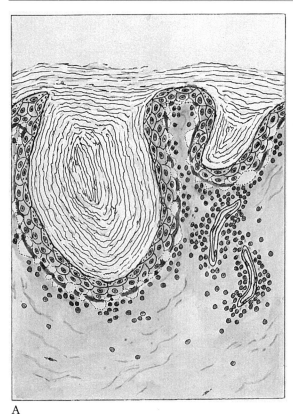

A

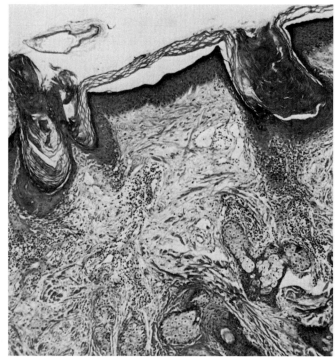

B

Fig. **12-3.** *Lupus erythematosus.*
A, B. *Follicular plugging, epidermal atrophy, a predominantly lymphocytic infiltrate dispersed about appendages and vessels, vacuolization, and thickening of the basement membrane zone characterize the mature chronic lesions.*

C, D. Similar changes but with edema, vascular ectasia, and sometimes smudged fibrinoid material about vessels are more typical of the lesions of systemic lupus erythematosus. A clear-cut distinction, however, between discoid and systemic erythemotosus cannot be made on the basis of routine histopathology.

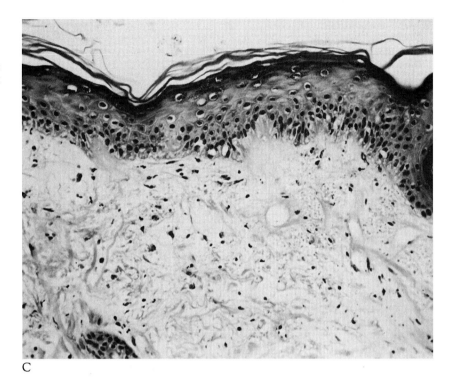

C

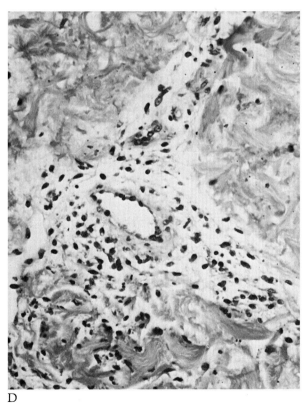

D

Fig. **12-3.** (continued)
E.   Notice the bandlike perifollicular
     infiltrate and thickened basement
     membrane.
F.   PAS-D stain highlights the
     thickened basement membrane.

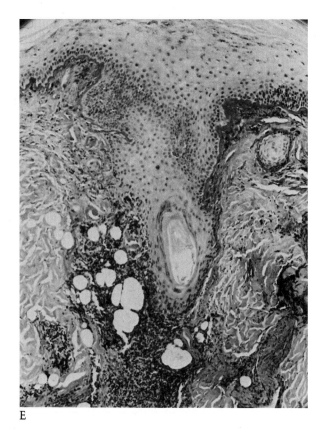

E

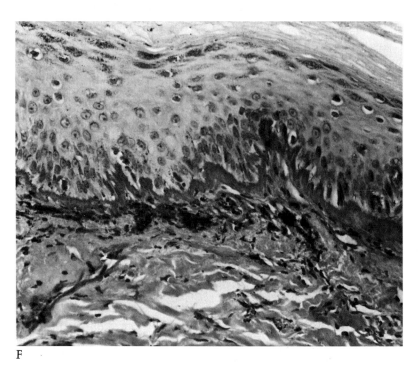

F

IV. Arthropod bite reaction (see Fig. 16-2)

1. Variable epidermal spongiosis and microvesicle formation
2. Epidermal necrosis or ulceration occasionally observed at site of bite
3. Bandlike lymphocytic and **eosinophilic infiltrate** may extend into upper reticular dermis; plasma cells may be noted
4. Perivascular infiltrate may extend into deep reticular dermis and subcutaneous tissue
5. **Endothelial cell swelling** often present
6. Extravasation of erythrocytes common

The polymorphous infiltrate of insect bites may be bandlike, nodular, perivascular, diffuse, or any combination of these patterns
See also Ch. 5, III.A; Ch. 13, I.F; Ch. 16, I.A.2; Ch. 19, II

V. Lichen planus–like drug eruption

1. Variable amount of hyperkeratosis
2. Parakeratosis common
3. Hypergranulosis may not be present
4. Variable number of Civatte bodies
5. Vacuolization and squamatization of basal layer may be focal
6. Hyperplastic epidermis assumes sawtooth rete pattern
7. Dermal infiltrate containing **eosinophils** and rare neutrophils in addition to mononuclear cells
8. Infiltrate may extend more prominently about superficial venules and mid-dermal small veins than along dermoepidermal junction

VI. Some persistent light eruptions, including actinic reticuloid

1. Occasional dyskeratotic cell
2. Occasional epidermal hyperplasia
3. Focal vacuolization of basal cell layer
4. Bandlike dermal infiltrate composed predominantly of lymphocytes
5. Infiltrate may extend into subcutaneous fat

See also Ch. 11, II.N

In actinic reticuloid, the lymphocytes may appear atypical; at times histiocytes, eosinophils, and plasma cells may be observed (see also Ch. 11, II.N)

VII. Acrodermatitis chronica atrophicans

1. **Epidermal atrophy**
2. Grenz zone of normal papillary dermis
3. Lymphocytic bandlike infiltrate often striking
4. Dermal edema

See also Ch. 8, IV; Ch. 20, XI

Special stains may identify causative organisms, *Borrelia burgdorferi*

5. **Decreased amount of collagen and elastic fibers**
6. Atrophy of pilosebaceous units

VIII. Poikiloderma vasculare atrophicans (see Fig. 8-2)

1. Hyperkeratosis
2. Focal parakeratosis
3. **Epidermal atrophy** with flattening of rete ridges
4. Dyskeratosis
5. Vacuolization along dermoepidermal interface
6. Bandlike lymphocytic dermal infiltrate
7. Vascular ectasia
8. Melanin incontinence may be prominent

Poikiloderma may be:

Congenital
Idiopathic
Associated with dermatomyositis
Associated with mycosis fungoides

Poikiloderma vasculare atrophicans should lack lymphocytic atypism. When lymphocytic atypism is present, we identify the lesion as mycosis fungoides
See also Ch. 8, V; Ch. 10, VI

IX. Parapsoriasis

As noted in Chapter 8, the nosology of parapsoriasis is confusing. In this chapter the term *parapsoriasis* is used in a general fashion to refer to a group of cutaneous disorders characterized by erythematous patches and plaques of variable size and configuration previously subclassified as listed in Chapter 8.

The histology described here contains features common to many of the subclassified disorders. We use the term *parapsoriasis* for lesions in which we cannot confidently identify cytologic atypia. When atypia is present, we identify these lesions as mycosis fungoides or as suggestive of or consistent with mycosis fungoides.

1. Marked hyperkeratosis
2. **Mounds of parakeratotic scale** either closely adherent to or separated in toto from the underlying epidermis
3. Epidermis may be normal, slightly hyperplastic, or even atrophic
4. Invasion of epidermis by lymphocytes
5. Delicate linear fibrosis of papillary dermis
6. Bandlike lymphohistiocytic infiltrate
7. Spongiosis variable

Careful clinicopathologic correlation, including multiple and sequential biopsies, is recommended
See also Ch. 5, I.E; Ch. 8, II

X. Cutaneous T-cell lymphoma, mycosis fungoides variant, patch or plaque (see Fig. 5-6)

1. Psoriasiform epidermal hyperplasia
2. Intercellular edema typically absent, but the presence of intercellular edema does not exclude the diagnosis of mycosis fungoides
3. **Epidermal invasion by atypical lymphocytes, which may form Pautrier microabscesses**
4. Bandlike, nodular, or perivascular infiltrate of variably atypical mononuclear cells admixed with eosinophils, neutrophils, and plasma cells

See also Ch. 5, III.B; Ch. 18, VII.A.2

XI. Lichenoid actinic keratosis (Fig. 12-4)

1. Hyperkeratosis
2. Parakeratosis
3. **Keratinocytic atypia**
4. Loss of cellular polarity
5. Solar elastosis
6. Dense, bandlike infiltrate composed of lymphocytes and plasma cells

See also Ch. 7, III.A.4

XII. Lichenoid keratosis

See also Ch. 7, III.A.4

Fig. **12-4.** *Lichenoid actinic keratosis. Parakeratosis overlies atypical proliferating epidermis. The lymphocytic infiltrate is described as lichenoid because of its close apposition to the lower epidermis.*

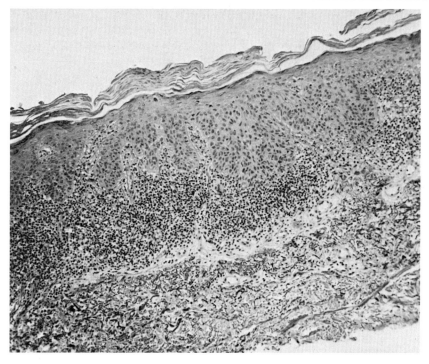

XIII. Secondary syphilis (Fig. 12-5; see also Fig. 5-7)

1. Hyperkeratosis and parkeratosis
2. **Psoriasiform epidermal hyperplasia and vacuolization** along the dermoepidermal junction
3. Perivascular **lymphocytic and plasma cell** infiltrate at times in a bandlike disposition
4. **Endothelial swelling proliferation**
5. Nodular, granuloma-like aggregates formed by endothelial and inflammatory cells sometimes present
6. Occasional epithelioid cell granulomas with or without giant cells
7. Involvement of venules at all levels of the dermis and subcutaneous tissue may be noted

Condylomata lata are mucosal lesions of secondary syphilis with prominent perivascular, lymphocytic, and plasma cell infiltrate, and marked epithelial hyperplasia (see also Ch. 5, III.C)

Silver stain may demonstrate spirochetes in epidermis and around vessels (Ch. 3)

XIV. Urticaria pigmentosa: papular lesion (see Fig. 18-8)

1. Epidermis normal to flattened
2. Increased melanin in basal layer
3. Bandlike infiltrate of **cuboidal or oval mast cells,** often containing visible dark cytoplasmic granules, fills papillary dermis, extending into upper or mid-reticular dermis
4. Variable numbers of eosinophils admixed with mast cells
5. Subepidermal bulla containing mast cells and eosinophils occurs rarely

Grenz zone of uninvolved papillary dermis occasionally observed
Diagnostic metachromatic mast cell granules stain with Leder, Giemsa, or toluidine blue

See also Ch. 11, II.O; Ch. 13, IV; Ch. 18, IV

XV. Progressive pigmented purpura (Fig. 12-6)

1. Epidermis normal
2. Bandlike infiltrate of lymphocytes filling papillary dermis but sparing dermoepidermal junction
3. Scattered **red blood cells in upper dermis**
4. Numerous macrophages containing green-brown granules
5. Venules often obscured by endothelial cell swelling

Differential diagnosis: Stasis dermatitis

Appropriate stains for iron show variable staining within the infiltrate and upper dermis

See also Ch. 13, III.D

Fig. **12-5.** *Secondary syphilis. An infiltrate of mononuclear cells is disposed in a handlike array in the upper dermis. Basal vacuolization and exocytosis are noted.*

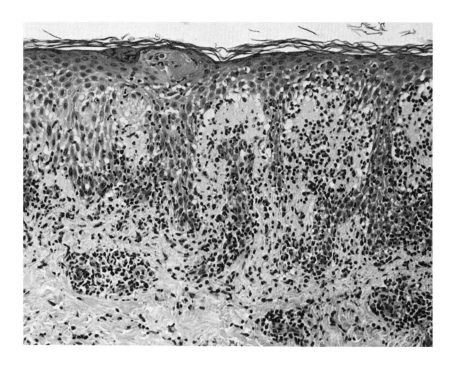

Fig. **12-6.** *Progressive pigmented purputa. Lymphocytes are present around capillaries and in the interstitial papillary dermis. Erythrocytes (arrows) are extravasated.*

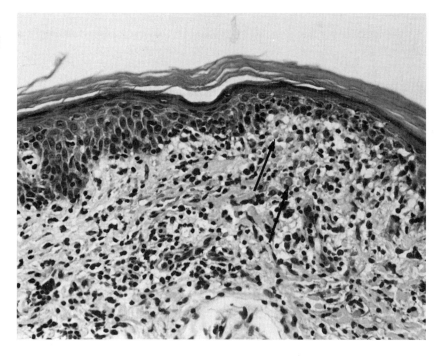

Fig. **12-7.** *Lichen nitidus. The lymphocytic and histiocytic lichenoid infiltrate expands a dermal papilla. The rete ridges on either side sometimes appear to encircle or "hug" the infiltrate partially.*

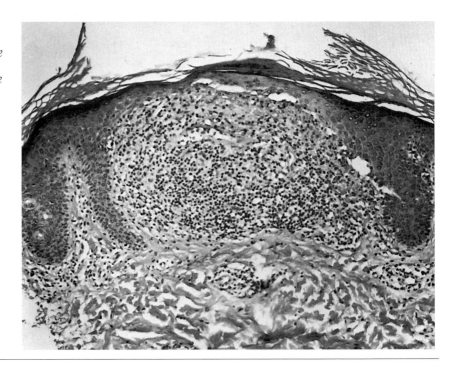

XVI. Graft-versus-host reaction, lichenoid stage

1. Variable epidermal hyperplasia
2. Exocytosis of lymphocytes into epidermis and follicular epithelium
3. Dyskeratotic keratinocytes
4. Basal vacuolization
5. Bandlike upper dermal lymphocytic infiltrate partially obscuring the dermal-epidermal junction

A lichenoid graft-versus-host reaction contains fewer lymphocytes than lichen planus but is otherwise indistinguishable

See also Ch. 10, II; Ch. 11, I.D; Ch. 20, IV

XVII. Lichen nitidus (Fig. 12-7)

1. Epidermis variably thinned over infiltrate
2. Rete ridges adjacent to dermal infiltrate typically elongated and infolding **("ball and claw")**
3. Discrete focus of inflammatory cells **(lymphocytes and histiocytic cells)** fill and expand papillary dermis

Suggested Reading

Lichen Planus

Ellis, F. A. Histopathology of lichen planus based on analysis of one hundred biopsy specimens. *J. Invest. Dermatol.* 48:143, 1967.

Ragaz, A., and Ackerman, A. B. Evolution, maturation and regression of lesions of lichen planus: New observations and correlations of clinical and histologic findings. *Am. J. Dermatopathol.* 3:5, 1981.

Shiohara, T., Moriya, N., Mochizuki, T., et al. Lichenoid tissue reaction (LTR) induced by local transfer of Ia-reactive T-cell clones. II. LTR by epidermal invasion of cytotoxic lymphokine-producing autoreactive T cells. *J. Invest. Dermatol.* 89:8–14, 1987.

Shiohara, T., Moriya, N., Tsuchiya, K., et al. Lichenoid tissue reaction induced by local transfer of Ia-reactive T-cell clones. J. Invest. Dermatol. 87:33–38, 1986.

Weedon, D., Searle, J., and Kerr, J. F. R. Apoptosis: Its nature and implications for dermatology. Am. J. Dermatopathol. 4:133–144, 1979.

Lichen Sclerosus et Atrophicus

Bergfeld, W. F., and Lesowitz, S. A. Lichen sclerosus et atrophicus. Arch. Dermatol. 101:247, 1970.

Steigleder, G. K., and Raab, W. P. Lichen sclerosus et atrophicus. Arch. Dermatol. 84:219, 1961.

Lupus Erythematosus

Brown, M. M., and Yount, W. J. Skin immunopathology in systemic lupus erythematosus. JAMA 243:38, 1980.

Clark, W. H., Reed, J. R., and Mihm, M. C., Jr. Lupus erythemtosus: Histopathology of cutaneous lesions. Hum. Pathol. 4:157, 1973.

Connelly, M. G., and Winkelmann, R. K. Coexistence of lichen sclerosus, morphea, and lichen planus. J. Am. Acad. Dermatol. 12:844, 1985.

Dubois, E. L. *Lupus Erythematosus: A Review of the Current Status of Discoid and Systemic Lupus Erythematosus and Their Variants* (2nd ed.). Los Angeles: University of Southern California Press, 1974.

Jerdan, M. S., Hood, A. F., Moore, W., et al. Histopathologic comparison of the subsets of lupus erythematosus. Arch. Dermatol. 126:52, 1990.

McCreight, W. G., and Montgomery, H. Cutaneous changes in lupus erythematosus. Arch. Dermatol. Syphilol. 61:1, 1950.

Provost, T. T., Zone, J. J., Synkowski, D., et al. Unusual cutaneous manifestations of systemic lupus erythematosus: I. Urticaria-like lesions. Correlation with clinical and serological abnormalities. J. Invest. Dermatol 75:495, 1980.

Prunieras, M., and Montgomery, H. Histopathology of cutaneous lesions in systemic lupus erythematosus. Arch. Dermatol. 74:177, 1956.

Prystowsky, S. D., and Gilliam, J. N. Discoid lupus erythematosus as part of a larger disease spectrum. Arch. Dermatol. 111:1448, 1975.

Synkowski, D. R., Reichlin, M., and Provost, T. T. Serum autoantibodies in systemic lupus erythematosus and correlation with cutaneous features. J. Rheumatol. 9:380, 1982.

Tuffanelli, D. L., Kay, D., and Fukuyama, K. Dermal–epidermal junction in lupus erythematosus. Arch. Dermatol. 99:652, 1969.

Winkelmann, R. K. Spectrum of lupus erythematosus. J. Cutan. Pathol. 6:457, 1979.

Lichen Planus–Like (Lichenoid) Drug Eruption

Almeyda, J., and Levantine, A. Lichenoid drug eruptions. Br. J. Dermatol. 85:604–607, 1971.

Fry, L. Skin disease from colour developers. Br. J. Dermatol. 77:456, 1965.

Maltz, B. L., and Becker, L. E. Quinidine-induced lichen planus. Int. J. Dermatol. 19:96–97, 1980.

Penneys, N. S., Ackerman, A. B., and Gottlieb, N. L. Gold dermatitis: A clinical and histopathological study. Arch. Dermatol. 109:372, 1974.

Winer, L. H., and Leeb, A. J. Lichenoid eruptions: A histopathological study. Arch. Dermatol. Syphilol. 70:274, 1954.

Persistent Light Reactions

Ive, F. A., Magnus, I. A., Warin, R. P., and Jones, E. W. Actinic reticuloid: A chronic dermatosis associated with severe photosensitivity and the histological resemblance to lymphoma. Br. J. Dermatol. 81:469, 1969.

Johnson, S. C., Cripps, D. J., and Norback, D. H. Actinic reticuloid: A clinical, pathologic, and action spectrum study. Arch. Dermatol. 15:1078, 1979.

Acrodermatitis Chronica Atrophicans

Asbrink, E., Brehmer-Andersson, E., and Hovmark, A. Acrodermatitis chronica atrophicans—a spirochetosis. Am. J. Dermatopathol. 8:209, 1986.

Bangert, J., Freeman, R., Sontheimer, R. D., and Gilliam, J. N. Subacute cutaneous lupus erythematosus and discoid lupus erythematosus. Comparative histologic findings. Arch. Dermatol. 120:332–337, 1984.

Burgdorf, W. H. C., Worret, W. I., and Schultka, O. Acrodermatitis chronica atrophicans. Int. J. Dermatol. 18:595, 1979.

de Koning, J., Tazelaar, D. J., Hoogkamp-Korstanje, J. A., and Elema, J. D. Acrodermatitis chronica atrophicans: A light and electron microscopic study. J. Cutan. Pathol. 22:23–32, 1995.

Poikiloderma Vasculare Atrophicans

Watsky, M. S., and Lynfield, Y. L. Poikiloderma vasculare atrophicans. *Cutis* 17:938, 1976.

Wolf, D. J., and Selmanowitz, V. J. Poikiloderma vasculare atrophicans. *Cancer* 25:682, 1970.

Parapsoriasis

Bonvalet, D. The different forms of parapsoriasis en plaques. A report of 90 cases. *Acta Derm. Venereol. (Stockh.)* 104:18, 1977.

Hu, C. H., and Winkelmann, R. K. Digitate dermatosis. A new look at symmetrical, small plaque parapsoriasis. *Arch. Dermatol.* 107:65, 1973.

Samman, P. D. The natural history of parapsoriasis en plaques (chronic superficial dermatitis) and prereticulotic poikiloderma. *Br. J. Dermatol.* 87:405, 1972.

Mycosis Fungoides

Degreef, H., Holvoet, C., Van Vloten, W. A., et al. Woringer-Kolopp disease. An epidermotropic variant of mycosis fungoides. *Cancer* 138:2154, 1976.

Jimbow, K., Chiba, M., and Horikoshi, T. Electron microscopic identification of Langerhans cells in the dermal infiltrates of mycosis fungoides. *J. Invest. Dermatol.* 78:102, 1982.

Lutzner, M., Edelson, R., Schein, P., et al. Cutaneous T-cell lymphomas: The Sézary syndrome, mycosis fungoides and related disorders. *Ann. Intern. Med.* 83:534, 1975.

McMillan, E. M., Wasik, R., and Everett, M. A. In situ demonstration of T cell subsets in atrophic parapsoriasis. *J. Am. Acad. Dermatol.* 6:32, 1982.

McNutt, N. S., and Crain, W. R. Quantitative electron microscopic comparison of lymphocyte nuclear contours in mycosis fungoides and in benign infiltrates in skin. *Cancer* 47:698, 1981.

Picker, L. J., Weiss, L. M., Medeires, L. J., et al. Immunophenotypic criteria for the diagnosis of non-Hodgkin's lymphoma. *Am. J. Pathol.* 128:181, 1987.

Smoller, B. R., Bishop, K., Glusac, E. J., Kim, Y. H., and Hendrickson, M. R. Re-evaluation of histologic parameters in diagnosing mycosis fungoides. *Am. Surg. Pathol.* 19:1423–1430, 1995.

Waldorf, D. S., Ratner, A. C., and Van Scott, E. J. Cells in lesions of mycosis fungoides lymphoma following therapy. Changes in number and type. *Cancer* 21:264, 1968.

Weiss, L. M., Hu, E., Wood, G. S., et al. Clonal rearrangements of T-cell receptor genes in mycosis fungoides and dermatopathic lymphadenopathy. *N. Engl. J. Med.* 313:539, 1985.

Actinic Keratosis

Ackerman, A. B., and Reed, R. J. Epidermolytic variant of solar keratosis. *Arch. Dermatol.* 107:104, 1973.

Shapiro, L., and Ackerman, A. Solarity lichen planus–like keratosis. *Dermatologica* 132:386, 1966.

Secondary Syphilis

Abell, E., Marks, R., and Wilson-Jones, E. Secondary syphilis: A clinicopathological review. *Br. J. Dermatol.* 93:53, 1955.

Alessi, E., Innocenti, M., and Ragusa, G. Secondary syphilis: Clinical morphology and histopathology. *Am. J. Dermatopathol.* 5:11–17, 1983.

Engelkens, H. J., ten Kate, F. J., Vuzevski, V. D., van der Sluis, J. J., and Stolz, E. Primary and secondary syphilis: A histopathological study. *Int. J. STD AIDS* 2:280–284, 1991.

Jeerapaet, P., and Ackerman, A. B. Histologic patterns of secondary syphilis. *Arch. Dermatol.* 107:373, 1973.

Pandhi, R. K., Singh, N., and Ramam, M. Secondary syphilis: A clinicopathologic study. *Int. J. Dermatol.* 34:240–243, 1995.

Primary and secondary syphilis—United States, 1997. MMWR *Morb. Mortal. Wkly. Rep.* 47:493–497, 1998.

Urticaria Pigmentosa

Burgoon, C. F., Graham, J. H., and McCaffree, D. L. Mast cell disease. A cutaneous variation with multisystem involvement. *Arch Dermatol.* 98:590, 1968.

Monheit, G. D., Murad, I., and Conrad, M. Systemic mastocytosis and the mastocytosis syndrome. *J. Cutan. Pathol.* 6:42, 1979.

Chapter 13

Predominantly Perivascular Infiltrate of the Upper Dermis

I. Mixed infiltrate without evidence of vascular damage
   A. Urticaria
   B. Erythema multiforme
   C. Acute lupus erythematosus
   D. Pityriasis rosea—cell poor
   E. Drug eruptions
      1. Urticarial
      2. Eczematous
      3. Morbilliform
   F. Arthropod bite reaction, early
   G. Secondary syphilis
II. Mixed infiltrate with vascular damage (fibrinoid necrosis)
   A. Cutaneous necrotizing vasculitis (leukocytoclastic vasculitis; allergic cutaneous vasculitis)
   B. Urticarial vasculitis
III. Predominantly lymphocytic infiltrate
   A. Superficial annular and figurate erythemas
      1. Erythema annulare centrifugum
   B. Morbilliform viral exanthem
   C. Cytomegalovirus (CMV) infection
   D. Progressive pigmented purpura
   E. Pityriasis lichenoides et varioliformis acuta (PLEVA, Mucha–Habermann), early lesions
   F. Stasis dermatitis
IV. Mast cell infiltrate
   A. Urticaria pigmentosa
      1. Telangiectasia macularis eruptiva perstans and erythrodermic mastocytosis
      2. Macular and papular lesions

The Reactive Process and the Disease	Histopathology	Comments
I. Mixed infiltrate without evidence of vascular damage		
A. Urticaria (Fig. 13-1)	1. Epidermis normal 2. **Edema** of papillary dermis, demonstrated by separation of collagen bundles and widening of papillary dermis 3. Scant perivascular inflammatory infiltrate 4. Ectasia of lymphatic vessels	The histologic features of urticaria vary markedly with regard to the intensity and composition of the infiltrate; some lesions exhibit predominantly neutrophils, some predominantly eosinophils, some only lymphocytes, and some a mixture of these inflammatory cells A true necrotizing vasculitis may occasionally be seen in urticarial lesions and is designated urticarial vasculitis Urticaria is listed in the differential diagnosis of "nothing lesions" (see table, inside front cover, and Ch. 16, I.A)
B. Erythema multiforme	1. Intercellular edema and mild to moderate **dyskeratosis** 2. Vacuolization at the dermoepidermal junction; occasional **subepidermal bulla** 3. **Lymphocytes** in superficial dermis principally about blood vessels, but also **along the dermoepidermal junction** 4. Endothelial cell swelling	See also Ch. 6, II.L; Ch. 10, I; Ch. 11, II.I The presence of eosinophils in the infiltrate may suggest a drug-related erythema multiforme
C. Acute lupus erythematosus	1. Perivascular lymphocytic infiltrate 2. Minimal to absent basal vacuolization 3. Edema of papillary dermis	The early lesion of acute lupus erythematosus may lack significant epidermal and adnexal involvement See also Ch. 12, III; Ch. 16, I.B.1
D. Pityriasis rosea-cell poor (Fig. 13-2)	1. Slight hyperkeratosis 2. **Focal parakeratosis** ("skipping scale") overlying focal areas of mild intercellular epidermal edema 3. Irregular, mild psoriasiform epidermal hyperplasia 4. Slight exocytosis of lymphocytes in areas of intercellular edema 5. Slight perivascular lymphocytic infiltrate with a few eosinophils	See also inflammatory pityriasis rosea, Ch. 5, I.H

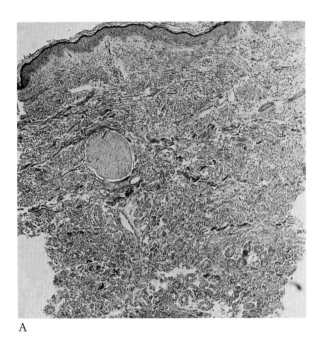

A

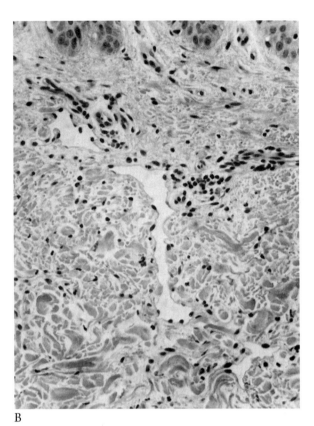

B

Fig. **13-1.** Urticaria.
A. *Low magnification reveals little change. Mild dermal edema and vascular dilatation are present.*
B. *Higher magnification shows an ectatic vessel surrounded by a few lymphocytes and granulocytes.*

Fig. **13-2.** *Pityriasis rosea. "Skipping" parakeratosis (foci of well-circumscribed, tight parakeratotic scale that frequently appear to be lifting off the epidermis) and a mild superficial perivascular lymphocytic infiltrate are typical but not diagnostic of this disorder. Focal spongiosis and mononuclear cell aggregates within the epidermis are not uncommon.*

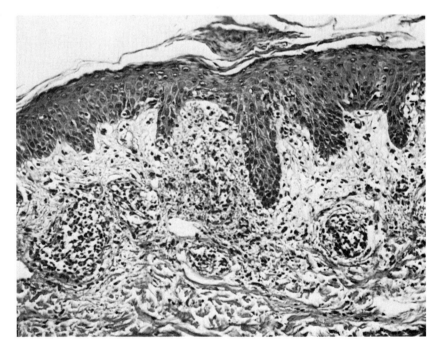

E. Drug eruptions

1. Urticarial

1. Epidermis normal
2. **Papillary dermal edema**
3. Slight perivascular infiltrate of lymphocytes, eosinophils, and a few polymorphonuclear leukocytes
4. In any drug eruption, the perivascular infiltrate may extend to deep venules

See also Ch. 16, I.A.3

2. Eczematous

1. Hyperkeratosis
2. Focal parakeratosis
3. Irregular **epidermal hyperplasia** with **variable spongiosis**
4. Perivascular infiltrate of lymphocytes, histiocytic cells, eosinophils, and neutrophils

3. Morbilliform

1. Basal vacuolization
2. Mild to moderately intense perivascular infiltrate, predominantly composed of **lymphocytes** with variable numbers of **eosinophils** and **neutrophils**
3. Variable extravasation of erythrocytes

Morbilliform drug eruptions in thrombocytopenic patients often show erythrocyte extravasation

F. Arthropod bite reaction, early (see Fig. 16-2)

1. Epidermal hyperplasia with variable spongiosis
2. Ulceration or epidermal necrosis may occur at punctum site
3. Edema of the papillary dermis
4. Moderate to dense perivascular lymphocytic and eosinophilic infiltrate

See also Ch. 5, III.A

The polymorphous infiltrate may occasionally be bandlike, nodular, perivascular, diffuse, or any combination, depending on the age of the lesion, the initiating arthropod, and the host response (see Ch. 12, IV; Ch. 16, I.A.2; Ch. 19, II)

G. Secondary syphilis (see Fig. 5-7)

In some lesions of secondary syphilis, the infiltrate may be predominantly superficial and perivascular

See also Ch. 5, III.C; Ch. 12, XIII; Ch. 16, I.A.6

II. Mixed infiltrate with vascular damage (fibrinoid necrosis)

A. Cutaneous necrotizing vasculitis (leukocytoclastic vasculitis; allergic cutaneous vasculitis) (Fig. 13-3)

1. Perivascular infiltrate predominantly of **neutrophils,** sometimes admixed with lymphocytes, and eosinophils

Minimal histologic requirements for diagnosis of cutaneous necrotizing vasculitis:
  Fibrin deposition
  Neutrophils
  Hemorrhage

Fig. **13-3.** (A, B) *Cutaneous necrotizing vasculitis. The hallmarks of this disorder include fibrinoid change about vessel walls, intramural neutrophilic infiltrates, often with leukocytoclasis, and extravasation of erythrocytes.*

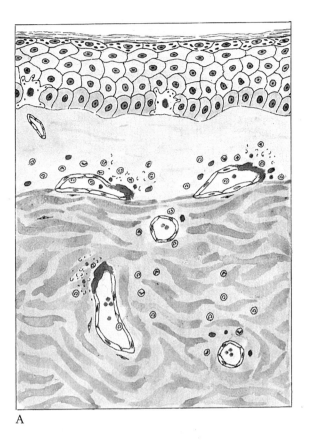

A

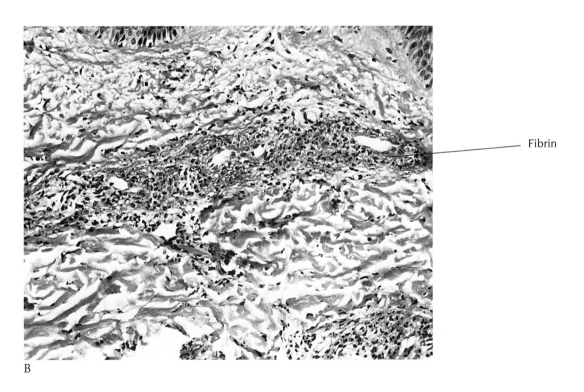

Fibrin

B

2. Neutrophils in vessel walls
3. **Nuclear "dust"** (karyorrhexis, nuclear debris from fragmented, necrotic polymorphonuclear leukocytes)

> *Necrotizing vasculitis* may occur idiopathically or may be seen in association with:
>
> Henoch–Schönlein purpura syndrome
> Serum sickness
> Rheumatoid arthritis, lupus erythematosus, and other collagen-vascular disorders
> Lymphoproliferative disorders
> Infections, especially herpes virus and chronic meningococcemia

4. Deposition of brightly eosinophilic **fibrinoid material** in and about affected cells
5. Endothelial cell swelling
6. **Extravasation of erythrocytes**

B. Urticarial vasculitis

1. Epidermis normal
2. Marked **papillary dermal edema**
3. Perivascular neutrophils, occasional lymphocytes and scattered nuclear debris
4. Fibrinoid necrosis of superficial venules focally present
5. Extravasation of erythrocytes

> Fibrinoid necrosis is often subtle, multiple sections may be necessary to demonstrate this feature

III. Predominantly lymphocytic infiltrate

A. Superficial annular and figurate erythemas

I. Erythema annulare centrifugum (Fig. 13-4)

1. Focal parakeratosis
2. Slight intercellular edema and vacuolization at the dermoepidermal junction
3. **Tight cuff of lymphocytes about vessels** without endothelial swelling

> *Erythema annulare centrifugum* may occur with:
>
> Dermatophytosis
> Candidal infections
> Malignant neoplasms
> Medications

Fig. **13-4.** *Erythema annulare centrifugum. A tightly perivascular lymphocytic infiltrate in the upper dermis is characteristic of this figurate erythema.*

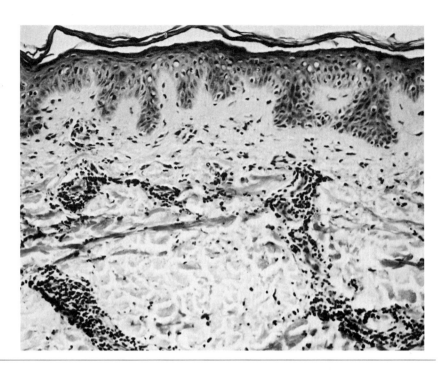

B. Morbilliform viral exanthem

1. Focal dyskeratosis
2. Multinucleate keratinocytes may be present, depending on the causative agent
3. Vacuolization along dermoepidermal junction
4. Focal, scant lymphocytic perivascular infiltrate
5. Focal extravasation of erythrocytes may be present

Except for multinucleate keratinocytes, this pattern is nonspecific

In the absence of multinucleate giant cells, a morbilliform drug eruption should be considered

See also Ch. 10, III

C. Cytomegalovirus (CMV) infection (Fig. 13-5)

1. Superficial perivascular lymphocytic infiltrate often found
2. Characteristic cells showing cytopathic effects consisting of **cellular enlargement, nuclear enlargement, a basophilic nuclear inclusion** with halo ("owl's eye"), and occasionally finely stippled basophilic cytoplasmic inclusions
3. Involved cells include endothelial cells, eccrine epithelium, and inflammatory cells

Necrotizing vasculitis has been described with CMV

The presence of CMV does not necessarily identify the cause of the lesion

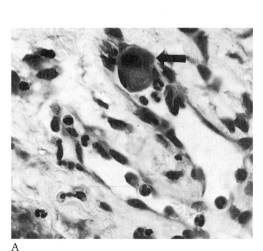

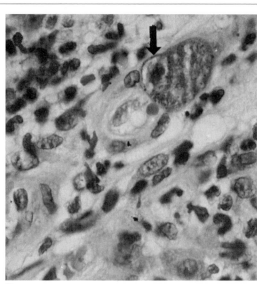

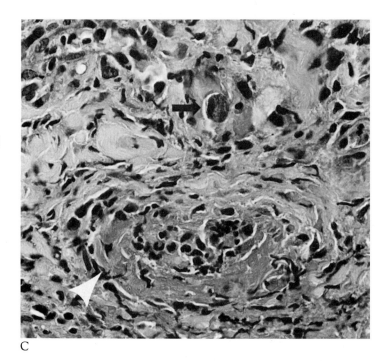

Fig. **13-5.** *Cytomegalovirus.*
A. *Typical cytopathic effect is seen in this perivascular cell (arrow).*
B. *The cytopathic effect in these cells is further advanced. The perinuclear halo imparts an "owl's eye" appearance (arrow). Cytoplasmic basophilic stippling represents viral particles.*
C. *Cytomegalovirus (arrow) associated with vasculitis. The vessel (arrowhead) displays thrombosis and fibrin deposition.*

A

B

C

D. Progressive pigmented purpura (Fig. 13-6)

1. Fairly discrete clusters of perivascular lymphocytic inflammation around upper dermal capillaries (capillaritis)
2. Erythrocyte extravasation

The upper dermal lymphocytic infiltrate may be primarily perivascular or perivascular and interstitial (bandlike). See also Ch. 12, XV

Fig. **13-6.** *Progressive pigmented purpura. Superficial perivascular lymphocytic infiltrates with erythrocyte extravasation, endothelial cell swelling, and occasionally perivascular thickening are typical.*

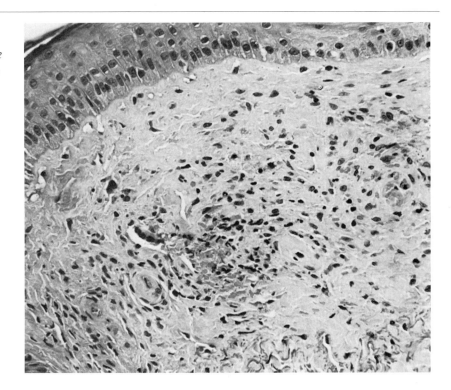

E. Pityriasis lichenoides et varioliformis acuta (PLEVA, Mucha-Habermann), early lesions (Fig. 13-7)

Early lesions of PLEVA may have a superficial perivascular infiltrate

See also Ch. 16, I.B.5

Fig. **13-7.** *Pityriasis lichenoides et varioliformis acuta.*
A. *Low magnification reveals a superficial and middermal lymphocytic perivascular infiltrate with exocytosis.*
B. *Dyskeratosis, extravasation of erythrocytes and leukocytes into the epidermis and dermis, vacuolization and inflammation at the dermoepidermal junction, and "lymphocytic vasculitis" (vessel lumens appear compromised because of endothelial cell swelling and lymphoid infiltrates) are characteristic.*

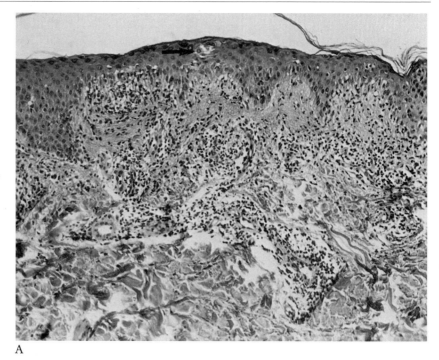

A

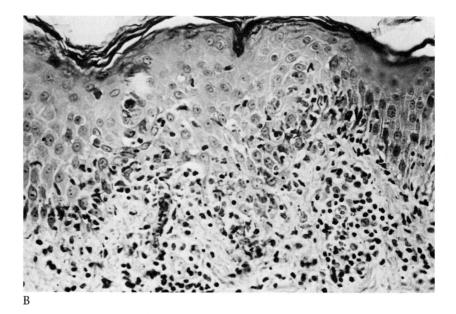

B

F. Stasis dermatitis (see Fig. 22-11)

1. Hyperkeratosis and variable parakeratosis
2. Atrophic or acanthotic epidermis with flattened rete
3. Mild to moderate intercellular edema
4. Perivascular lymphocytic infiltrate, which may be superficial but at times extends into the deep reticular dermis or panniculus
5. **Vascular ectasia; vessel proliferation**
6. **Thickened vessel walls**
7. **Erythrocyte extravasation with hemosiderin deposition**
8. **Fibrosis of the reticular dermis** with entrapped hemosiderin-laden macrophages

See also Ch. 16, I.B.7; Ch. 22, II.A

Differential diagnosis: Progressive pigmented purpura

Fig. **13-8.** Urticaria
pigmentosa (papular lesion).
A. *An increased number of
mononuclear cells is present in the
upper dermis.*
B. *Giemsa stain reveals the cytoplasmic
granules (arrows) at higher
magnification.*

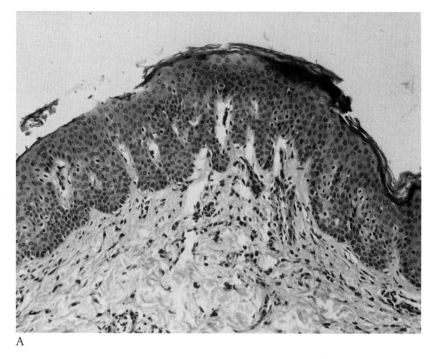

A

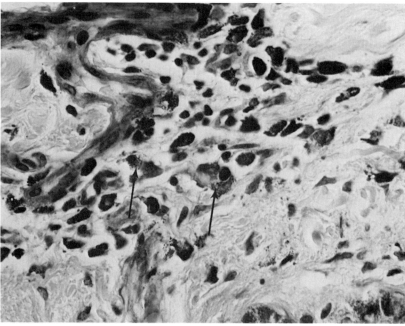

B

IV. Mast cell infiltrate

    A. Urticaria pigmentosa
       (Fig. 13-8)

1. Telangiectasia macularis eruptiva perstans and erythrodermic mastocytosis	1. Increased basal cell layer melanin 2. Perivascular and interstitial spindle-shaped **mast cells** 3. Vascular ectasia	As a rule of thumb, the number of mast cells around a given blood vessel in cross section is normally not more than five; the finding of more than five perivascular mast cells strongly suggests the diagnosis of mast cell hyperplasia, as can be seen in telangiectasia macularis eruptiva perstans
2. Macular and papular lesions (see Fig. 18-8)	1. Perivascular, oval or spindleshaped mast cells in papillary and upper reticular dermis 2. Variable number of eosinophils 3. Increased melanin in basal layer 4. Fibrosis of papillary dermis	See also Ch. 11, II.O; Ch. 12, XIV; Ch. 18, IV

Suggested Reading

Erythema Multiforme

Ackerman, A. B., Penneys, N. S., and Clark, W. H., Jr. Erythema multiforme exudativum: Distinctive pathological process. *Br. J. Dermatol.* 84:554, 1971.

Bedi, R. R., and Pinkus, H. Histopathological spectrum of erythema multiforme, *Br. J. Dermatol.* 95:243, 1976.

O'Loughlin, S., Schroeter, A. L., and Jordon, R. E. Chronic urticaria-like lesions in systemic lupus erythematosus. A review of 12 cases. *Arch. Dermatol.* 114:879, 1978.

Orfanos, C. E., Schaumburg-Lever, G., and Lever, W. F. Dermal and epidermal types of erythema multiforme. *Arch. Dermatol.* 109:682, 1974.

Pityriasis Rosea

Bunch, L. W., and Tilley, J. C. Pityriasis rosea. A histologic and serologic study. *Arch. Dermatol.* 84:79, 1961.

Lipman Cohen, E. Pityriasis rosea. *Br. J. Dermatol.* 79:533, 1967.

Drug Eruptions

Alanko, K., Stubb, S., and Kauppinen, K. Cutaneous drug reactions: Clinical types and causative agents. *Acta Derm. Venereol.* (Stockh.) 69:223–226, 1989.

Burrows, N. P., and Russell Jones, R. Pustular drug eruptions: A histopathologic spectrum. *Histopathology* 22:569–573, 1993.

Callot, V., Roujeau, J.-C., Bagot, M., Wechsler, J., Chosidow, O., Souteyrand, P., Morel, P., et al. Drug-induced pseudolymphoma and hypersensitivity syndrome. Two different clinical entities. *Arch. Dermatol.* 132:1315–1321, 1996.

Fitzpatrick, J. E. New histopathologic findings in drug eruptions. *Dermatol. Clin.* 10:19–36, 1992.

Halvey, S., and Shai, A. Lichenoid drug eruptions. *J. Am. Acad. Dermatol.* 29:249–255, 1993.

Horn, T. D., Beveridge, R. A., Egorin, M. J., et al. Observations and proposed mechanism of N, N', N''-triethylenethiophosphamide (Thiotepa)-induced hyperpigmentation. *Arch. Dermatol.* 125:524–527, 1989.

Kauppinen, K., and Stubb, S. Drug eruptions: Causative agents and clinical types. *Acta Derm. Venereol.* 64:320–324, 1984.

Mullick, F. G., McAllister, H. A., Jr., Wagner, B. M., and Fenoglio, J. J. Drug related vasculitis. Clinicopathologic correlations in 30 patients. *Hum. Pathol.* 10:313, 1979.

Arthropod Bite Reactions

Fernandez, N., Torres, A., and Ackerman, A. B. Pathologic findings in human scabies. *Arch. Dermatol.* 113:320, 1977.

Goldman, L., Rockwell, E., and Richfield, D. F., III. Histopathological studies on cutaneous reactions to the bites of various arthropods. *Am. J. Trop. Med. Hyg.* 1:514, 1952.

Horen, W. P. Insect and scorpion sting. JAMA 221:894, 1972.

Larrivee, D. H., Benjamini, E., Feingold, B. F., et al. Histologic studies of guinea pig skin: Different stages of allergic reactivity to flea bites. *Exp. Parasicol.* 15:491, 1964.

Steffen, C. Clinical and histopathologic correlation of midge bites. *Arch. Dermatol.* 117:785, 1981.

Thomson, J., Cochran, T., Cochran, R., and McQueen, A. Histology simulating reticulosis in persistent nodular scabies. *Br. J. Dermatol.* 90:421, 1974.

Cutaneous Nearotizing Vasculitis

Claudy, A. Pathogenesis of leukocytoclastic vasculitis. *Eur. J. Dermatol.* 8:75–79, 1998.

Copeman, P. W. M., and Ryan, T. J. The problems of classification of cutaneous angiitis with reference to histopathology and pathogenesis. *Br. J. Dermatol.* 82 (Suppl. 5):2, 1970.

Cream, J. J., Gumpel, J. M., and Peachy, R. D. Schönlein-Henoch purpura in the adult: A study of 77 adults with anaphylactoid or Schönlein-Henoch purpura. *Q. J. Med.* 39:461, 1970.

Fauci, A. S., Haynes, B. F., and Katz, P. The spectrum of vasculitis: Clinical, pathologic, immunologic, and therapeutic considerations. *Ann. Intern. Med.* 89:660–676, 1978.

Fox, B. C., and Peterson, A. Leukocytoclastic vasculitis after pneumococcal vaccination. *Am. J. Infect. Control* 26:365–366, 1998.

Grunwald, M. H., Avinoach, I., Amichai, B., and Halevy, S. Leukocytoclastic vasculitis—correlation between different histologic stages and direct immunofluorescence results. *Int. J. Dermatol.* 36:349–352, 1997.

Reed, R. J. *Cutaneous Vasculitides. Immunologic and Histologic Correlations.* Chicago: American Society of Clinical Pathologists, 1977.

Sais, G., Vidaller, A., Jucgla, A., Servitje, O., Condom, E., and Peyri, J. Prognostic factors in leukocytoclastic vasculitis: A clinicopathologic study of 160 patients. *Arch. Dermatol.* 134:309–315, 1998.

Sanchez, N. P., Van Hale, H. M., and Su, W. P. D. Clinical and histopathologic spectrum of necrotizing vasculitis. Report of findings in 101 cases. *Arch. Dermatol.* 121:220–224, 1985.

Soter, N. A. Chronic urticaria as a manifestation of necrotizing venulitis. *N. Engl. J. Med.* 296:1440, 1977.

Annular and Figurate Erythemas

Ellis, F. A., and Friedmap, A. A. Erythema annulare centrifugum (Darier's): Clinical and histologic study. *Arch. Dermatol. Syphilol.* 70:496, 1954.

Harrison, P. V. The annular erythemas. *Int. J. Dermatol.* 18:282, 1979.

Maciejewski, W. Annular erythema as an unusual manifestation of chronic disseminated lupus erythematosus. *Arch. Dermatol.* 116:450, 1980.

Thomson, J., and Stankler, L. Erythema gyratum repens: Reports of two further cases associated with carcinoma. *Br. J. Dermatol.* 82:406, 1970.

White, J. W., and Perry, H. O. Erythema perstans. *Br. J. Dermatol.* 81:641, 1969.

Pigmented Purpura

Randall, S. J., Kierland, R. R., and Montgomery, H. Pigmented purpuric eruptions. *Arch. Dermatol. Syphilol.* 94:626, 1966.

Stell, J. S., and Moyer, D. G. Schamberg's disease. *Arch. Dermatol.* 94:626, 1966.

Pityriasis Lichenoides et Varioliformis Acuta

Black, M. M., and Marks, R. The inflammatory reaction in pityriasis lichenoides, *Br. J. Dermatol.* 87:533, 1972.

Hood, A. F., and Mark, E. J. Histopathologic diagnosis of pityriasis lichenoides et varioliformis acuta and its clinical correlation. *Arch. Dermatol.* 118:478, 1982.

Marks, R., Black, M., and Wilson-Jones, E. Pityriasis lichenoides: A reappraisal. *Br. J. Dermatol.* 86:215, 1972.

Szymanski, F. J. Pityriasis lichenoides et varioliformis acuta: Histopathological evidence that it is an entity distinct from parapsoriasis. *Arch. Dermatol.* 79:7, 1959.

Statis Dermatitis   Graham, J. H., et al. Stasis Dermatitis. In J. H. Graham, W. C. Johnson, and W. B.
Helwig (Eds.), *Dermal Pathology*. Hagerstown, Md.: Harper & Row, 1972.
Kulwin, M. H., and Hines, E. A., Jr. Blood vessels of the skin in chronic venous
insufficiency: Clinical pathologic study. *Arch. Dermatol Syphilol.* 62:293, 1950.

Mast Cell Infiltrate   Monheit, G. D., Murad, T., and Conrad, M. Systemic mastocytosis and the mastocytosis syndrome. *J. Cutan. Pathol.* 6:42, 1979.
Parkes-Weber, F. Telangiectasia macularis eruptiva perstans. *Br. J. Dermatol.* 24:372,
1940.

Chapter 14

Deposition in and Alteration of the Papillary Dermis

235

Deposition of abnormal tissue elements in the papillary dermis may occur subtly with minor tinctorial changes, for example, focally increased eosinophilia. Clues to the presence of macular amyloidosis are the identification of melanophages in the papillary dermis and dyskeratotic keratinocytes in the epidermis. In other instances, large accumulations of refractile, fractured amyloid, or colloid are readily discerned. Careful observation of tissue sections at low magnification will help to direct attention to areas with minimal change.

The Reactive Process and the Disease	Histopathology	Comments
I. Amyloidosis		
A. Macular amyloidosis (Fig. 14-1)	1. Variable hyperkeratosis 2. Deposition of **eosinophilic acellular globules** of varying sizes in the dermal papillae, occasionally extending to the superficial vascular plexus 3. Melanophages in the papillary dermis	Apple-green dichroism of Congophilic deposits examined by polaroscopy is characteristic of amyloid Amyloid stains best with Congo red or thioflavine-T applied to frozen sections of unfixed skin Amyloid fibrils demonstrated by electron microscopy are the most specific findings for the diagnosis of amyloidosis

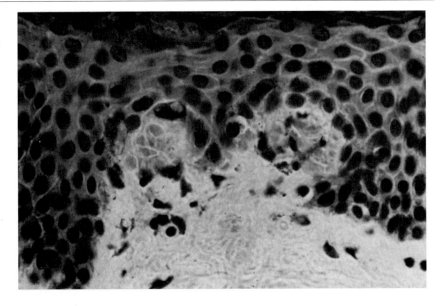

Fig. **14-1**. *Macular amyloidosis. Deposits of glassy eosinophilic and Congophilic cytoid bodies within dermal papillae are associated with melanin-laden macrophages.*

B. Lichen amyloidosis

Pathophysiology: *The amyloid is derived from keratin filaments in macular and lichen amyloidosis; these forms display numerous dyskeratotic keratinocytes. In nodular amyloidosis, the amyloid is from immunoglobulin light chains; this form is associated with numerous surrounding plasma cells.*

1. Hyperkeratosis

2. **Acanthosis;** elongated rete may be laterally displaced by deposition of **amorphous eosinophilic globules** in papillary dermis and around venules of the superficial plexus
3. Dermal melanin, free and within macrophages

Differential diagnosis:
Colloid milium
Solar elastosis

See also Ch. 21, I.B

II. Colloid milium

1. Hyperkeratosis
2. Flattened to atrophic epidermis
3. Deposition of faintly eosinophilic, amorphous, and homogeneous material that is often **fissured**
4. Material fills and distends dermal papillae
5. Solar elastosis commonly present beneath and adjacent to deposition

Colloid deposits are usually larger than those of amyloidosis but may be histologically and histochemically indistinguishable from amyloid

Fig. **14-2.** *Erythropoietic proto-porphyria. Waxy, eosinophilic deposits (arrows) encircle the vessels of the upper dermis.*

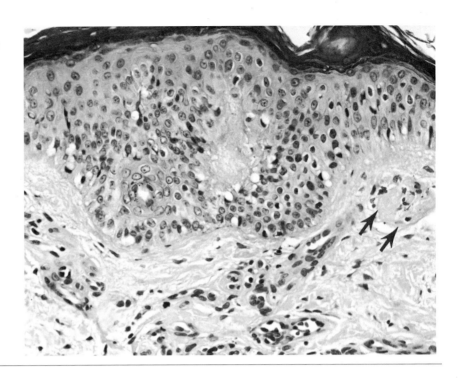

| **III.** Erythropoietic protoporphyria (Fig. 14-2) | 1. Epidermal hyperplasia, variable
2. Prominent **perivascular and intervascular deposition of amorphous pale, slightly refractile eosinophilic material**
3. Affected vessels have round to irregular shapes due to deposited material
4. Papillary dermal fibrosis sometimes entraps eosinophilic deposits | Hyalin material contains type IV collagen |
| **IV.** Lichen sclerosus et atrophicus | Homogenization of upper dermis with sclerosis of collagen | See also Ch. 8, I, Ch. 11, II.L |

Suggested Reading

Amyloidosis

Breathnach, S. M. Amyloid and amyloidosis. J. Am. Acad. Dermatol. 18:1, 1988.

Habermann, M. C., and Montenegro, M. R. Primary cutaneous amyloidosis: Clinical, laboratorial and histopathological study in 25 cases. *Dermatologica* 160:240, 1980.

Hashimoto, K. Nylon brush macular amyloidosis. *Arch. Dermatol.* 123:633, 1987.

Hashimoto, K. Diseases of amyloid, colloid, and hyalin. J. *Cutan. Pathol.* 12:322, 1985.

Kyle, R. A., and Gertz, M. A. Primary systemic amyloidosis: Clinical and laboratory features in 474 cases. *Semin. Hematol.* 32:45–59, 1995.

Kobayashi, H., and Hashimoto, K. Amyloidogenesis in organ-limited cutaneous amyloidosis: An antigenic identity between epidermal keratin and skin amyloid. J. *Invest. Dermatol.* 80:66, 1983.

Poh-Fitzpatrick, M. B. The erythropoietic porphyrias. *Dermatol. Clin.* 4:291, 1986.

Robert, C., Aractingi, S., Prost, C., Verola, O., Blanchet-Bardon, C., Blanc, F., et al. Bullous amyloidosis. *Medicine* 24:124–138, 1994.

Vasily, D. B., Bhatia, S. G., and Uhlin, S. R. Familial primary cutaneous amyloidosis. Clinical, genetic, and immunofluorescent studies. *Arch. Dermatol.* 114:1173, 1978.

Westermark, P. Amyloidosis of the skin: a comparison between localized and systemic amyloidosis. *Acta Derm. Venereol. (Stockh.)* 80:341–345, 1979.

Chapter 15

Hyperplasia of the
Papillary Dermis

Fig. **15-1.** *Fibrous papule.*
A,B. *Perifollicular fibrosis, numerous small vessels, and fibrosis are characteristic.*

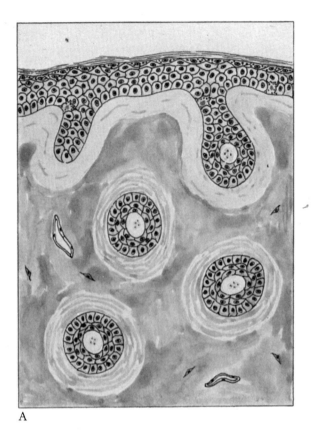

A

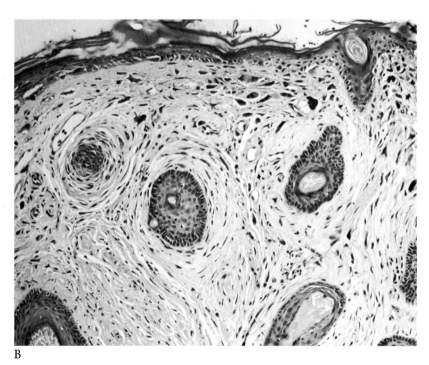

B

C. *Stellate fibroblasts are characteristic.*

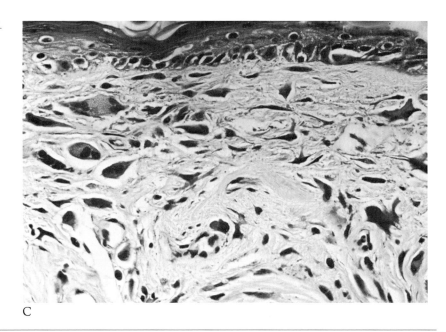

C

The entities considered here are characterized by an increased amount and/or altered quality of papillary dermal collagen.

The Reactive Process and the Disease	Histopathology	Comments
I. Fibrous papule (Fig. 15-1)	1. Intraepidermal melanocytic hyperplasia 2. Papillary dermal fibrosis with **concentric perifollicular fibrosis** 3. Increased number of spindle-shaped fibroblasts and stellate fibrohistiocytic cells 4. Vascular ectasia and proliferation	Antibodies to anticoagulation Factor XIIIa and to S-100 protein stain the stellate fibrocytic cells

II. Angiofibroma	1. Fibrovascular hyperplasia of the upper dermis
	2. May be histologically indistinguishable from a fibrous papule, usually the concentric perifollicular fibrosis and bizarre cells in the dermis are absent
		Differential diagnosis:
		  Fibrous papule
		  Scar
		  Regressed nevus
		  Connective tissue nevus

III. Perifollicular fibroma	Dense concentric fibrosis of perifollicular adventitia	

IV. Pleomorphic fibroma

1. Dome-shaped papule or polyp
2. Slight increase in fibroblasts within **myxoid matrix** in papillary and reticular dermis
3. Striking nuclear atypia of fibroblasts
4. Many **multinucleated giant cells**
5. Occasional mitoses
6. Collagen bundles in haphazard array

Suggested Reading

Fibrous Papule

Meigel, W. N., and Ackerman, A. B. Fibrous papule of the face. *Am. J. Dermatopathol.* 1:329, 1979.

Willis, W. F., and Garcia, R. L. Giant angiofibroma in tuberous sclerosis. *Arch. Dermatol.* 114:1843, 1978.

Nemeth, A. J., Penneys, N. S., and Bernstein, H. B. Fibrous papule: A tumor of fibrohistiocytic cells that contain Factor XIIIa. *J. Am. Acad. Dermatol.* 19:1102, 1988.

Perifollicular Fibroma

Zackheim, H. S., and Pinkus, H. Perifollicular fibroma. *Arch. Dermatol.* 82:913, 1960.

Part IV

Reticular Dermis

Chapter 16

Predominantly
Perivascular Infiltrate
of the Reticular
Dermis

I. Perivascular infiltrate without vascular damage
   A. Mixed infiltrate
      1. Urticaria/angioedema
      2. Arthropod bite reaction
      3. Drug reaction
      4. Photoallergic reaction
      5. Acute febrile neutrophilic dermatosis (Sweet's syndrome)
      6. Secondary syphilis
   B. Lymphocytic infiltrates
      1. Lupus erythematosus
      2. Polymorphous light eruption
      3. Lymphocytic infiltration of the skin (Jessner–Kanof)
      4. Deep figurate or gyrate erythemas
      5. Pityriasis lichenoides et varioliformis acuta (PLEVA, Mucha–Habermann)
      6. Lymphomatoid papulosis
      7. Stasis dermatitis
      8. Indeterminate leprosy
II. Perivascular infiltrate with vascular damage—vasculitis
   A. Cutaneous necrotizing vasculitis
   B. Focal embolic lesions in gonococcemia
   C. Acute meningococcemia
   D. Erythema elevatum diutinum
      1. Early stage
      2. Late stage
   E. Granuloma faciale
   F. Periarteritis nodosa
      1. Degenerative stage
      2. Inflammatory stage
      3. Granulation stage
      4. Fibrotic stage
   G. Lymphocytic vasculitis
   H. Allergic granulomatosis (of Churg and Strauss)
   I. Wegener's granulomatosis
      1. Necrotizing granulomatous inflammation
      2. Necrotizing vasculitis
   J. Giant-cell (temporal) arteritis
   K. Erythema nodosum leprosum
   L. Tertiary syphilis
   M. Palisaded neutrophilic and granulomatous dermatitis of rheumatoid arthritis
   N. Angiocentric T-cell lymphoma
III. Perivascular inflammation with thrombosis
   A. Bacterial sepsis
   B. Disseminated intravascular coagulation (DIC)
   C. Superficial migratory thrombophlebitis
   D. Cryoglobulinemia/macroglobulinemia
IV. Prominent vascular damage—minimal inflammatory infiltrate
   A. Degos' disease (malignant atrophic papulosis)
   B. Atrophie blanche
   C. Lupus anticoagulant

In this chapter, we discuss inflammatory cell infiltrates involving the reticular dermis that are predominantly perivascular in distribution. Some disorders, such as the figurate erythemas, are characterized by an infiltrate that is tightly arrayed about dermal venules. Other perivascular infiltrates, such as photoallergic and drug eruptions, contain infiltrates with some degree of extension into the interstitial dermis. In some diseases, the inflammatory cells are predominantly situated in the upper dermis (urticaria), while others are superficial and deep or mainly deep (lupus erythematosus). Determining the predominant type of inflammatory cell is crucial. Neutrophils characterize necrotizing vasculitis, eosinophils occur commonly in dermal hypersensitivity reactions (e.g., insect bite reactions), while most infiltrates contain mononuclear cells. Immunophenotypic analysis has revealed that most mononuclear cells, in the disorders discussed in this chapter, are lymphocytes.

The Reactive Process and the Disease	Histopathology	Comments
I. Perivascular infiltrate without vascular damage		
A. Mixed infiltrate		
1. Urticaria/angioedema (Fig. 16-1)	1. Epidermis normal 2. **Edema** of papillary and reticular dermis often striking 3. Superficial and deep perivascular infiltrate composed of a variable number and a variable mixture of lymphocytes, neutrophils, and eosinophils	See papillary dermis, Ch. 11, I.A; angioedema exhibits these changes in the deep dermis and subcutis
2. Arthropod bite reaction (Fig. 16-2)	1. Epidermal changes may include focal spongiosis, hyperplasia, dyskeratosis, necrosis, and ulceration at site of puncta 2. Slight to marked **edema** of the papillary dermis 3. Moderate to heavy **perivascular infiltrate composed of lymphocytes and eosinophils** extending into deep reticular dermis; neutrophils and plasma cells may be observed 4. **Endothelial cell swelling prominent** 5. Vascular proliferation common in older lesions	See also Ch. 5, III.A; Ch. 12, IV; Ch. 13, I.F; Ch. 19, II Fibrin deposition, even fibrin thrombi, may be seen in spider bites Rarely, insect parts may be observed in the epidermis or dermis (for example, scabies, tungiasis, myiasis, and hymenoptera stings)
3. Drug reaction	1. Normal epidermis 2. Edema of papillary dermis 3. Perivascular infiltrate composed of lymphocytes, eosinophils, a few neutrophils, and plasma cells	See also Ch. 13, I.E Some reactions (e.g., Dilantin) may have extensive dermal infiltrates

Fig. **16-1.** Urticaria. Dermal edema as manifested here by separation of collagen bundles is the hallmark of urticaria. Perivascular infiltrates, lymphocytic and eosinophilic, vary from minimal to heavy. Cutaneous necrotizing vasculitis also has been observed in some cases of chronic urticaria.

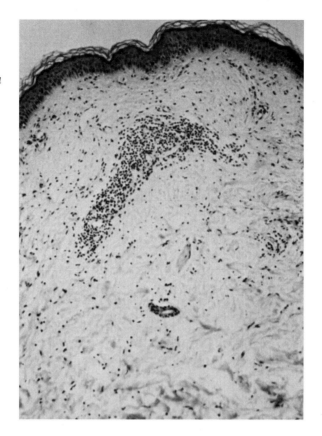

Fig. **16-2.** Perivascular infiltrate consistent with arthropod bite reaction. Epidermal hyperplasia and spongiosis with a deep and superficial perivenular infiltrate composed of lymphocytes, histiocytes, and eosinophils. Similar findings can be observed in drug reaction.

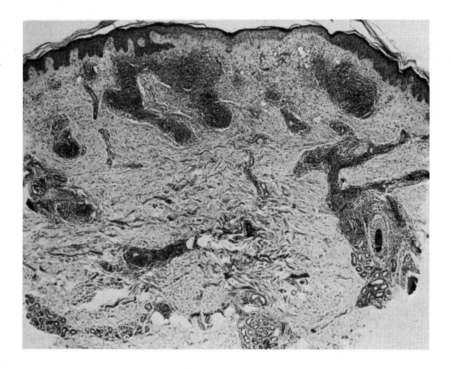

4. Photoallergic reaction

1. Focal intercellular edema **(spongiosis)**
2. Dyskeratosis
3. Basal vacuolization, variable
4. Loose perivascular lymphocytic infiltrate with rare neutrophils
5. Infiltrate predominantly in upper but may extend with decreasing intensity to midreticular dermis
6. Slight extravasation of erythrocytes
7. Endothelial cell swelling and vacuolization

This is a type IV delayed hypersensitivity reaction mediated by ultraviolet light to topically applied (and occasionally orally ingested) agents

5. Acute febrile neutrophilic dermatosis (Sweet's syndrome) (Fig. 16-3)

1. Epidermal hyperplasia
2. Intercellular edema
3. Migration of neutrophils into epidermis, sometimes forming microabscesses
4. **Edema of papillary dermis, often severe**
5. **Dense perivascular** and diffuse infiltrate composed **predominantly of neutrophils** with lymphocytes
6. **Nuclear "dust"**
7. Vascular ectasia

Epidermal changes may be absent

See also Ch. 18, V.C

The lack of fibrin deposition, hemorrhage, and invasion of blood vessel walls by neutrophils (i.e., necrotizing vasculitis) help distinguish this entity from cutaneous necrotizing vasculitis

6. Secondary syphilis (see Figs. 5-7 and 12-5)

1. Hyperkeratosis and parakeratosis
2. Epidermal hyperplasia and vacuolization at the dermoepidermal junction
3. Dense perivascular lymphocytic and **plasma cell infiltrate,** which may extend to form a bandlike infiltrate in the papillary dermis
4. **Endothelial cell swelling** with nodular pseudogranulomatous aggregates formed by endothelial cells and inflammatory cells
5. Occasional epithelioid cell granulomas with or without giant cells

See also Ch. 5, III.C; Ch. 12, XIII; Ch. 13, I.G
Silver stains may demonstrate spirochetes in the epidermis and around vessel walls (see Ch. 3)

Fig. **16-3.** Acute febrile neutrophilic dermatosis (Sweet's syndrome).
A. Low magnification reveals marked upper dermal edema and a dense infiltrate of neutrophils. Spongiosis is present.
B. Higher magnification shows the diffuse neutrophils and absence of specific vascular damage.

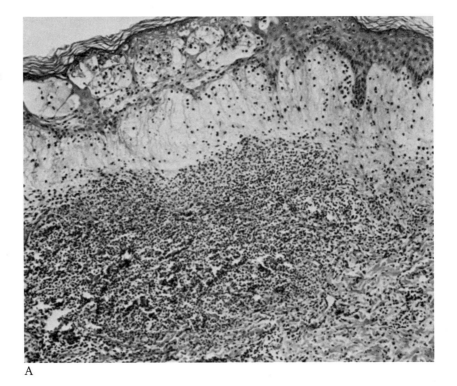

A

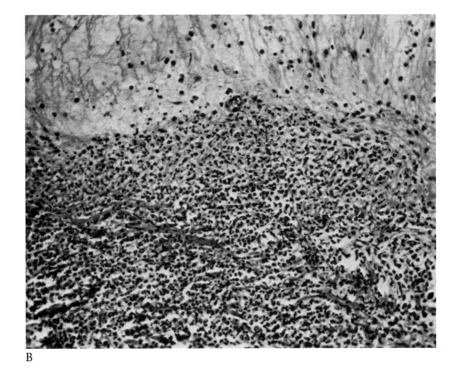

B

B. Lymphocytic infiltrates

1. Lupus erythematosus (see Fig. 12-3)

1. Hyperkeratosis
2. Epidermal **atrophy**
3. Keratin-filled epidermal invaginations
4. Dyskeratotic cells
5. **Vacuolization and squamatization of basal layer**
6. Basement membrane thickened in older lesions
7. Edema of papillary dermis
8. Vascular ectasia
9. **Perivascular, periappendageal, and occasionally bandlike lymphocytic infiltrate**
10. Extravasation of erythrocytes

See also Ch. 8, VI; Ch. 11, II.D; Ch. 12, III; Ch. 13, I.C; Ch. 24, I,K; Ch. 26, I.B.1

Special stains (see Ch. 3) may demonstrate widened basement membrane zone and acid mucopolysaccharide deposition in the dermis

2. Polymorphous light eruption (Fig. 16-4)

1. Focal parakeratosis
2. Intercellular edema (spongiosis)
3. Dyskeratosis
4. Slight basal vacuolization
5. Edema of papillary dermis, variable
6. Predominantly lymphocytic infiltrate with occasional neutrophils, nuclear debris, and rare eosinophils may extend with decreasing intensity into lower dermis and perifollicularly
7. Extravasated erythrocytes
8. Endothelial cell swelling and often prominent endothelial cell vacuolization

Differential diagnosis:
   Lupus erythematosus
   Photoallergic reaction
   Drug eruption

In polymorphous light eruption, lymphocytes surround appendages, but appendageal exocytosis is not seen. In lupus erythematosus, appendageal exocytosis is common.

3. Lymphocytic infiltration of the skin (Jessner–Kanof)

1. Epidermis may appear normal or have flattened rete ridges
2. **Dense, circumscribed aggregates of lymphocytes around vessels and appendages** of the papillary and reticular dermis
3. Lymphocytes may extend in single-cell array between collagen fibers of the dermis
4. Little or no endothelial cell swelling

Differential diagnosis:
   Lupus erythematosus
   Lymphoma cutis, chronic lymphocytic type
   Polymorphous light eruption

Special stains demonstrate increased acid mucopolysaccharide deposition between collagen fibers in the upper reticular dermis
Normal epidermis helpful in differentiating lymphocytic infiltrate from lupus erythematosus

Fig. **16-4.** *Lymphocytic infiltrate consistent with polymorphous light eruption. Perivascular lymphocytic infiltrates disposed somewhat loosely about venules with edema of the papillary dermis and rare dyskeratotic cells within the epidermis (the latter not evident at this power) are characteristic of this disorder.*

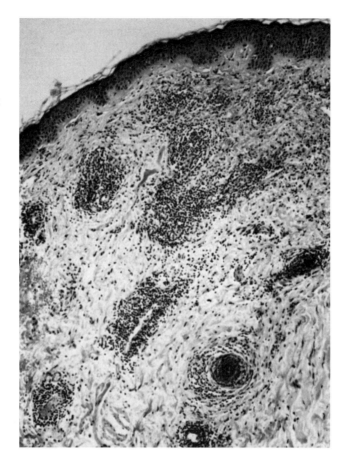

4. Deep figurate or gyrate erythemas (Fig. 16-5)	1. Usually normal epidermis 2. Moderately intense, **tight perivascular lymphocytic infiltrate** throughout the reticular dermis 3. Occasional eosinophils and extravasated erythrocytes may be present; plasma cells are present in the advancing border of erythema chronicum migrans	This term refers to persistent figurate erythemas such as erythema annulare centrifugum, erythema gyratum repens, and erythema chronicum migrans Epidermal changes including parakeratosis, spongiosis, and exocytosis may be present in erythema annulare centrifugum; the epidermis in the center of erythema chronicum migrans may be acanthotic with spongiosis The term *coat-sleeve infiltrate* refers to the tight perivascular array characteristic of figurate erythemas Erythema chronicum migrans may be associated with Lyme disease; Warthin–Starry stains may demonstrate spirochetes (*Borrelia burgdorferi*) within the dermis
5. Pityriasis lichenoides et varioliformis acuta (PLEVA, Mucha–Habermann) (see Fig. 13-7)	1. Focal parakeratosis and scale crust 2. Variable hyperkeratosis 3. Focal **dyskeratosis** may be prominent 4. Exocytosis of lymphocytes 5. **Extravasation of erythrocytes into epidermis and dermis** 6. Perivascular infiltrate of lymphocytes 7. Infiltrate often extends to deep reticular dermis 8. Marked **endothelial cell swelling**	See also Ch. 13, III.E Top-heavy infiltrate gives low power, wedge-shaped appearance to the infiltrate

Red blood cells in the epidermis may be observed in:

Pityriasis lichenoides et varioliformis acuta
Allergic contact dermatitis
Lymphomatoid papulosis
Pityriasis rosea, inflammatory
Arthropod bite reaction
Leukocytoclastic vasculitis

Fig. **16-5.** *Erythema chronicum migrans.*
A. At *low magnification, there is a superficial and deep perivascular and periadnexal inflammatory cell infiltrate.*
B. *Higher magnification reveals numerous plasma cells within the infiltrate.*

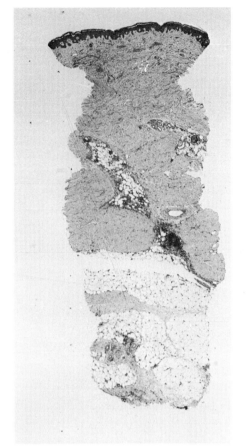

A

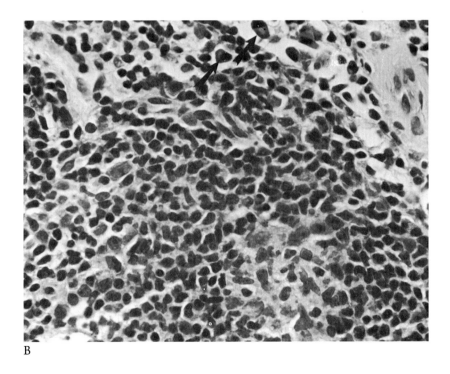

B

6. Lymphomatoid papulosis (Fig. 16-6)

1. Erosion or ulceration may be seen

2. Parakeratosis, acanthosis, and spongiosis of epidermis
3. Variable exocytosis and basal vacuolization
4. Dense, polymorphous dermal infiltrate, often perivascular, composed of lymphocytes, and prominent **atypical mononuclear cells**
5. These cells have extremely bizarre, large nuclei, mitotic figures, and prominent nucleoli
6. Prominent endothelial cell swelling
7. Variable erythrocyte extravasation

Differential diagnosis:
  Hodgkin's disease
  Non-Hodgkin's large cell lymphoma
  Cutaneous T-cell lymphoma
  Arthropod bite reaction
  Lymphomatoid granulomatosis

Atypical mononuclear cells occur in two patterns. Type A resemble Reed–Sternberg cells of Hodgkin's disease, while type B with cerebriform nuclei resemble the smaller cells of mycosis fungoides, cutaneous T cell lymphoma

Pathophysiology: *The large cells in type A disease are CD_{30} positive (like Reed-Sternberg cells) but do not reliably show T-cell receptor gene rearranged bands (i.e., clonality). In contrast, type B cells generally exhibit clonal cell population(s) using the T-cell receptor gene.*

7. Stasis dermatitis (see Fig. 22-11)

1. Atrophic or acanthotic epidermis with flattened rete
2. Mild to moderate intercellular edema may be present
3. Perivascular lymphocytic infiltrate, which may extend into the subcutaneous tissue
4. **Vascular ectasia and proliferation**
5. **Vessel walls often thickened**
6. Dermal **hemorrhage and hemosiderin** deposition
7. **Fibrosis** of reticular dermis

See also Ch. 13, III.F; Ch. 22, II.A

Differential diagnosis:
  Progressive pigmented purpura
  Kaposi's sarcoma

8. Indeterminate leprosy

1. Normal epidermis
2. Slight lymphocytic perivascular and **perineural** infiltrate

Special acid-fast stains (see Ch. 3) may demonstrate organisms within nerves

II. Perivascular infiltrate with vascular damage—vasculitis

A. Cutaneous necrotizing vasculitis (see Fig. 13-3)

See Ch. 13, II.A

Fig. **16-6.** *Lymphomatoid papulosis. The mix of small, dark lymphocytes and large, extremely atypical lymphoid cells (type A) associated with endothelial swelling is typical. These infiltrates frequently are extensive and may be associated with ulceration of the epidermis.*

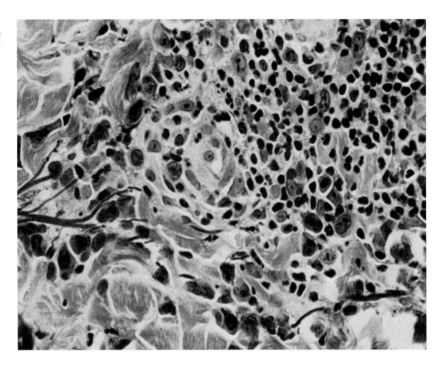

B. Focal embolic lesions in gonococcemia (Fig. 16-7)

1. Necrotic epidermis may be present
2. **Subepidermal pustules characteristic**
3. **Vasculitis** with variable fibrinoid necrosis of venules and striking inflammatory infiltrate of lymphocytes, histiocytes, neutrophils, and "nuclear dust"
4. **Fibrin thrombi in involved vessels**
5. Extravasation of erythrocytes

Fibrin thrombi occur with and without endothelial cell necrosis in disseminated intravascular coagulation (DIC) and may be associated with variable neutrophilic infiltrate

The presence of fibrin thrombi is helpful in distinguishing septic embolic phenomenon from purely allergic cutaneous vasculitis

Organisms are rarely demonstrated in acute gonococcemia

C. Acute meningococcemia

1. Extensive fibrin thrombi throughout dermis and subcutis
2. Massive hemorrhage with variable epidermal necrosis
3. Variable neutrophilic infiltrate with neutrophilic debris ("nuclear dust")

Gram-negative intracellular and extracellular organisms are easily demonstrated with special stains (see Ch.3)

D. Erythema elevatum diutinum

1. Early stage

1. Epidermal hyperplasia and invasion by neutrophils
2. Papillary dermal edema with occasional subepidermal bulla
3. **Heavy aggregates** of inflammatory cells with up to 90% **neutrophils**
4. **Leukocytoclastic vasculitis** involving superficial and deep vessels of dermis with fibrin deposition in and around vessels, nuclear debris, and extravasation of erythrocytes

Lack of grenz zone and predominance of neutrophils separate erythema elevatum diutinum from granuloma faciale

2. Late stage

1. Infiltrate less pronounced but still predominantly neutrophils
2. Fibrin deposition may be replaced by fibrous thickening of vessel walls
3. Extracellular and/or intracellular **lipid (cholesterol) deposition** in dermis

Polaroscopic examination of formalin-fixed frozen sections will reveal doubly refractile cholesterol esters in the dermis

Fig. **16-7.** *Septic embolus (gonococcemia)*

A. *Neutrophils surround vessels in the dermis. Overlying epidermal necrosis with additional neutrophils is present.*

B. *The vessels are occluded by fibrin thrombi and are surrounded by neutrophils.*

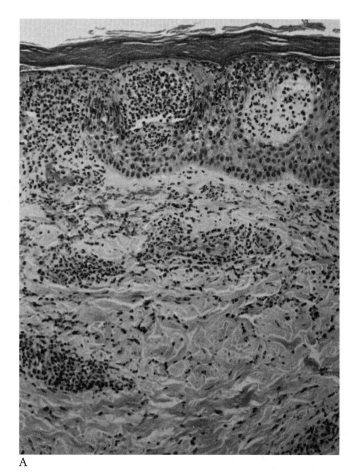

A

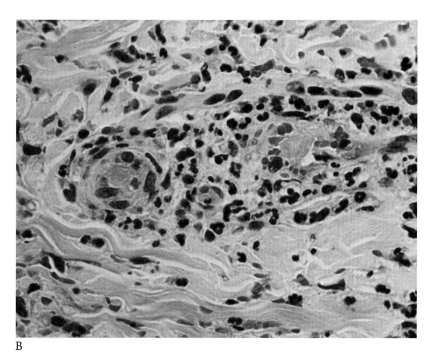

B

E. Granuloma faciale (see Fig. 18-9)

1. Normal epidermis
2. **Grenz zone** of uninvolved papillary and adventitial dermis separates epidermis and adnexal structures from infiltrate
3. Perivascular nodular and diffuse aggregates of lymphocytes and variable but usually **prominent eosinophils** (up to 90%) plus neutrophils, plasma cells, and mast cells
4. Infiltrate usually confined to upper and middle dermis but may extend to subcutaneous tissue
5. Typical changes of leukocytoclastic vasculitis may be seen but vessels are often obscured by dense infiltrate
6. Extravasation of erythrocytes
7. Hemosiderin-laden macrophages
8. Variable fibrosis

Grenz zone commonly seen in:

Granuloma faciale
Leukemia cutis
Lymphoma cutis (B cell)
Acrodermatitis chronica atrophicans
Lepromatous leprosy

See Ch. 18, V. A

F. Periarteritis nodosa (Fig. 16-8)

Small- and medium-sized vessels at junction of dermis and subcutaneous fat are affected

1. Degenerative stage

Segmental medial necrosis sometimes extending into the intima

2. Inflammatory stage

Necrotic area densely infiltrated by neutrophils, eosinophils, and mononuclear cells; thrombosis may occur

Vessels of the superficial vascular plexus may show vasculitis

3. Granulation stage

Granulation tissue replaces the necrotic areas; intimal proliferation leads to partial or complete luminal occlusion

Cutaneous ulceration may follow arterial occlusion

4. Fibrotic stage

Scarring of vascular wall; lumen shows narrowing, obliteration, or recanalization; sometimes aneurysmal deformity of vessel occurs

Subcutaneous hemorrhage may occur secondarily to aneurysm formation

If granulomas are seen, consider allergic granulomatosis, Wegener's granulomatosis, or sarcoidal vasculitis

Vasculitis affecting arterioles, venules, and veins:

Periarteritis nodosa
Henoch–Schönlein purpura
Drug reaction (e.g., Dilantin)
Wegener's granulomatosis

Fig. **16-8.** *Periarteritis nodosa.*
A. *An arteriole at the junction of the dermis and subcutis is affected.*
B. *Thrombosis and inflammatory cells within the vessel wall are seen.*

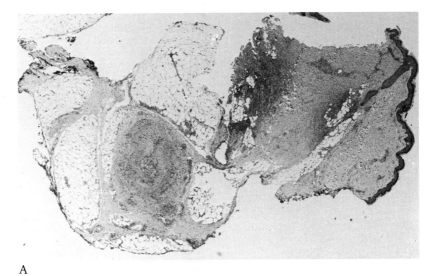

A

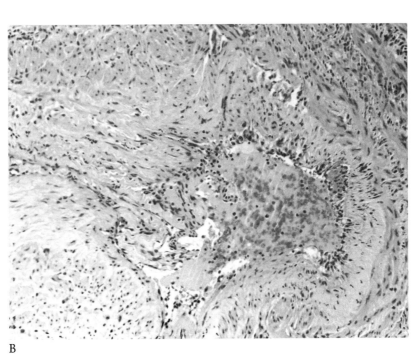

B

G. Lymphocytic vasculitis

1. Epidermal necrosis may occur but is unusual
2. Perivascular and intramural lymphocytic infiltrate
3. Brightly eosinophilic material deposited in and about vessel walls
4. Extravasated erythrocytes
5. Fibrin thrombi may be present

Lymphocytic vasculitis may occur as an idiopathic entity or may be associated with the following disorders:

Sjögren's syndrome
Rheumatoid arthritis
Lupus erythematosus
Drug reactions
Lymphocytic dyscrasias
Malignant atrophic papulosis (Degos' disease)
Atrophie blanche
Pemiosis
Pityriasis lichenoides of varioliformis acuta (PLEVA)

H. Allergic granulomatosis (of Churg and Strauss)

1. The type of vessels involved and the histopathology are similar to those of periarteritis nodosa with the addition of intramural and extravascular granulomatous inflammation.
2. **Granulomatous inflammation** consists of a central core of collagen admixed with fibrinoid material and **eosinophilic cellular debris;** a radial arrangement of epithelioid and giant cells surrounds the necrotic area

The following are necessary findings for the diagnosis of allergic granulomatosis:
1. Respiratory involvement, i.e., pulmonary infiltrates or involvement of lung
2. Eosinophilia circulating and within lesions

Differential diagnosis:
  Eosinophilic cellulitis
  Periarteritis nodosa
  Wegener's granulomatosis

I. Wegener's granulomatosis

1. Necrotizing granulomatous inflammation

1. Confluent, variably sized areas of **vessel wall necrosis**
2. **Granulomatous inflammation** with giant cells and an infiltrate of neutrophils, lymphoid cells, and plasma cells surrounds necrotic vessels
3. Few eosinophils are present

Differential diagnosis:
  Periarteritis nodosa
  Allergic granulomatosis
  Vasculitis related to infection

2. Necrotizing vasculitis (see Fig. 13-3)

1. Deep and/or superficial small arteries and veins in the dermis are affected
2. Fibrinous exudate and polymorphous infiltrate
3. Thrombosis of the lumen may be seen
4. Intimal proliferation may be marked

Epidermal ulcers may form as a result of vascular obliteration and/or granulomatous inflammation

Necrotizing vasculitis is seen often in biopsies from patients with Wegener's granulomatosis but is *not* diagnostic; more specific (but less commonly observed) are the granulomatous inflammation and necrosis described above

J. Giant-cell (temporal) arteritis

1. Degeneration of internal elastic lamina with phagocytosis by macrophages and multinucleated foreign-body giant cells
2. Intimal fibrosis and fibrinoid degeneration
3. Mononuclear and plasma cell infiltrate between intima and media

Elastic tissue stains demonstrate fragmentation of internal elastic lamella

K. Erythema nodosum leprosum

1. Deep dermal vessels show neutrophilic vasculitis with endothelial cell swelling, fibrinoid material in and around vessel walls, and the perivascular disposition of neutrophils and macrophages
2. Special stains (see Ch. 3) disclose many bacilli in macrophages, vessel walls, and lumens

L. Tertiary syphilis

1. Deep dermal vessels show endothelial cell swelling and an infiltrate of intramural plasma cells and lymphoid cells
2. Caseation necrosis is marked in tissue adjacent to vessels

Spirochetes difficult to demonstrate

See also Ch. 17, III.I; Ch. 19, V

M. Palisaded neutrophilic and granulomatous dermatitis of rheumatoid arthritis (Fig. 16-9)

1. Spongiotic epidermis with variable intraepidermal vesicles
2. Dense dermal neutrophilic infiltrate
3. Degenerating collagen bundles
4. Later lesions with palisaded granulomas and fibrosis

Comment: Most observers fail to note overt vasculitis in this entity, but it has been described in some early cases.

Differential diagnosis of palisaded neutrophilic and granulomatous dermatitis of rheumatoid arthritis

1. Acute febrile neutrophilic dermatosis (Sweet's)
2. Granuloma annulare
3. Leukocytoclastic vasculitis
4. Necrobiosis lipoidica diabeticorum
5. Wegener's granulomatosis

N. Angiocentric T-cell lymphoma

1. Epidermis often ulcerated and necrotic
2. Dermis with areas of infarction and dense perivascular and diffuse dermal infiltrate of lymphocytes
3. **Vessels thrombosed** with **transmural infiltration** of **atypical lymphocytes**
4. Lymphocytes enlarged with irregular nuclear contours
5. Rare eosinophils

Fig. **16-9.** *Palisaded neutrophilic and granulomatous dermatitis.*
A. *Perivascular infiltrate extends throughout the reticular dermis.*
B. *Lymphohistiocytic and neutrophilic infiltrate surrounds altered collagen bundle.*

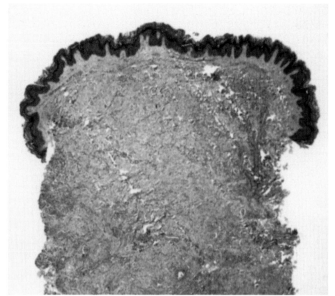

A

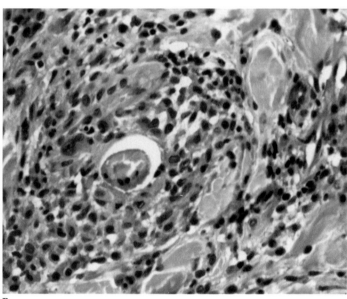

B

III. Perivascular inflammation
with thrombosis

A. Bacterial sepsis	1. **Intraepidermal and subepidermal nustules,** frequently with necrosis of overlying epidermis 2. **Leukocytoclastic vasculitis** with fibrin deposition, neutrophils within vessel walls, nuclear debris, and extravasation of erythrocytes 3. **Fibrin thrombi**	Examples include gonococcemia, acute meningococcemia, staphylococcemia
B. Disseminated intravascular coagulation (DIC) (Fig. 16-10).	**Fibrin thrombi** occur with and without endothelial cell necrosis and variable neutrophilic infiltrate	See Table 16-1
C. Superficial migratory thrombophlebitis	1. Normal epidermis 2. Inflammation around and within walls of a large vessel in the deep reticular dermis; infiltrate may be predominantly neutrophilic or mononuclear cells depending on age of lesion 3. **Occlusion of lumen by thrombus**	
D. Cryoglobulinemia/ macroglobulinemia	1. Waxy, clefted, brightly eosinophilic thrombi fill and distort cutaneous venules and small veins 2. Variable neutrophilic infiltrate surrounds affected vessels 3. Extensive extravasation of erythrocytes	Clefting of thrombus is unique to cryoglobulin deposits

Table **16-1.** *Differential Diagnosis
of Cutaneous Thrombosis*

Inflammatory Vasculitis	Perivascular Mixed Infiltrate	Noninflammatory[a]
Gonococcemia Sepsis Hypercoagulable states	Macroglobulinemia Cryoglobulinemia Disseminated intravascular coagulation Thrombophlebitis	Macroglobulinemia Cryoglobulinemia Disseminated intravascular coagulation Thrombotic thrombocyto-penic purpura Phlebothrombosis

[a]Any inflammation present is secondary to tissue necrosis.

Fig. **16-10.** (A,B) *Disseminated intravascular coagulation. Thrombosis and erythrocyte extravasation are prominent. Note the absence of significant inflammation.*

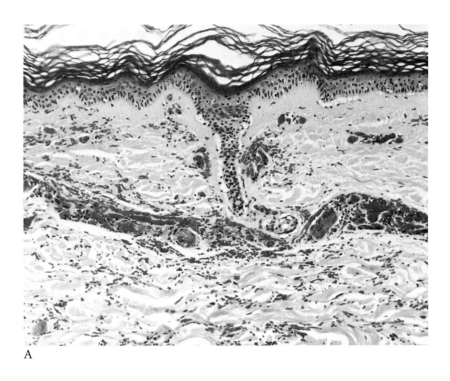

A

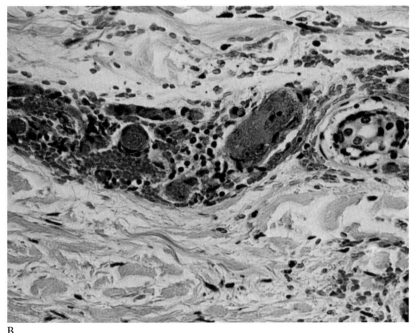

B

IV. Prominent vascular damage—minimal inflammatory infiltrate

A. Degos' disease (malignant atrophic papulosis)

Fully evolved lesion

1. Marked epidermal atrophy overlying
2. **Zone of altered reticular dermal collagen** (loss of refractile nature of collagen fibers)
3. Scattered pyknotic fibroblasts amid deposits of **acid mucopolysaccharides**
4. Scattered lymphocytes at depth of and surrounding zone of altered collagen
5. Venules and arterioles surrounded by lymphocytes show endothelial cell vacuolization
6. Perineural and intraneural lymphocytes easily demonstrated

> *Perineural and intraneural lymphocytes* may be seen in:
>
> Leprosy
> Dego's disease
> Atopic dermatitis

B. Atrophie blanche

1. Epidermis flattened or ulcerated
2. Superficial vessels with prominent smudged **eosinophilic hyalinized** (fibrin) walls
3. Thrombosis, variable
4. Perivascular lymphocytic infiltrate, variable
5. Dermal sclerosis may be prominent

These changes may vary according to the evolution of the lesion

C. Lupus anticoagulant (Fig. 16-11)

1. Epidermis unremarkable in early lesions
2. Later lesions may demonstrate epidermal necrosis
3. **Occlusion of vessels** throughout the dermis by fibrin
4. Minimal inflammation

> Differential diagnosis of obstructive vasculopathy
>
> 1. Coumadin necrosis
> 2. Cryoglobulinemia (monoclonal)
> 3. Disseminated intravascular coagulopathy
> 4. Hyperfibrinogenemia
> 5. Protein C or protein S deficiency
> 6. Purpura fulminans
> 7. Septic emboli
> 8. Sneddon syndrome
> 9. Thrombotic thrombocytopenic purpura

Fig. **16-11.** Lupus anticoagulant.
A. Normal epidermis overlying a
   dermis with multiple occluded
   vessels.
B. Vessels are occluded with fibrinoid
   material and erythrocytes. There is
   only a slight perivascular infiltrate.

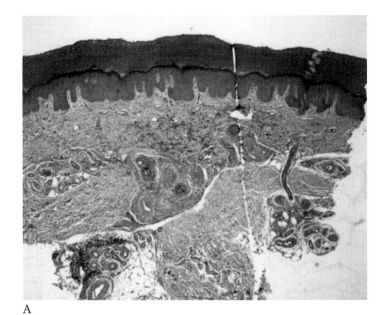

A

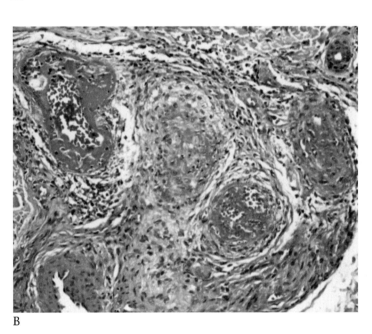

B

Suggested Reading

Urticaria

Monroe, E. W., Schulz, C. I., Maize, J. C., and Jordan, R. E. Vasculitis in chronic urticaria: An immunopathologic study. *J. Invest. Dermatol.* 76:103, 1981.

Arthropod Bite Reaction

Goldman, L., Rockwell, E., and Richfield, D. F. Histopathological studies on cutaneous reactions to the bites of various arthropods. *Am. J. Trop. Med. Hyg.* 1:514, 1952.

Thomson, J., Cochrane, T., Cochran, R., and McQueen, A. Histology simulating reticulosis in persistent nodular scabies. *Br. J. Dermatol.* 90:421, 1974.

Winer, L. H., and Strakosch, E. A. Tick bite—*Dermacentor variabilis* (Say). *J. Invest. Dermatol.* 4:249, 1941.

Photoallergic Reaction

Emmett, E. A. Drug photoallergy. *Int. J. Dermatol.* 17:370, 1978.

Tanaka, M., Niizeki, H., Shimizu, S., and Miyakawa, S. Photoallergic drug eruption due to pyridoxine hydrochloride. *J. Dermatol.* 23:708–709, 1996.

Acute Febrile Neutrophilic Dermatosis

Benton, E. C., Butherford, D., and Hunter, J. A. Sweet's syndrome and pyoderma gangrenosum associated with ulcerative colitis. *Acta. Derm. Venereol. (Stockh.)* 65:77–80, 1985.

Callen, J. P. Acute febrile neutrophilic dermatosis (Sweet's syndrome) and the related conditions of "bowel bypass" syndrome and bullous pyoderma gangrenosum. *Dermatol. Clin.* 3:153–163, 1985.

Cooper, P. H., Innes, D. J., Jr., and Greer, K. E. Acute febrile neutrophilic dermatosis (Sweet's syndrome) and myeloproliferative disorders. *Cancer* 51:1518, 1983.

Kemmett, D., and Hunter, J. A. A. Sweet's syndrome: A clinicopathologic review of 29 cases. *J. Am. Acad. Dermatol.* 23:503–607, 1990.

Sweet, R. D. An acute febrile neutrophilic dermatosis. *Br. J. Dermatol.* 76:349, 1964.

Secondary Syphilis

Abell, E., Marks, R., and Wilson-Jones, E. Secondary syphilis: A clinicopathological review. *Br. J. Dermatol.* 93:53, 1975.

Alessi, E., Innocenti, M., and Ragusa, G. Secondary syphilis: Clinical morphology and histopathology. *Am. J. Dermatopathol.* 2–2:200–203, 1983.

Carbia, S. G., Lagodin, C., Abbruzzese, M., Sevinsky, L., Casco, R., Casas, J., and Woscoff, A. Lichenoid secondary syphilis. *Int. Dermatol.* 38:53–55, 1999.

Engelkens, H. J., ten Kate, F. J., Vuzevski, V. D., van der Sluis, J. J., and Stolz, E. Primary and secondary syphilis: A histopathological study. *Int. J. STD AIDS* 2:280–284, 1991.

Jeerapaet, P., and Ackerman, A. B. Histologic patterns of secondary syphilis. *Arch. Dermatol.* 107:373, 1973.

Lawrence, P., and Saxe, N. Bullous secondary syphilis. *Clin. Exp. Dermatol.* 17:44–46, 1992.

Lupus Erythematosus

Bangert, J., Freeman, R., Santheimer, R. D., and Gilliam, J. N. Subacute cutaneous lupus erythematosus and discoid lupus erythematosus: Comparative histologic findings. *Arch. Dermatol.* 120:332–337, 1984.

Bielsam, I., Herrero, C., Collado, A., Cobos, A., Palou, J., and Mascaro, J. M. Histopathologic findings in cutaneous lupus erythematosus. *Arch. Dermatol.* 130:54–58, 1994.

Brown, M. M., and Yount, W. J. Skin immunopathology in systemic lupus erythematosus. *JAMA* 243:38, 1980.

Callen, J. P., and Klein, J. Subacute cutaneous lupus erythematosus. Clinical, serologic, immunogenetic, and therapeutic considerations in 72 patients. *Arthritis Rheum.* 31:1007–1013, 1998.

Clark, W. H., Reed, R. J., and Mihm, M. C., Jr. Lupus erythematosus: Histopathology of cutaneous lesions. *Hum. Pathol.* 4:157, 1973.

Connelly, M. G., and Winkelmann, R. K. Coexistence of lichen sclerosus, morphea, and lichen planus. *J. Am. Acad. Dermatol.* 12:844, 1985.

Dubois, E. L. *Lupus Erythematosus: A Review of the Current Status of Discoid and Systemic Lupus Erythematosus and Their Variants* (2nd ed.). Los Angeles: University of Southern California Press, 1974.

Jerdan, M. S., Hood, A. F., Moore, W., et al. Histopathologic comparison of the subsets of lupus erythematosus. *Arch. Dermatol.* 126:52, 1990.

McCreight, W. G., and Montgomery, H. Cutaneous changes in lupus erythematosus. *Arch. Dermatol. Syphilol.* 61:1, 1950.

Provost, T. T., Zone, J. J., Synkowski, D., et al. Unusual cutaneous manifestations of systemic lupus erythematosus: I. Urticaria-like lesions. Correlation with clinical and serological abnormalities. *J. Invest. Dermatol.* 75:495, 1980.

Prunieras, M., and Montgomery, H. Histopathology of cutaneous lesions in systemic lupus erythematosus. *Arch. Dermatol.* 74:177, 1956.

Prystowsky, S. D., and Gilliam, J. N. Discoid lupus erythematosus as part of a larger disease spectrum. *Arch. Dermatol.* 111:1448, 1975.

Sitjas, D., Puig, L., Cuatrecasas, M., and De Moragas, J. M. Acute febrile neutrophilic dermatosis (Sweet's syndrome). *Int. J. Dermatol.* 32:261–268, 1993.

Synkowski, D. R., Reichlin, M., and Provost, T. T. Serum autoantibodies in systemic lupus erythematosus and correlation with cutaneous features. *J. Rheumatol.* 9:380, 1982.

Tuffanelli, D. L., Kay, D., and Fukuyama, K. Dermal–epidermal junction in lupus erythematosus. *Arch. Dermatol.* 99:652, 1969.

Winkelmann, R. K. Spectrum of lupus erythematosus. *J. Cutan. Pathol.* 6:457, 1979.

Polymorphous Light Eruption

Elpern, D. J., Morison, W. L., and Hood, A. F. Papulovesicular light eruption: A defined subset of polymorphous light eruption. *Arch. Dermatol.* 121:1286, 1985.

Hood, A. F., Elpern, D. J., and Morison, W. L. Histopathologic findings in papulovesicular light eruption. *J. Cutan. Pathol.* 13:13, 1986.

Panet-Raymond, G., and Johnson, W. C. Lupus erythematosus and polymorphous light eruption: Differentiation by histochemical procedures. *Arch. Dermatol.* 108:785, 1973.

Stern, W. K. Evolution of an abnormal light test reaction. *Arch. Dermatol.* 103:154, 1971.

Lymphocytic Infiltration of the Skin (Jessner–Kanof)

Clark, W. H., Mihm, M. C., Jr., Reed, R. J., and Ainsworth, A. M. The lymphocytic infiltrates of the skin. *Hum. Pathol.* 5:25, 1974.

Jessner, M., and Kanof, N. B. Lymphocytic infiltration of the skin. *Arch. Dermatol. Syphilol.* 68:447, 1953.

Ten Have Opbroek, A. A. W. On the differential diagnosis between chronic discoid lupus erythematodes and lymphocytic infiltration of the skin with emphasis on fluorescence microscopy. *Dermatologica* 132:109, 1966.

Wantzin, G. L., Hov-Jensen, K., Nielsen, M., et al. Cutaneous lymphocytomas: Clinical and histologic aspects. *Acta. Dermatol. Venereol. (Stockh).* 62:119, 1982.

Figurate Erythema

Berger, B. W. Erythema chronicum migrans of Lyme disease. *Arch. Dermatol.* 120:1017, 1984.

Berger, B. W., Clemmensen, O. J., and Ackerman, A. B. Lyme disease is a spirochetosis: A review of the disease and evidence for its cause. *Am. J. Dermatopathol.* 5:111, 1983.

Ellis, F. A., and Friedman, A. A. Erythema annulare centrifugum (Darier's): Clinical and histologic study. *Arch. Dermatol. Syphilol.* 70:496, 1954.

Harrison, P. V. The annular erythemas. *Int. J. Dermatol.* 18:282, 1979.

Thomson, J., and Stankler, L. Erythema gyratum repens: Reports of two further cases associated with carcinoma. *Br. J. Dermatol.* 83:406, 1970.

Pityriasis Lichenoides et Varioliformis Acuta

Black, M. M., and Marks, R. The inflammatory reaction in pityriasis lichenoides. *Br. J. Dermatol.* 87:533, 1972.

Hood, A. F., and Mark, E. J. Histopathologic diagnosis of pityriasis lichenoides et varioliformis acuta and its clinical correlation. *Arch. Dermatol.* 118:478–482, 1982.

Marks, R., Black, M. M., and Wilson-Jones, E. Pityriasis lichenoides: A reappraisal. *Br. J. Dermatol.* 86:215, 1972.

Nigra, T. P., and Soter, N. A. Pityriasis lichenoides. In T. B. Fitzpatrick et al. (Eds.), *Dermatology in General Medicine* (2nd ed.), New York: McGraw-Hill, 1979.

Szymanski, F. J. Pityriasis lichenoides et varioliformis acuta: Histopathological evidence that it is an entity distinct from parapsoriasis. *Arch. Dermatol.* 79:7, 1959.

Lymphomatoid Papulosis

Black, M. M., and Wilson Jones, E. Lymphomatoid pityriasis lichenoides; a variant with histological features simulating a lymphoma. *Br. J. Dermatol.* 86:329, 1972.

Kadin, M. E., Vonderheid, E. C., Sako, D., Clayton, L. K., and Olbricht, S. Clonal composition of T cells in lymphomatoid papulosis. *Am. J. Pathol.* 126:13–17, 1987.

Karp, D. L., and Horn, T. D. Lymphomatoid papulosis. *J. Am. Acad. Dermatol.* 30:379–395, 1994.

Sina, B., and Burnett, J. W. Lymphomatoid papulosis. Case reports and literature review. *Arch. Dermatol.* 119:189, 1983.

Valentino, L. A., and Helwig, E. B. Lymphomatoid papulosis. *Arch. Pathol.* 96:409, 1973.

Weinman, V. F., and Ackerman, A. B. Lymphomatoid papulosis: A critical review and new findings. *Am. J. Dermatopathol.* 3:129, 1981.

Whittaker, S., Smith, N., Jones, R. R., and Luzzatto, L. Analysis of B, V, and S-T cell receptor genes in lymphomatoid papulosis: Cellular basis of two distinct histologic subsets. *J. Invest. Dermatol.* 96:786, 1991.

Willemze, R., Meyer, C. J., van Vloten, W. A., and Scheffer, E. The clinical and histological spectrum of lymphomatoid papulosis. *Br. J. Dermatol.* 107:131–144, 1982.

Leprosy

Azulay, R. D. Histopathology of skin lesions in leprosy. *Int. J. Lepr.* 39:244, 1971.

Liu, T-C., Yen, L-Z., Ye, G-Y., and Dung, G. L. Histology of indeterminate leprosy. *Int. J. Lepr.* 50:172, 1982.

Modlin, R. L., Hofman, F. M., Taylor, C. R., and Rea, T. H. T lymphocyte subsets in the skin lesions of patients with leprosy. *J. Am. Acad. Dermatol.* 8:182, 1983.

Ridley, D. S. Histological classification and the immunological spectrum of leprosy. *Bull. W.H.O.* 51:451, 1974.

Ridley, D. S., and Jopling, W. H. Classification of leprosy according to immunity. A five-group system. *Int. J. Lepr.* 34:255, 1966.

Sehgal, V. N. *Clinical Leprosy* (3rd ed.). New Delhi: Jaypee Brothers, 1993.

Sehgal, V. N. Leprosy. *Dermatol. Clin.* 12:629–644, 1994.

Van Voorhis, W. C., Kaplan, G., Nunes Sarno, E., Horowitz, M. A., Steinman, R. M., Levis, W. R., Nogueira, N., et al. The cutaneous infiltrates of leprosy. Cellular characteristics and the predominant T-cell phenotypes. *N. Engl. J. Med.* 307:1593–1597, 1982.

Cutaneous Necrotizing Vasculitis

Claudy, A. Pathogenesis of leukocytoclastic vasculitis. *Eur. J. Dermatol.* 8:75–79, 1998.

Copeman, P. W. M., and Ryan, T. J. The problems of classification of cutaneous angiitis with reference to histopathology and pathogenesis. *Br. J. Dermatol.* 82 (Suppl. 5):2, 1970.

Cream, J. J., Gumpel, J. M., and Peachey, R. D. Schönlein–Henoch purpura in the adult: A study of 77 adults with anaphylactoid or Schönlein–Henoch purpura. *Q. J. Med.* 39:461, 1970.

Fauci, A. S., Haynes, B. F., and Katz, P. The spectrum of vasculitis: Clinical, pathologic, immunologic, and therapeutic considerations. *Ann. Intern. Med.* 86:660, 1978.

Fox, B. C., and Peterson, A. Leukocytoclastic vasculitis after pneumococcal vaccination. *Am. J. Infect. Control* 26:365–366, 1998.

Gower, R. G., Sams, W. M., Jr., Thorne, E. G., et al. Leukocytoclastic vasculitis: Sequential appearance of immunoreactants and cellular changes in serial biopsies. *J. Invest. Dermatol.* 69:477, 1977.

Grunwald, M. H., Avinoach, I., Amichai, B., and Halevy, S. Leukocytoclastic vasculitis—correlation between different histologic stages and direct immunofluorescence results. *Int. J. Dermatol.* 36:349–352, 1997.

Reed, R. J. *Cutaneous Vasculitides. Immunologic and Histologic Correlations.* Chicago: American Society of Clinical Pathologists, 1977.

Sais, G., Vidaller, A., Jucgla, A., Servitje, O., Condom, E., and Peyri, J. Prognostic factors in leukocytoclastic vasculitis: A clinicopathologic study of 160 patients. *Arch. Dermatol.* 134:309–315, 1998.

Soter, N. A. Chronic urticaria as a manifestation of necrotizing venulitis. *N. Engl. J. Med.* 296:1440, 1977.

Gonococcemia and Meningococcemia

Ackerman, A. B., Miller, R. C., and Shapiro, L. Gonococcemia and its cutaneous manifestations. *Arch. Dermatol.* 91:227, 1965.

Al-Suleiman, S. A., Grimes, E. M., and Jonas, H. S. Disseminated gonococcal infections. *Obstet. Gynecol.* 61:48–51, 1983.

English, J. C., and Monk, J. S. Gonococcal dermatitis–arthritis syndrome. *Am. Fam. Physician* 34:77–79, 1986.

Nielsen, T. Chronic meningococcemia. *Arch. Dermatol.* 102:97, 1970.

Shapiro, L., Teisch, J. A., and Brownstein, M. H. Dermatohistopathology of chronic gonococcal sepsis. *Arch. Dermatol.* 107:403, 1973.

Silva, J., and Wilson, K. Disseminated gonococcal infections (DGI). *Cutis* 24:601–606, 1979.

Erythema Elevatum Diutinum

Cream, J. J., Levene, G. M., and Calnan, C. D. Erythema elevatum diutinum. *Br. J. Dermatol.* 84:393, 1971.

Laymon, C. W. Erythema elevatum diutinum. *Arch. Dermatol.* 85:22, 1962.

Wolf, H. H., Scherer, R., Maciejewski, W., et al. Erythema elevatum diutinum: I. Electron microscopy of a case with extracellular cholesterolosis. *Arch. Dermatol. Res.* 261:7, 1978.

Granuloma Faciale

Johnson, W. C., Higdon, R. S., and Helwig, E. B. Granuloma faciale. *Arch. Dermatol.* 79:42, 1959.

Okun, M. R., Bauman, L., and Minor, D. Granuloma faciale with lesions on the face and hand. *Arch. Dermatol.* 92:78, 1965.

Pedace, F. J., and Perry, H. O. Granuloma faciale: A clinical and histopathologic review. *Arch. Dermatol.* 94:387, 1966.

Periarteritis Nodosa

Borrie, P. Cutaneous polyarteritis nodosa. *Br. J. Dermatol.* 87:87, 1972.

Cohen, R. D., Conn, D. L., and Ilstrup, D. M. Clinical features, prognosis, and response to treatment in polyarteritis. *Mayo Clin. Proc.* 55:146, 1980.

Diaz-Perez, J. L., and Winkelmann, R. K. Cutaneous periarteritis nodosa. *Arch. Dermatol.* 110:407, 1974.

Daoud, M. S., Hutton, K. P., and Gibson, L. E. Cutaneous periarteritis nodosa: A clinicopathologic study of 79 cases. *Br. J. Dermatol.* 136:706–713, 1997.

Minkowitz, G., Smoller, B. R., and McNutt, N. S. Benign cutaneous polyarteritis nodosa: Relationship to systemic polyarteritis nodosa and hepatitis B infection. *Arch. Dermatol.* 127:1520–1523, 1991.

Rodgers, H., Guthrie, J. A., Brownjohn, A. M., and Turney, J. H. Microscopic polyarteritis: Clinical features and treatment. *Postgrad. Med. J.* 65:515–518, 1989.

Zeek, P. M., Smith, C. C., and Weeter, J. C. Studies on periarteritis nodosa. III. The differentiation between the vascular lesions of periarteritis nodosa and of hypersensitivity. *Am. J. Pathol.* 24:889, 1948.

Allergic Granulomatosis

Chumbley, L. C., Harrison, E. G., and DeRemee, R. A. Allergic granulomatosis and angiitis (Churg–Strauss syndrome). *Mayo Clin. Proc.* 52:477, 1977.

Churg, J., and Strauss, L. Allergic granulomatosis, allergic angiitis and periarteritis nodosa. *Am. J. Pathol.* 27:277, 1951.

Crotty, C. P., DeRemee, R. A., and Winkelmann, R. K. Cutaneous clinicopathologic correlation of allergic granulomatosis. *J. Am. Acad. Dermatol.* 5:571, 1981.

Lie, J. T. The classification of vasculitis and a reappraisal of allergic granulomatosis and angiitis (Churg–Strauss syndrome). *Mt. Sinai J. Med.* 53:429–439, 1986.

Wegener's Granulomatosis

Barksdale, S. K., Hallahan, C. W., Kerr, G. S., Fauci, A. S., Stern, J. B., and Travis, W. D. Cutaneous pathology in Wegener's granulomatosis. A clinicopathologic study of 75 biopsies in 46 patients. *Am. J. Surg. Pathol.* 19:161–172, 1995.

Daoud, M. S., Gibson, L. E., DeRemee, R. A., Specks, U., el-Azhar, R. A., and Su, W. P. D. Cutaneous Wegener's granulomatosis: Clinic, histopathologic, and immunopathologic features of thirty patients. *J. Am. Acad. Dermatol.* 31:605–612, 1994.

Fauci, A. S., Haynes, B. F., Katz, P., and Wolf, S. M. Wegener's granulomatosis: Prospective clinical and therapeutic experience with 85 patients for 21 years. *Ann. Intern. Med.* 98:76, 1983.

Frunza Patten, S., and Tomecki, K. J. Wegener's granulomatosis: Cutaneous and oral mucosal disease. *J. Am. Acad. Dermatol.* 28:710–718, 1993.

Godman, G. C., and Churg, J. Wegener's granulomatosis: Pathology and review of the literature. *Arch. Pathol.* 58:533, 1954.

Reed, W. B., Jenson, A. K., Konwaler, B. E., et al. The cutaneous manifestations in Wegener's granulomatosis. *Acta. Derm. Venereol.* (Stockh.) 43:250, 1968.

Rottem, M., Fauci, A. S., Hallahan, C. W., Kerr, G. S., Lebovics, R., Leavitt, R. Y., and Hoffman, G. S. Wegener granulomatosis in children and adolescents: Clinical presentation and outcome. *J. Pediatr.* 122:26–31, 1993.

Erythema Nodosum Leprosum

Jolliffe, D. S. Leprosy reactional states and their treatment. *Br. J. Dermatol.* 97:345, 1977.

Modlin, R. L., Bakke, A. C., Vaccaro, S. A., et al. Tissue and blood T-lymphocyte subpopulations in erythema nodosum leprosum. *Arch. Dermatol.* 121:216, 1985.

Ridley, D. S. Reactions in leprosy. *Lepr. Rev.* 40:77, 1969.

Ridley, M. J., and Ridley, D. S. The immunopathology of erythema nodosum leprosum: The role of extravascular complexes. *Lepr. Rev.* 54:95, 1983.

Tertiary Syphilis

Johnson, W. C. Venereal Diseases and Treponemal Infections. In J. H. Graham, W. C. Johnson, and W. B. Helwig (Eds.), *Dermal Pathology.* Hagerstown, MD.: Harper & Row, 1972.

Varela, P., Alves, R., Velho, G., Santos, C., Massa, A., and Sanches, M. Two recent cases of tertiary syphilis. *Eur. J. Dermatol.* 9:300–302, 1999.

Bacterial Sepsis

Alpert, J. S., Krous, H. F., Dalen, J. E., et al. Pathogenesis of Osler's nodes. *Ann. Intern. Med.* 85:471, 1976.

Disseminated Intravascular Coagulation

DiCato, M. A., and Ellman, L. Coumadin-induced necrosis of breast, disseminated intravascular coagulation, and hemolytic anemia. *Ann. Intern. Med.* 83:233, 1975.

Robboy, S. J., Mihm, M. C., Jr., Colman, R. W., et al. The skin in disseminated intravascular coagulation: Prospective analysis of thirty-six cases. *Br. J. Dermatol.* 88:221, 1973.

Superficial Migratory Thrombophlebitis

Blum, F., Gilkeson, G., Greenberg, C., and Murray, J. Superficial migratory thrombophlebitis and the lupus anticoagulant. *Int. J. Dermatol.* 29:190–192, 1990.

Fiehn, C., Pezzuto, A., and Hunstein, W. Superficial migratory thrombophlebitis in a patient with reversible protein C deficiency and anticardiolipin antibodies. *Ann. Rheum. Dis.* 53:843–844, 1994.

Rossman, R. E., and Freeman, R. G. Chest wall thrombophlebitis (Monder's disease). *Arch. Dermatol.* 87:475, 1963.

Samlaska, C. P., James, W. D., and Simel, D. L. Superficial migratory thrombophlebitis and factor XII deficiency. *J. Am. Acad. Dermatol.* 22:939–943, 1990.

Chapter 17

Granulomas and Granulomatous Inflammation

I. Palisading granulomas
  A. Granuloma annulare
  B. Necrobiosis lipoidica
  C. Rheumatoid nodule
  D. Rheumatic fever nodule
  E. Subcutaneous granuloma annulare (pseudorheumatoid nodule)
  F. Necrobiotic xanthogranuloma with paraproteinemia
II. Epithelioid cell granulomas
  A. Sarcoidosis
  B. Granulomatous rosacea
  C. Cheilitis granulomatosa (Miescher-Melkersson-Rosenthal)
  D. Cutaneous Crohn's disease
  E. Tuberculoid leprosy
  F. Tuberculosis
    1. Primary inoculation
    2. Lupus vulgaris
    3. Tuberculosis verrucosa cutis
    4. Scrofuloderma
    5. Miliary tuberculosis
  G. "Tuberculids"
    1. Papulonecrotic tuberculid
    2. Lichen scrofulosorum
    3. Nodular vasculitis (erythema induratum)
  H. Zirconium granuloma and cutaneous lesions of systemic berylliosis
  I. Inoculation (local) beryllium granuloma
  J. Miscellaneous foreign-body granulomas
III. Granulomatous inflammation
  A. North American blastomycosis (cutaneous nodule or verrucous plaque associated with systemic infection)
  B. South American blastomycosis (mucosal or cutaneous lesions)
  C. Chromomycosis
    1. Dermal lesions
    2. Subcutaneous lesions
  D. Phaeohyphomycosis
  E. Sporotrichosis
    1. Primary lesion
    2. Secondary cutaneous nodules
  F. Coccidioidomycosis
    1. Early primary cutaneous lesions
    2. Late primary cutaneous lesions; secondary (disseminated) cutaneous lesions
    3. Subcutaneous abscesses
  G. Cryptococcosis
    1. Granulomatous reaction
    2. Gelatinous reaction
  H. Atypical mycobacteriosis
    1. Early lesions
    2. Late lesions
  I. Tertiary syphilis
  J. Cat-scratch disease

K. Other infections with granulomatous inflammation
   1. Leishmaniasis
   2. Histoplasmosis
L. Protothecosis

Histologically, a granuloma is defined as a space-occupying lesion composed of aggregates of histiocytic cells. Granulomatous disorders are divided into three categories according to the disposition and arrangement of the histiocytic cells within the dermis: (1) palisading granulomas: histiocytic cells and lymphocytes with long axes arranged perpendicular to ("palisading") areas of altered collagen; (2) epithelioid cell granulomas: focal aggregates of epithelioid histiocytic cells with or without necrosis; and (3) granulomatous inflammation: diffuse infiltration of histiocytic cells admixed with other inflammatory cells without discrete granuloma formation.

The Reactive Process and the Disease	**Histopathology**	**Comments**
I. Palisading granulomas		
A. Granuloma annulare (Fig. 17-1)	1. Normal epidermis (except in perforating variant) 2. Small or large foci of altered collagen, most frequently in upper and mid dermis but occasionally in deep dermis or subcutaneous tissue	See Table 17-1 for comparison of various palisading granulomas Very earliest lesions are said to have leukocytoclastic vasculitis in area of collagen alteration

Table **17-1.** *Comparison of Histologic Findings in Palisading Granulomas*

Disease	Area of Collagen Alteration "Necrobiosis"	Type and Degree of Collagen Alteration	Acid Mucopoly-saccharide Deposition	Lipid in Dermis	Vascular Changes
Granuloma annulare	Upper to midreticular dermis; rarely, subcutaneous tissue	Focally altered collagen	Common	Rare	Rare
Necrobiosis lipoidica	Entire reticular dermis	Larger confluent areas of altered collagen	Rare	Common	Endothelial cell hypertrophy and proliferation
Rheumatoid nodule	Deep reticular dermis; subcutaneous tissue	Large areas with fibrinoid alteration	Variable	Variable	Variable
Rheumatic fever nodule	Subcutaneous tissue	Large areas of fibrinoid alteration	Variable	Variable	Vessel proliferation
Subcutaneous granuloma annulare (pseudorheumatoid nodule)	Mid- to deep reticular dermis and subcutaneous tissue	Large confluent areas of altered colagen	Common	Variable	Variable

Fig. **17-1.** *Granuloma annulare. A central zone of necrobiotic collagen is surrounded by histiocytic cells, lymphocytes, and a few scattered multinucleate giant cells. A portion of another palisading granuloma is present at the extreme right of the field.*

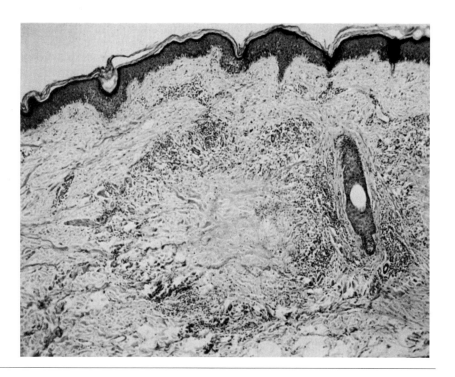

3. Early lesion consists of:
   a. Subtle collagen alteration characterized by splaying and fragmentation of collagen fibers
   b. Deposition of granular and/or wispy bluish substance **(acid mucopolysaccharides)** on and between collagen fibers
   c. **Infiltration of histiocytic cells and lymphocytes between collagen bundles**
4. Later lesions show well-defined areas of **dermal degeneration** characterized by foci of relatively acellular, homogeneous, or amorphous collagen
5. Variable numbers of histiocytic cells and lymphocytes surround abnormal collagen
6. Giant cells and/or aggregates of epithelioid cells occasionally present
7. Variants include
   a. Perforating granuloma annulare with extrusion of granulomatous and connective tissue through the epidermis

Identifying acid mucopolysaccharide with alcian blue or colloidal iron stains is often helpful in identifying areas of altered collagen

Differential diagnosis: Papular mucinosis

b. Subcutaneous granuloma annulare may be indistinguishable from rheumatoid nodule, particularly in children and young adults

B. Necrobiosis lipoidica (Fig. 17-2)

1. Epidermal **atrophy,** occasionally with ulceration
2. Ectatic venules in compressed papillary dermis
3. One or more areas of altered collagen that initially show fragmentation and clumping of collagen fibers and later become **hyalinized, eosinophilic, and relatively acellular**
4. Altered collagen surrounded by a zone of palisading histiocytic cells, epithelioid cells, and lymphocytes
5. Patchy perivascular inflammatory infiltrate composed of lymphocytes, plasma cells, lipid-laden histiocytic cells, and giant cells is present scattered throughout dermis and extending into the subcutis
6. **Vessel walls thickened** by endothelial proliferation

Frozen sections stained for fat (see Ch. 3) often reveal lipid within areas of collagen alteration

Epidermal atrophy, thickened vessel walls, broad zones of collagen alteration, extracellular fat in the dermis, and the presence of plasma cells in the infiltrate help differentiate necrobiosis lipoidica from granuloma annulare; however, at times it may be impossible to histologically distinguish these two entities, and the use of the generic term palisading granuloma is preferable

Vascular changes are often prominent in lesions from the leg but may be absent or mild in lesions from other areas

C. Rheumatoid nodule (Fig. 17-3)

1. Normal epidermis
2. In the subcutaneous tissue and/or deep reticular dermis, there are large, well-demarcated areas of eosinophilic, **relatively amorphous (fibrinoid) material**
3. A zone of histiocytic cells and lymphocytes surrounds fibrinoid material
4. Vascular proliferation often observed peripheral to altered collagen

Special stains (see Ch. 3) reveal fibrin deposition in areas of collagen degeneration

Differential diagnosis: Other palisading granulomas Epithelioid cell sarcoma

D. Rheumatic fever nodule

In the deep dermis and subcutaneous tissue are areas of edematous altered collagen admixed with **neutrophils** and surrounded by loosely aggregated palisading histiocytic cells and other mononuclear cells

E. Subcutaneous granuloma annulare (pseudorheumatoid nodule)

Deep dermal or subcutaneous areas of altered collagen with peripheral palisading of histiocytic cells and lymphocytes

Most commonly appearing in young individuals without any evidence of rheumatoid disease

Fig. **17-2.** *Necrobiosis lipoidica. Lymphohistiocytic infiltrates with multinucleate cells surround large areas of collagen necrobiosis. The palisading granulomas and necrobiosis extend well beyond the field of this micrograph.*

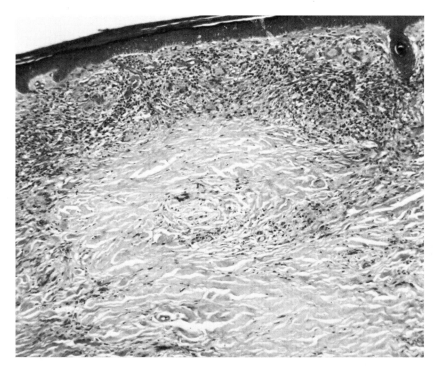

Fig. **17-3.** *Rheumatoid nodule. This biopsy from the subcutis exhibits palisading of histiocytic cells admixed with lymphocytes about a central zone of fibrinoid necrosis. Only a portion of the rheumatoid nodule is present in this field.*

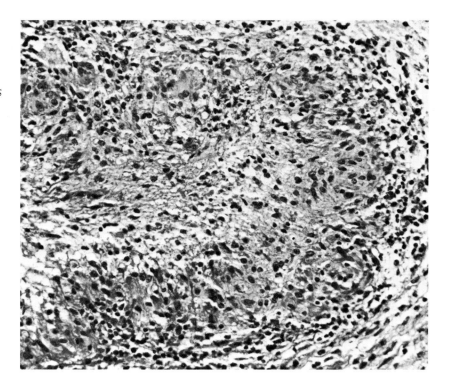

F. Necrobiotic xanthogranuloma with
paraproteinemia
(Fig. 17-4)

1. Atrophic to normal epidermis
2. **Large areas of necrobiosis**
   and pallor in reticular dermis
3. Palisade of histiocytes and
   multinucleated giant cells
   surrounding degenerating
   collagen

There is more extensive
necrobiosis and cellular
response than is seen in
necrobiosis lipoidica.

Fig. **17-4.** *Necrobiotic xanthogranuloma.*
A. *Zones of altered collagen in the
reticular dermis surrounded by a
lymphohistiocytic infiltrate.*
B. *Lymphoid follicles in the deep
reticular dermis.*

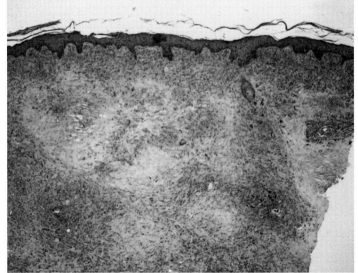

A

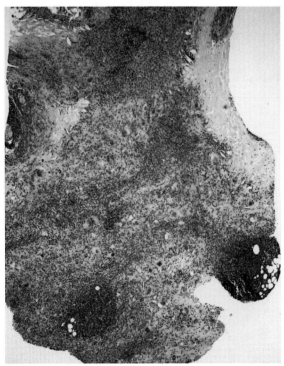

B

C. *Cholesterol clefts.*
D. *Large, and sometimes bizarre, multinucleated giant cells.*

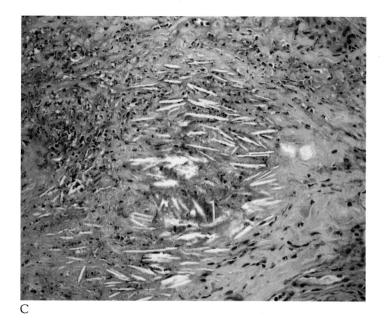

C

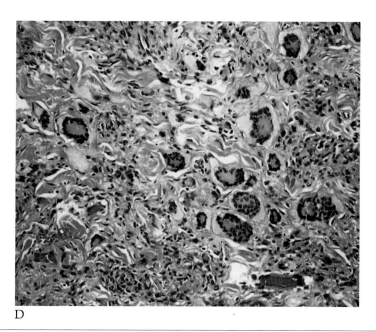

D

4. Abundant lipid within histiocytes and giant cells
5. **Cholesterol clefts** in dermis
6. **Lymphoid nodules** variably present in deep reticular dermis

II. Epithelioid cell granulomas

A. Sarcoidosis (Figs. 17-5, 17-6)

1. Epidermis usually normal but may show parakeratosis, atrophy, or even basal vacuolization
2. **Epithelioid cell granulomas** of variable size scattered throughout the papillary dermis, reticular dermis, and/or subcutaneous tissue
3. Granulomas and granulomatous inflammation may extend upward to hug the epidermis
4. Granulomas often contain giant cells and lymphocytes
5. The associated lymphocytic infiltrate is usually sparse, hence the term *naked tubercle*
6. Central "caseation" or necrosis may be present but is rarely extensive
7. Schaumann bodies (round, laminated, calcified inclusions) and asteroid bodies (stellate eosinophilic inclusions surrounded by a clear zone) occasionally present in giant cells

Differential diagnosis:
Silica and certain other foreign bodies
Tuberculoid leprosy
Cheilitis granulomatosa
Crohn's disease
Rosacea
Some infections with fungi, mycobacteria, and spirochetes

Histologic changes observed in a positive Kveim test are similar to those of sarcoid

---

Schaumann and *asteroid* bodies may be found in:

Sarcoidosis
Tuberculosis
Leprosy
Berylliosis
Foreign-body reaction

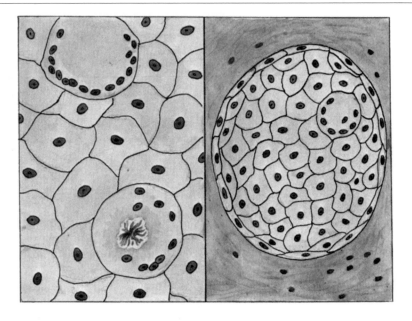

Fig. **17-5.** Granulomas. Aggregates of epithelioid histiocytic cells and multinucleate giant cells (as well as an asteroid body, left) can be seen in a variety of granulomatous disorders, including sarcoidosis.

Fig. **17-6.** (A,B). Sarcoidosis. Granulomas within the dermis are associated with numerous etiologies such as infections, physical agents, and so on. These causes must be ruled out and the clinical status of the patient evaluated before a diagnosis of sarcoidosis can be rendered.

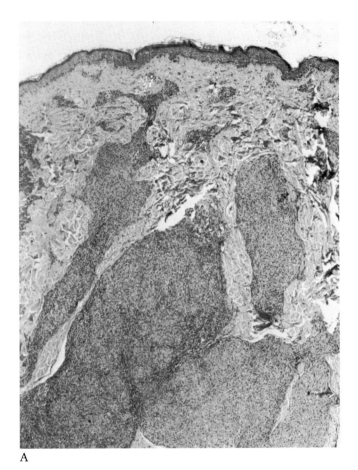

A

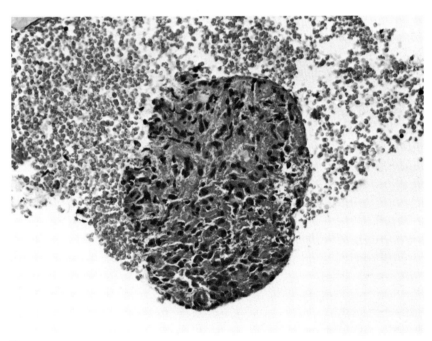

B

B. Granulomatous rosacea

1. Epidermis may be normal or atrophic
2. Small, epithelioid cell granulomas with or without focal necrosis frequently present around follicles
3. Variable infiltrate of lymphocytes and histiocytes

Similar changes with caseation are seen with lupus miliaris disseminatus faciei

Differential diagnosis:
   Lupus vulgaris
   Sarcoidosis

C. Cheilitis granulomatosa (Miescher–Melkersson–Rosenthal)

1. Epidermis and mucosal epithelium normal
2. Edema of dermis and submucosa
3. Epithelioid cell granulomas
4. Infiltrate of plasma cells and lymphocytes

By definition this disorder usually occurs on the lip and consists of a triad of findings including swelling of the lip, facial nerve paralysis, and scrotal tongue

Granulomas may occasionally be absent

Differential diagnosis: sarcoidosis

D. Cutaneous Crohn's disease

1. Epidermis normal
2. Dermal infiltrate composed of lymphocytes, histiocytic cells, epithelioid cells, giant cells, and noncaseating granulomas
3. Granulomas sometimes angiocentric
4. Fibrinoid necrosis variable

Usual sites of involvement are intraoral (pyostomatitis vegetans), perioral, and perianal

Differential diagnosis:
   Orificial tuberculosis
   Sarcoidosis
   Cheilitis granulomatosa
   Rosacea

E. Tuberculoid leprosy (Fig. 17-7)

1. Epidermis usually normal
2. Epithelioid cell granulomas throughout entire dermis admixed with lymphocytes, and occasional giant cells
3. **Tubercles (granulomas) often arranged in "cords" around nerves and vessels**
4. Granulomatous infiltrate often extends upward and "hugs" the epidermis
5. Invasion of nerve and/or arrector pili muscle by granulomatous infiltrate common
6. Atrophy of pilosebaceous units

Acid-fast bacilli, when present, are found more frequently within granulomas, nerves, or arrector pili muscles

Differential diagnosis: sarcoidosis

Nerve involvement is quite characteristic of tuberculoid leprosy; silver stains or immunoperoxidase (S-100) techniques may demonstrate a nerve in the center of a granuloma

F. Tuberculosis

1. Primary inoculation

1. 1 to 14 days: suppurative inflammation of dermis
2. 1 to 6 weeks: appearance of epithelioid cells with subsequent granuloma formation and chronic inflammation

In early suppurative lesions, numerous tubercle bacilli may be observed with acid-fast stains; in the granulomatous phase, organisms may be more difficult to demonstrate

Fig. **17-7.** *Leprosy, tuberculoid or borderline type. Numerous tuberculoid granulomas are present throughout the dermis*

A. *Some of these granulomas appear elongated or sausage-shaped*

B. *Presumably because of their disposition along nerves (arrows).*

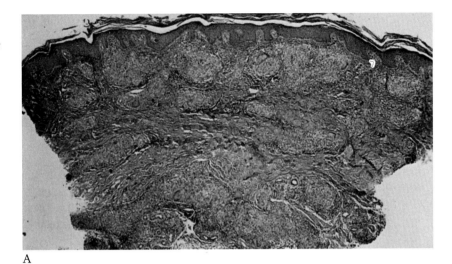

A

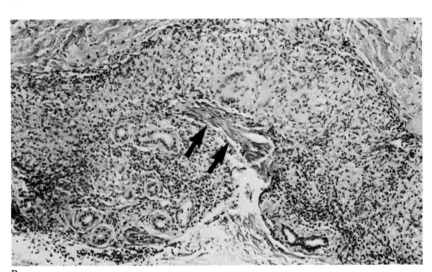

B

2. Lupus vulgaris

1. Epidermal changes vary from atrophy and ulceration to marked hyperplasia
2. Sharply demarcated epithelioid cell granulomas with Langhans giant cells are located in upper third of dermis
3. Numerous histiocytic cells and lymphocytes surround granulomas
4. **Caseation** variably present
5. Fibrosis of reticular dermis variably present

Lupus vulgaris is reactivation of infection in a sensitized individual. Skin lesions commonly occur on the face

Differential diagnosis:
Sarcoidosis
Rosacea
Lupus miliaris disseminatus faciei
Foreign-body reaction (e.g., zirconium)
Deep fungal infection

Acid-fast bacilli difficult to demonstrate with special stains

3. Tuberculosis verrucosa cutis

1. Hyperkeratosis and epidermal hyperplasia with papillomatosis
2. Intraepidermal microabscesses containing neutrophils may be present
3. Edema of papillary and upper reticular dermis
4. Diffuse inflammatory infiltrate in upper dermis composed of neutrophils, lymphocytes, and histiocytic cells
5. Dermal abscesses often present
6. Epithelioid cell granulomas in mid-dermis admixed with neutrophils and lymphocytes
7. Variable caseation

Tuberculosis verrucosa cutis is a result of inoculation of M. *tuberculosis* in a sensitized individual. Lesions typically appear as acrally located warty papules and in the past were commonly referred to as *prosector's warts*.

Differential diagnosis:
　Atypical mycobacteria
　　(especially M. *marinum*)
　Sporotrichosis
　Deep fungal infections

Acid-fast bacilli often difficult to demonstrate

4. Scrofuloderma

1. Epidermal ulceration
2. Track of necrotic tissue lined by an inflammatory infiltrate composed of lymphocytes, histiocytic cells, neutrophils, and occasional plasma cells extending from lymphoid tissue to skin
3. **Caseating epithelioid cell granulomas**
4. Fibrosis of adjacent dermis

Scrofuloderma refers to tuberculous lymphadenitis extending to overlying skin. It appears as a draining sinus tract typically located overlying cervical lymph nodes

Differential diagnosis:
　Actinomycosis
　Gummatous tertiary syphilis

Acid-fast bacilli readily demonstrable

5. Miliary tuberculosis

Focal zone of neutrophils, debris, epithelioid cells, and histiocytic cells in mid-dermis

Numerous acid-fast bacilli present

G. "Tuberculids"

A *tuberculid* is a cutaneous manifestation of sensitivity to M. *tuberculosis* and is defined by the following:
　Occult focus of
　　M. *tuberculosis*
　High degree of immunologic
　　sensitivity to M. *tuberculosis*
　No evidence of M. *tuberculosis*
　　in cutaneous lesions

1. Papulonecrotic tuberculid

1. Focal epidermal necrosis and ulceration
2. Aggregates of histiocytic cells and epithelioid cells sometimes observed at base of ulcer
3. Perivascular lymphocytic and histiocytic infiltrate
4. Endothelial swelling often marked
5. Scattered erythrocytes in dermis
6. Dermal fibrosis

Differential diagnosis:
　Pityriasis lichenoides et
　　varioliformis acuta
　Allergic granulomatosis

2. Lichen scrofulosorum

1. Parakeratosis, epidermal atrophy, and occasionally follicular plugs
2. Noncaseating epithelioid cell granulomas
3. Langhans giant cells and lymphocytes around and between hair follicles

3. Nodular vasculitis (erythema induratum)

See Ch. 26, I.C

H. Zirconium granuloma and cutaneous lesions of systemic berylliosis

1. Epidermis usually normal
2. Noncaseating epithelioid cell granulomas accompanied by a few giant cells and slight lymphocytic infiltrate

Polaroscopy is negative in these disorders; however, spectrographic analysis identifies both zirconium and beryllium

Differential diagnosis:
Sarcoidosis
Silica granuloma

I. Inoculation (local) beryllium granuloma

1. Acanthosis
2. Epithelioid cell granulomas throughout dermis and subcutaneous fat
3. Eosinophilic, **hyalinized necrosis** of dermis is prominent

Diffuse hyalinization of granulomas is specific for this disorder

Differential diagnosis:
Necrobiosis lipoidica
Rheumatoid nodule

J. Miscellaneous foreign-body granulomas (Fig. 17-8)

1. Diffuse epithelioid cell granulomas and granulomatous inflammation
2. Granulomas or giant cells may contain **foreign bodies** such as suture material, talc, starch, keratin, hair, tattoo pigment

Silica particles (soil, talc), wood, and suture material are birefringent with polarized light

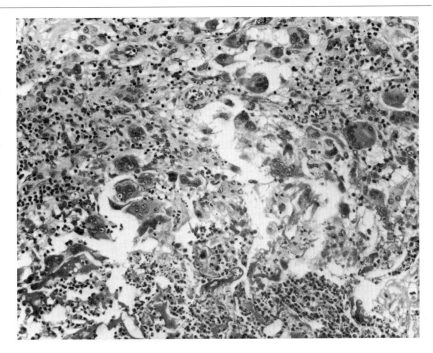

Fig. **17-8.** *Foreign-body reaction. Multinucleated giant cells are interspersed with neutrophils and necrotic debris. The haphazardly placed nuclei in several giant cells are characteristic of the response to a foreign body—here, a ruptured follicle.*

III. Granulomatous inflammation (Fig. 17-9)

A. North American blastomycosis (cutaneous nodule or verrucous plaque associated with systemic infection) (Fig. 17-10)

1. **Marked epidermal hyperplasia** with papillomatosis (pseudoepitheliomatous hyperplasia)

   Causative organism: *Blastomyces dermatitidis*

   Thick-walled spores measure 8 to 15 μm with budding forms occasionally seen; the neck where budding occurs is wide, in contrast to the narrow neck of cryptococcus and paracoccidioidomycosis; although organisms can be seen in H&E-stained sections, visualization is facilitated by use of PAS stain or Gomori's methenamine silver stain

2. **Intraepidermal neutrophilic microabscesses**
3. Dense dermal infiltrate composed of histiocytic cells, epithelioid cells, giant cells, lymphocytes, and many neutrophils
4. Collections of dermal neutrophils frequently surrounded by epithelioid and giant cells
5. Organisms usually numerous and found within neutrophilic abscesses, within giant cells, or free in dermis

---

Intraepidermal neutrophilic microabscesses with epidermal hyperplasia may be seen in:

Deep fungal infections
Granuloma inguinale
M. *marinum* infections
Tuberculosis verrucosa cutis
Halogenodermas
Psoriasis and Reiter's disease

Primary cutaneous inoculation blastomycosis is characterized by a predominantly neutrophilic dermal infiltrate with numerous organisms

Fig. **17-9.** *Granulomatous inflammation. Acanthosis, often approaching pseudoepitheliomatous hyperplasia, overlies the granulomatous dermal infiltrate.*

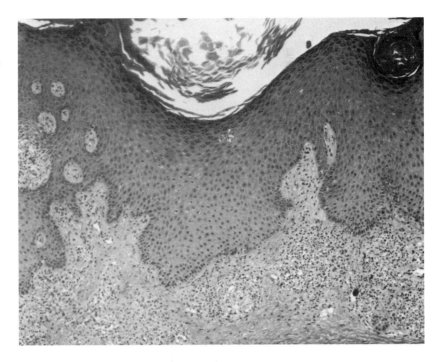

Fig. **17-10.** *North American blastomycosis.*

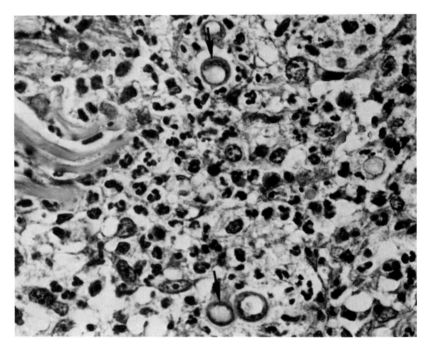

B. South American blastomycosis (mucosal or cutaneous lesions) (Fig. 17-11)

1. **Marked epidermal or epithelial hyperplasia**
2. Granulomatous infiltrate with epithelioid and giant cells admixed with **neutrophilic abscesses**
3. Organisms are numerous and found within abscesses and giant cells
4. Diagnostic multiple budding organisms, so-called **marine pilot's wheel**, may be difficult to detect

Causative organism: *Paracoccidioides brasiliensis*

Spherules with or without budding measure 5 to 20 μm in diameter; those with multiple narrow-based buds measure up to 60 μm; PAS or methenamine silver stains helpful in identifying organism

Differential diagnosis:
North American blastomycosis
Coccidioidomycosis
Cryptococcosis
Tuberculosis verrucosa cutis

C. Chromomycosis (Fig. 17-12)

1. Dermal lesions

1. **Marked epidermal hyper-plasia** with papillomatosis (pseudoepitheliomatous hyperplasia)
2. Spongiosis
3. **Intraepidermal abscesses** filled with neutrophils and mononuclear cells
4. Dense dermal infiltrate composed of histiocytic cells, giant cells, epithelioid cells, lymphocytes, plasma cells, and neutrophils
5. Dermal neutrophilic abscesses common
6. Epithelioid cell granulomas sometimes present
7. **Brown, thick-walled "copper penny" organisms** are present in giant cells and in abscesses or are free in tissue

Causative organisms include:
Phialophora verrucosa
Cladosporium carrionii
Fonsecaea pedrosoi
Fonsecaea compactum

Special stains *not* required to see organism

The spores are also known as *Medlar bodies* and *sclerotic bodies*

2. Subcutaneous lesions

1. Subcutaneous abscess composed of necrotic debris and eosinophils
2. Epithelioid and giant cells surround abscesses
3. Fibrous capsule
4. Organisms found within abscess or in giant cells

Causative organism: *Cladosporium gougerotti*

D. Phaeohyphomycosis

1. Variable acanthosis, pseudo-epitheliomatous hyperplasia
2. Mixed inflammatory cell infiltrate in dermis and subcutis
3. Organisms are **brown budding spores and/or hyphae**

Causative organisms include:
Exophiala jeanselmei
Wangiella dermatitidis

Fig. **17-11.** *South American blastomycosis.*

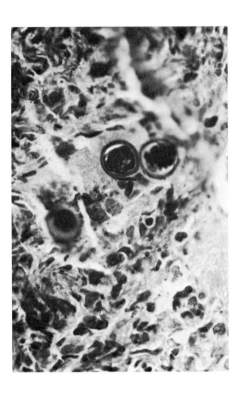

Fig. **17-12.** *Chromomycosis.*

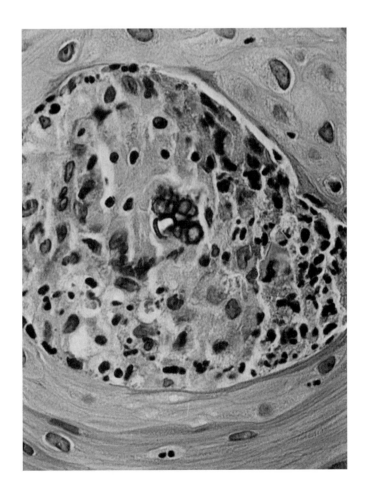

E. Sporotrichosis
(Fig. 17-13)

1. Primary lesion

1. Epidermal hyperplasia with papillomatosis adjacent to ulceration
2. Intraepidermal neutrophilic microabscesses
3. Dermal infiltrate composed of many lymphocytes, plasma cells, and variable numbers of giant and epithelioid cells
4. Small dermal neutrophilic abscesses often present
5. Organism notoriously difficult to find

Causative organism: *Sporotrichum schenckii*

Organisms best visualized with PAS stain after diastase digestion; round to oval budding spores measure 3 to 8 μm in diameter; characteristic cigar-shaped oval organism measures 4 to 5 μm in length and 1 to 2 μm in diameter

Asteroid spores with peripherally radiating eosinophilic extensions occasionally are seen in cases from tropical countries

Culture of lesions often necessary to confirm diagnosis

Very early lesions may show only a nonspecific lymphocytic infiltrate with plasma cells and neutrophils

2. Secondary cutaneous nodules

1. Epidermis usually normal but may be ulcerated
2. Deep dermal and/or subcutaneous infiltrate, characteristically with three zones of inflammation:
   a. Central zone: necrosis, debris, and neutrophils
   b. Middle zone: epithelioid cells and giant multinucleate cells
   c. Outer zone: lymphocytes and plasma cells with vascular proliferation

Secondary cutaneous nodules occur either locally over draining lymphatic channels or secondary to disseminated hematogenous or lymphatic spread

Differential diagnosis: tularemia

F. Coccidioidomycosis
(Fig. 17-14)

1. Early primary cutaneous lesions

1. Diffuse dermal infiltrate composed predominantly of neutrophils and lymphocytes
2. Epithelioid cells and giant cells rare to absent
3. Abundant organisms

Causative organism: *Coccidioides immitis*

Large, thick-walled spores measuring 10 to 80 μm in diameter contain either granular cytoplasm or a variable number of endospores; endospores measure 2 to 10 μm in diameter. Organisms may be visualized in H&E-stained sections but are better seen with PAS stain or silver stain

Fig. **17-13.** *Sporotrichosis.*

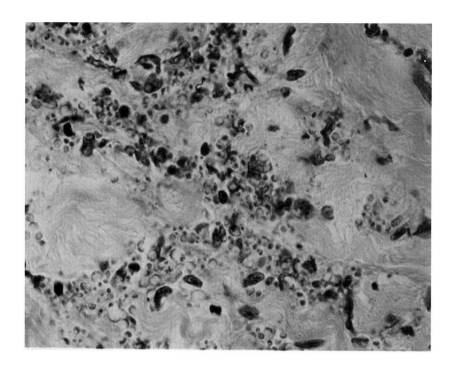

Fig. **17-14.** *Coccidioidomycosis.*

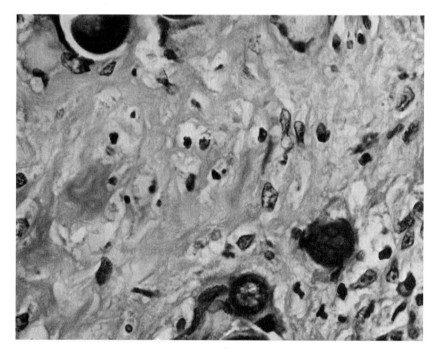

2. Late primary cutaneous lesions; secondary (disseminated) cutaneous lesions

1. Marked epidermal hyperplasia with papillomatosis (pseudoepitheliomatous hyperplasia)
2. Neutrophilic abscesses within the epidermis and dermis
3. Dense dermal infiltrate composed of lymphocytes, plasma cells, histiocytic cells, many neutrophils, with variable numbers of epithelioid and giant cells
4. Organisms present in histiocytic cells and giant cells or free in tissue

Number of organisms varies with host immunity

3. Subcutaneous abscesses

1. Central necrosis
2. Lymphocytes, histiocytic cells, plasma cells, epithelioid cells, and a few giant cells surrounding an area of necrosis
3. Numerous organisms

G. Cryptococcosis (Fig. 17-15)

1. Granulomatous reaction

1. Epidermal hyperplasia adjacent to ulceration
2. Dense dermal infiltrate of lymphocytes, histiocytic cells, epithelioid cells, giant cells, and plasma cells
3. Neutrophils uncommon
4. Organisms present within histiocytic and giant cells and free in tissue

Causative organism: *Cryptococcus neoformans*
Spherical to oval organism measures 5 to 10 μm in diameter and is surrounded by a clear halo; capsule visualized with special stains (see Ch. 3); staining tissue with both alcian blue and PAS results in organism with red cell wall and blue capsule; budding of yeast forms typically occurs with a narrow neck in comparison to broad-based neck of *Blastomyces dermatitidis*

2. Gelatinous reaction

Abundant numbers of organisms with prominent capsules and minimal inflammatory response

Both the granulomatous and gelatinous reactions to infection may be seen in the same lesion

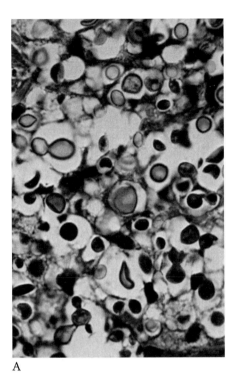 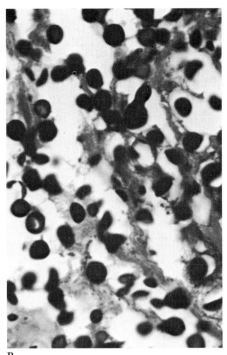

A   B

Fig. **17-15.** *Cryptococcosis.*
A. *Hematoxylin-eosin stain.*
B. *Periodic acid–Schiff stain.*

H. Atypical
mycobacteriosis

1. Early lesions	Dermal infiltrate of neutrophils admixed with variable numbers of lymphocytes and histiocytic cells	Causative organisms include: *Mycobacterium marinum* (most common) M. *scrofulaceum* M. *avium-intracellulare* M. *fortuitum* M. *chelonei* M. *kansasii*
2. Late lesions	1. Hyperkeratosis, parakeratosis 2. Epidermal hyperplasia often adjacent to ulceration 3. Neutrophilic epidermal microabscesses 4. Edema of papillary and upper reticular dermis 5. Diffuse dermal infiltrate composed of lymphocytes, histiocytic cells, plasma cells, epithelioid cells, and giant cells 6. Epithelioid cell granulomas frequently seen in lower reticular dermis of older lesions 7. Vascular ectasia and proliferation 8. Dermal fibrosis	*Mycobacterium avium-intercellulare* may be found in skin biopsy specimens from individuals infected with the human immunodeficiency virus. Its presence may be a coincidental finding, and the lesion biopsied may be due to another etiology. Because the number of organisms may be small, diagnosis may be difficult to establish without culture

I. Tertiary syphilis

1. Normal, flattened, or ulcerated epidermis
2. Edema of papillary dermis
3. Nodular or diffuse dermal infiltrate in reticular dermis composed of lymphocytes, histiocytic cells, epithelioid cells, giant cells, and **plasma cells**
4. Variable dermal necrosis
5. **Endothelial cell proliferation** may produce occlusion of vessel lumen
6. Proliferation of fibroblasts common in older lesions

Deep dermal infiltrate, extensive necrosis, and ulceration are characteristic of gummatous lesion
Plasma cell infiltrate usually prominent

See also Ch. 16, II.L; Ch. 19, V

Spirochetes not demonstrable

J. Cat-scratch disease

1. Variable epidermal changes, sometimes including necrosis
2. Dermal "granulomatous abscess," i.e., central necrosis peppered with neutrophils and karyorrhectic material is surrounded by histiocytic cells, giant cells, and lymphocytes
3. The dermal process is sometimes described as "stellate abscess" because the overall contours may appear folded or stellate rather than round or oval

Causative organism: *Bartonella henselae*

The histology within lymph nodes is identical

K. Other infections with granulomatous inflammation

1. Leishmaniasis
2. Histoplasmosis

See Ch. 18, VII.F
See Ch. 18, VII.E

L. Protothecosis

1. Epidermis variably ulcerated.
2. Dense, mixed inflammatory infiltrate throughout dermis
3. Abundant mulitnucleated giant cells
4. Characterstic morula present within cytoplasm of giant cells and extracellularly
5. Plasma cells common

It can be difficult to see the organisms on routine histologic sections, but PASD and methenamine silver stains highlight them.

Suggested Reading
Palisading Granulomas

Alegre, V. A., and Winkelmann, R. K. A new histopathologic feature of necrobiosis lipoidica diabeticorum: Lymphoid nodules. J. *Cutan. Pathol.* 15:75–77, 1988.
Bennett, G. A., Zeller, J. W., and Bauer, W. Subcutaneous nodules of rheumatoid arthritis and rheumatic fever: A pathologic study. *Arch. Pathol.* 30:70, 1940.
Binazzi, M., and Simonette, V. Granuloma annulare, necrobiosis lipoidica, and diabetic disease. *Int. J. Dermatol.* 27:576–579, 1988.
Cohen, I. J. K., Necrobiosis lipoidica and granuloma annulare. J. *Am. Acad. Dermatol.* 10:123–124, 1984.
Crosby, D. L., Woodley, D. T., and Leonard, D. D. Concomitant granuloma annulare and necrobiosis lipoidica. *Dermatologica* 183:225–229, 1991.
Dabski, K., and Winkelmann, R. K. Generalized granuloma annulare. Histopathology and immunopathology. J. *Am. Acad. Dermatol.* 20:28–39, 1989.
Dahl, M. V., Ullman, S., and Goltz, R. W. Vasculitis in granuloma annulare. *Arch. Dermatol.* 113:463, 1977.

Gray, H. R., Graham, J. H., and Johnson, W. C. Necrobiosis lipoidica: A histopathological and histochemical study. J. Invest. Dermatol. 44:369, 1965.

Kavanagh, G. M., Novelli, M., Hartog, M., and Kennedy, C. T. C. Necrobiosis lipoidica—involvement of atypical sites. Clin. Exp. Dermatol. 18:543–544, 1993.

Muller, S. A., and Winkelmann, R. K. Necrobiosis lipoidica diabeticorum: Histopathologic study of 98 cases. Arch. Dermatol. 94:1, 1966.

Owens, D. W., and Freeman, R. G. Perforating granuloma annulare. Arch. Dermatol. 103:64, 1971.

Reed, R. J., Clark, W. H., and Mihm, M. C. The cutaneous collagenoses. Hum. Pathol. 4:165, 1973.

Rubin, M., and Lynch, F. W. Subcutaneous granuloma annulare: Comment on familial granuloma annulare. Arch. Dermatol. 93:416, 1966.

Toro, J. R., Chu, P., Ben Yen, T-S. and LeBoit, P. E. Granuloma annulare and human immunodeficiency virus infection. Arch. Dermatol. 135:1341–1346, 1999.

Umbert, P., and Winkelmann, R. K. Histologic, ultrastructural, and histochemical studies of granuloma annulare. Arch. Dermatol. 113:1681, 1977.

Wood, M. G., and Beerman, H. Necrobiosis lipoidica, granuloma annulare and rheumatoid nodule. J. Invest. Dermatol. 34:139, 1960.

Epithelioid Cell Granulomas (Tuberculosis and Tuberculids):

Brown, F. S., Anderson, R. H., and Burnett, J. W. Cutaneous tuberculosis. J. Am. Acad. Dermatol. 6:101–106, 1982.

del Carmen Farina, M. Gezundez, I., Pique, E., Esteban, J., Martin, L., Requena, L., Barat, A., et al. Cutaneous tuberculosis: A clinical, histopathologic, and bacteriologic study. J. Am. Acad. Dermatol. 33:433–440, 1995.

Jetton, R. L., and Coker, W. L. Tuberculosis verrucosa cutis. Arch. Dermatol. 100:380, 1969.

Minkowitz, S., Brandt, L. J., Rapp, Y., and Raudlauer, C. B. "Prosector's wart" (cutaneous tuberculosis) in a medical student. Am. J. Clin. Pathol. 51:260, 1969.

Mitchell, P. C. Tuberculosis verrucosa cutis among Chinese in Hong Kong. Br. J. Dermatol. 66:444, 1954.

Montgomery, H. Histopathology of various types of cutaneous tuberculosis. Arch. Dermatol. Syphilol. 35:698, 1937.

Morrison, J. G. L., and Fourie, E. D. The papulonecrotic tuberculide. From arthus reaction to lupus vulgaris. Br. J. Dermatol. 91:263, 1974.

Nachbar, F., Classen, V., Nachbar, T., Meurer, M., Schirren, C. G., and Degitz, K. Orificial tuberculosis: Detection by polymerase chain reaction. Br. J. Dermatol. 135:106–109, 1996.

Schermer, D. R., Simpson, C. G., Haserick, J. R., et al. Tuberculosis cutis miliaris acuta generalisata. Arch. Dermatol. 99:64, 1969.

Smith, N. P., Ryan, T. J., Sanderson, K. V., et al. Lichen scrofulosorum. A report of four cases. Br. J. Dermatol. 94:319, 1976.

Tan, S. H., Tan, B. H., Goh, C. L., Tan, K. C., Tan, M. F., Ng, W. C., and Tan, W. C. Detection of mycobacterium tuberculosis DNA using polymerase chain reaction in cutaneous tuberculosis and tuberculids. Int. J. Dermatol. 38:122–127, 1999.

Wilson-Jones, E., and Winkelmann, R. K. Papulonecrotic tuberculid: A neglected disease in Western countries. J. Am. Acad. Dermatol. 14:815, 1986.

Wong, K. O., Lee, K. P., and Chiu, S. F. Tuberculosis of the skin in Hong Kong (a review of 160 cases). Br. J. Dermatol. 80:424, 1968.

Leprosy

Azulay, R. D. Histopathology of skin lesions in leprosy. Int. J. Lepr, 39:244, 1971.

Liu, T-C., Yen, L-Z., Ye, G-Y., and Dung, G. L. Histology of indeterminate leprosy. Int. J. Lepr. 50:172, 1982.

Modlin, R. L., Hofman, F. M., Taylor, C. R., and Rea, T. H. T lymphocyte subsets in the skin lesions of patients with leprosy. J. Am. Acad. Dermatol. 8:182, 1983.

Ridley, D. S. Histological classification and the immunological spectrum of leprosy. Bull. W.H.O. 51:451, 1974.

Ridley, D. S., and Jopling, W. H. Classification of leprosy according to immunity. A five group system. Int. J. Lepr. 34:255, 1966.

Sehgal, V. N. Clinical leprosy (3rd ed.). New Delhi: Jaypee Brothers, 1993.

Sehgal, V. N. Leprosy. Dermatol. Clin. 12:629–644, 1994.

Van Voorhis, W. C., Kaplan, G., Nunes Sarno, E., Horowitz, M. A., Steinman, R. M., Levis, W. R., Nogueira, N., et al. The cutaneous infiltrates of leprosy. Cellular characteristics and the predominant T-cell phenotypes. N. Engl. J. Med. 307:1593–1597, 1982.

Sarcoidosis

Banse-Kupin, L., and Pelachyk, J. M. Ichthyosiform sarcoidosis. Report of two cases and a review of the literature. *J. Am. Acad. Dermatol.* 17:616–620, 1987.

Callen, J. P. Sarcoidosis. In *Dermatologic Signs of Internal Disorders.* Chicago: Year Book Medical Publishers; 1980, pp. 311–332.

Elgart, M. L. Cutaneous lesions of sarcoidosis. *Primary Care* 5:249, 1978.

Garcia-Porrua, C., Gonzalez-Gay, M. A., Garcia-Pais, M. J., and Blanco, R. Cutaneous vasculitis: An unusual presentation of sarcoidosis in adulthood. *Scand. J. Rheumatol.* 27:80–82, 1998.

James, D. G., et al. Pathobiology of sarcoidosis. *Pathobiol. Annu.* 7:31, 1977.

Kataria, Y. P., and Holter, J. F. Immunology of sarcoidosis. *Clin. Chest. Med.* 18:719–739, 1997.

Mitchell, D. N., Scadding, J. G., Heard, B. E., and Hinson, K. F. W. Sarcoidosis: Histopathological definition and clinical diagnosis. *J. Clin. Pathol.* 30:395, 1977.

Sitzbach, L. E. (Ed.). Seventh international conference on sarcoidosis and other granulomatous disorders. *Ann. N.Y. Acad. Sci.* Vol. 278, 1976.

Steigleder, G. K., Silva, A., Jr., and Nelson, C. T. Histopathology of the Kveim test. *Arch. Dermatol.* 84:828, 1961.

Takemura, T., Shishiba, T., Akiyama, O., Oritsu, M., Matsui, Y., and Eishi, Y. Vascular involvement in cutaneous sarcoidosis. *Pathol. Int.* 47:84–89, 1997.

Vainsencher, D., and Winkelmann, R. K. Subcutaneous sarcoidosis. *Arch. Dermatol.* 120:1028, 1984.

Rosacea

Marks, R., and Harcourt-Webster, J. N. Histopathology of rosacea. *Arch. Dermatol.* 100:683, 1969.

Mullanax, M. G., and Kierland, R. R. Granulomatous rosacea. *Arch. Dermatol.* 101:206, 1970.

Cheilitis Granulomatosa (Miescher–Melkersson–Rosenthal Syndrome)

Hornstein, O. P. Melkersson–Rosenthal syndrome: A neuro-mucocutaneous disease of complex origin. *Curr. Probl. Dermatol.* 5:117, 1973.

Kintchkoff, D., and James, R. Cheilitis granulomatosa. *Arch. Dermatol.* 114:1203, 1978.

Laymon, C. W. Cheilitis granulomatosa and Melkersson–Rosenthal syndrome. *Arch. Dermatol.* 83:112, 1961.

Zirconium Granuloma

Epstein, W. L., and Allen, J. R. Granulomatous hypersensitivity after use of zirconium-containing poison oak lotions. *JAMA* 190:940, 1964.

Epstein, W. L., Skahen, J. R., and Krasnobrod, H. The organized epithelioid cell granuloma: Differentiation of allergic (zirconium) from colloidal (silica) types. *Am. J. Pathol.* 43:391, 1963.

Beryllium Granuloma

Grier, R. S., et al. Skin lesions in persons exposed to beryllium compounds. *J. Ind. Hyg. Toxicol.* 30:228, 1948.

Hardy, H. L., and Tabershaw, I. R. Delayed chemical pneumonitis occurring in workers exposed to beryllium compounds. *J. Ind. Hyg. Toxicol.* 28:197, 1946.

Neave, H. J., Frank, S. B., and Tolmach, J. A. Cutaneous granuloma following laceration by fluorescent light bulbs. *Arch. Dermatol. Syphilol.* 61:401, 1950.

Pyre, J., and Oatway, W. H., Jr. Beryllium granulomatosis. *Ariz. Med.* 4:21, 1947.

Granulomatous Inflammation

Binford, C. H., and Connor, D. H. *Pathology of Tropical and Extraordinary Diseases,* Vols. I and II. Washington, D.C.: Armed Forces Institute of Pathology, 1976.

Emmons, C. W., Binford, C. H., Utz, J. P., and Kwon-Chung, K. J. *Medical Mycology* (3rd ed.). Philadelphia: Lea & Febiger, 1977.

Blastomycosis

Bradsher, R. W. Clinical features of blastomycosis. *Semin. Respir. Infect.* 12:229–234, 1997.

Busey, J. F. Blastomycosis. I. A review of 198 collected cases in Veterans Administration hospitals. *Am. Rev. Respir. Dis.* 89:659, 1969.

Davies, S. F., and Sarosi, G. A. Epidemiological and clinical features of pulmonary blastomycosis. *Semin. Respir. Infect.* 12:206–218, 1997.

Hashimoto, K., Kaplan, R. J., Daman, L. A., et al. Pustular blastomycosis. *Int. J. Dermatol.* 16:277, 1977.

Landay, M. E., and Schwarz, J. Primary cutaneous blastomycosis. *Arch. Dermatol.* 104:408, 1971.

Mercurio, M. G., and Elewski, B. E. Cutaneous blastomycosis. *Cutis* 50:422–424, 1992.

Chromomycosis

Carrion, A. L. Chromoblastomycosis and related infections. *Int. J. Dermatol.* 14:27, 1975.

McGinnis, M. R. Chromoblastomycosis and phaeohyphomycosis: New concepts, diagnosis, and mycology. *J. Am. Acad. Dermatol.* 8:1, 1983.

Vollum, D. I. Chromomycosis: A review. *Br. J. Dermatol.* 96:454, 1977.

Sporotrichosis

Lurie, H. I. Histopathology of sporotrichosis. *Arch. Pathol.* 75:421, 1963.

Coccidioidomycosis

Basler, R. S., and Lagomarsino, S. L. Coccidioidomycosis: Clinical review and treatment update. *Int. J. Dermatol.* 18:104, 1979.

Harvey, W. C., and Greendyke, W. H. Skin lesions in acute coccidioidomycosis. *Am. Fam. Physician* 2:81, 1970.

Levan, N. E., and Huntington, R. W. Primary cutaneous coccidioidomycosis in agricultural workers. *Arch. Dermatol.* 92:215, 1965.

Vaz, A., Pineda-Roman, M., Thomas, A. R., and Carlson, R. W. Coccidiodomycosis: An update. *Hosp. Pract. (Off. Ed.)* 15:119–120, 1998.

Cryptococcosis

Ingleton, R., Koestenblatt, E., Don, P., Levy, H. Szaniawski, W., and Weinberg, J. M. Cutaneous cryptococcosis mimicking basal cell carcinoma in a patients with AIDS. *J. Cutan. Med. Surg.* 3:43–45, 1998.

Manfredi, R., Mazzoni, A., Nanetti, A. Mastroianni, A., Coronado, O., and Chiodo, F. Morphologic features and clinical significance of skin involvement in patients with AIDS-related cryptococcosis. *Acta Derm. Venereol.* 76:72–74, 1996.

Noble, R. C., and Fajardo, L. F. Primary cutaneous cryptococcosis: Review and morphologic study. *Am. J. Clin. Pathol.* 57:13, 1972.

Sarosi, G. A., Silberfarb, P. M., and Tosh, F. E.: Cutaneous cryptococcosis. A sentinel of disseminated disease. *Arch. Dermatol.* 104:1, 1971.

Schupbach, C. W., Wheeler, C. E., Briggaman, R. A., et al. Cutaneous manifestations of disseminated cryptococcosis. *Arch. Dermatol.* 112:1734, 1976.

Yantsos, V. A., Carney, J., and Greer, D. L. Review of the morphological variations in cutaneous cryptococcosis with a new case resembling varicella. *Cutis* 54:343–347, 1994.

Atypical Mycobacteriosis

Adams, R. M., Remington, J. S., Steinberg, J., et al. Tropical fish aquariums—A source of *Mycobacterium marinum* infection resembling sporotrichosis. *JAMA* 211:457, 1970.

Feldman, R. A., Long, M. W., and David, H. L. *Mycobacterium marinum*: A leisure-time pathogen. *J. Infect. Dis.* 129:618, 1974.

Hirsch, F. S., and Saffold, O. E. *Mycobacterium kansasii* infection with dermatologic manifestation. *Arch. Dermatol.* 112:706, 1976.

Owens, D. W. Atypical mycobacteria. *Int. J. Dermatol.* 17:180, 1978.

Philpott, J. A., Woodburne, A. R., Philpott, O. S., et al. Swimming pool granuloma—A study of 290 cases. *Arch. Dermatol.* 88:158, 1968.

Wallace, R. J., Swenson, J. M., Silcox, V. A. et al. Spectrum of disease due to rapidly growing mycobacteria. *Rev. Infect. Dis.* 5:657, 1983.

Zeligman, I. *Mycobacterium marinum* granuloma. *Arch. Dermatol.* 106:26, 1972.

Cat-Scratch Disease

Johnson, W. T., and Helwig, E. B. Cat-scratch disease. Histopathologic changes in the skin. *Arch. Dermatol.* 100:148, 1969.

Chapter 18

Diffuse Infiltrate

    I. Predominantly histiocytic cells
      A. Xanthelasma
      B. Eruptive xanthoma
      C. Tuberous and tendon xanthoma
      D. Lepromatous leprosy
      E. Langerhans cell histiocytosis
      F. Xanthogranuloma
      G. Reticulohistiocytosis
   II. Predominantly lymphocytes
      A. Lymphoma cutis
      B. Leukemia cutis (lymphocytic type)
  III. Predominantly plasma cells
      A. Plasmacytoma, primary lesions, and lesions associated with multiple myeloma
  IV. Predominantly mast cells
      A. Urticaria pigmentosa
   V. Predominantly neutrophils
      A. Granuloma faciale
      B. Erythema elevatum diutinum
      C. Acute febrile neutrophilic dermatosis (Sweet's syndrome)
      D. Cellulitis
      E. Leukemia cutis, granulocytic
  VI. Predominantly eosinophils
      A. Eosinophilic cellulitis (Wells' syndrome)
 VII. Mixed infiltrate
      A. Lymphoma cutis, polymorphous infiltrate
         1. Hodgkin's disease
         2. Cutaneous T-cell lymphoma, including mycosis fungoides
         3. Large cell anaplastic lymphoma
      B. Chancroid
      C. Primary syphilis
      D. Rhinoscleroma
      E. Histoplasmosis
      F. Leishmaniasis
      G. Granuloma inguinale

Recognition of a diffuse infiltrate of the skin requires identification of cells between collagen bundles (i.e., interstitial) or in a perivascular and interstitial array. Involvement of the subcutis may be present, but the entities described in this chapter are characterized by predominant dermal location of the infiltrate. At higher magnification, determination of infiltrating cell type as well as the presence or absence of cellular atypia are crucial in further classifying the process.

The Reactive Process and the Disease	Histopathology	Comments
I. Predominantly histiocytic cells		
A. Xanthelasma (Fig. 18-1)	1. Flattened, occasionally atrophic epidermis 2. Perivascular and diffuse infiltrate of **foam cells** in upper and middle reticular dermis 3. Inflammation and fibrosis minimal to absent	Lipid-laden histiocytic or foam cells have a round to oval, dark-staining nucleus surrounded by pale, vacuolated, or reticulated cytoplasm. Actual lipid is lost during routine processing
B. Eruptive xanthoma (Fig. 18-2)	1. Normal epidermis 2. **Lipid-laden histiocytic cells** admixed with lymphocytes, histiocytic cells, and neutrophils	

C. Tuberous and tendon xanthoma	1. Normal epidermis
	2. Sheets of **lipid-laden histiocytic cells** throughout the reticular dermis
	3. Multinucleate giant cells common
	4. Early lesions have variable lymphohistiocytic and neutrophilic infiltrates admixed with foam cells
	5. Older lesions characterized by dermal fibrosis
		Differential diagnosis:
		  Histiocytosis X
		  Granular cell tumor
		  Balloon cell nevus
		  Lepromatous leprosy

Fig. **18-1.** Xanthelasma. Histiocytic cells with foamy cytoplasm aggregate around vessels.

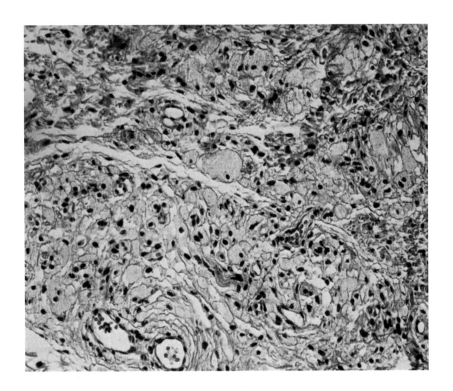

Fig. **18-2.** Eruptive xanthoma. Histiocytic aggregates (arrows), of foamy cells, are associated with inflammatory cells, including lymphocytes and neutrophils. Extracellular lipid present is not yet phagocytosed.

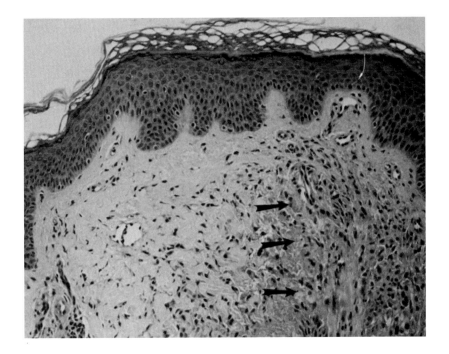

D. Lepromatous leprosy (Fig. 18-3)

1. Normal to flattened epidermis
2. Grenz zone of uninvolved papillary dermis
3. **Aggregates and sheets of foamy histiocytic cells** admixed with lymphocytes and occasional plasma cells extending throughout reticular dermis and into subcutaneous fat
4. **Destruction and loss of appendages**

Numerous acid-fast organisms found within foamy histiocytic cells, nerves, blood vessel walls, arrector pili muscles, and follicular epithelium

Modified acid-fast stains provide optimal visualization of organisms (see Ch. 3)

Fig. **18-3.** *Lepromatous leprosy.*
A. *These histiocytic cells with granular cytoplasm (called lepra cells) aggregate around vessels.*
B. *Wade-Fite stains usually are employed to demonstrate the lepra bacilli, which are often not as acid fast or alcohol resistant as other mycobacteria.*

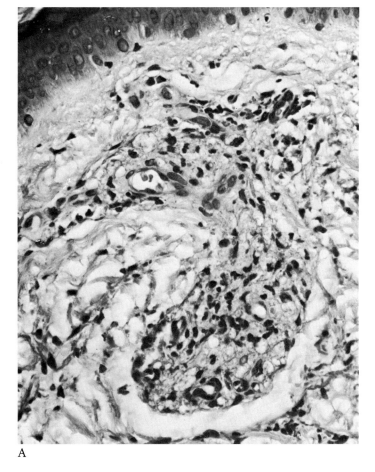

A

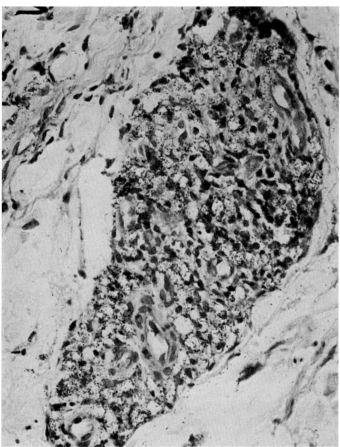

B

E. Langerhans cell histiocytosis (Fig. 18-4)

1. Epidermis may be normal, focally invaded by characteristic mononuclear cells, or ulcerated
2. The characteristic cell is a large histiocytic cell 15 to 25 μm in diameter with a round, oval, notched, or **bean-shaped nucleus** containing one or more fine, dotlike nucleoli; the abundant cytoplasm is pale pink or clear, and the cell margins may blend to form a syncytium; the cytoplasm of cells in older lesions is often quite foamy or vacuolated secondary to accumulation of lipid
3. Admixture of variable numbers of lymphocytes, **eosinophils,** neutrophils, plasma cells, and multinucleate giant cells of either foreign body or Touton type
4. Distribution of infiltrate may be:
   a. Perivascular, with extension into papillary dermis
   b. Bandlike and periappendageal
   c. Diffuse, extending from the epidermis into the subcutaneous fat
5. Proliferation of fibroblasts common
6. Extravasation of erythrocytes often present

Subclassification of the Langerhans cell histiocytosis group of diseases (Letterer–Siwe disease, Hand–Schüller–Christian disease, eosinophilic granuloma) depends on correlation of histologic and clinical findings

Electron microscope and immunohistochemical studies reveal that the infiltrating cell is related to the Langerhans cell, as confirmed by the presence of Birbeck granules, S-100 protein positivity, and characteristic pattern of staining for peanut agglutin

Differential diagnosis:
  Congenital self-healing reticulohistiocytosis
  Lymphoma cutis
  Xanthomas
  Nodular lesions of urticaria pigmentosa
  Histiocytic medullary reticulosis

Fig. **18-4.** *Langerhans cell histiocytosis. Histiocytic cells with mild atypia fill the papillary dermis and invade the epidermis.*

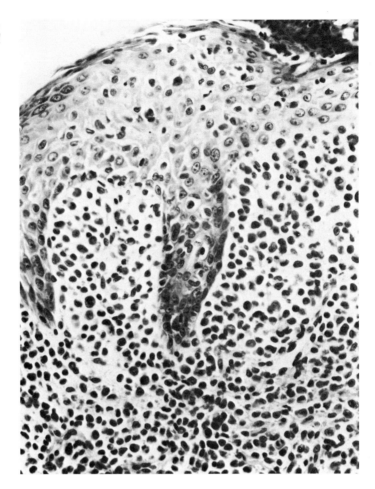

F. Xanthogranuloma
(Fig. 18-5)

1. Normal, acanthotic, or atrophic epidermis
2. Patchy or diffuse infiltrate composed of:
   a. Histiocytic cells, many of which are lipid laden and foamy
   b. Lymphocytes, eosinophils, fibroblasts, and multinucleate giant cells
   c. **Touton giant cells**

The presence of Touton giant cells with their "perfect wreath" of nuclei surrounded by foamy cytoplasm is a characteristic feature of xanthogranuloma

3. The infiltrate usually involves both the papillary and reticular dermis and rarely extends into subcutaneous tissue

Differential diagnosis:
Xanthoma
Dermatofibroma
Langerhans cell histiocytosis

G. Reticulohistiocytosis

1. Normal or acanthotic epidermis
2. Dense, diffuse dermal infiltrate composed of:
   a. Histiocytic cells, lymphocytes, neutrophils, some plasma cells, and eosinophils
   b. Characteristic giant cells with abundant homogeneous eosinophilic **ground glass or "muddy rose" cytoplasm** and one or more distinctive **vesicular nuclei** with prominent nucleoli

This entity occurs as a solitary lesion (reticulohistiocytic granuloma or reticulohistiocytoma) or as multiple nodules (multicentric reticulohistiocytosis)

Fig. **18-5.** *Xanthogranuloma.*
A. *The upper and middle dermis is filled with histiocytic cells (many with foamy cytoplasm), Touton giant cells, and lymphocytes.*
B. *Notice the foamy appearance of the cytoplasm and the "wreathed nuclei" of Touton giant cells. The latter are considered to be the distinctive cell of xanthogranuloma; however, similar giant cells can be seen in other disorders.*

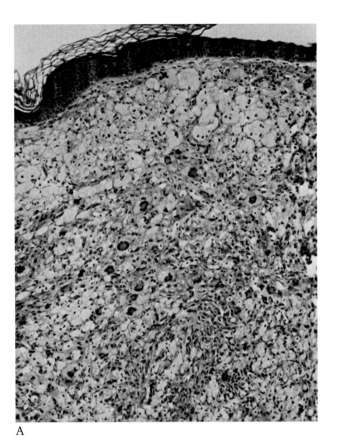

A

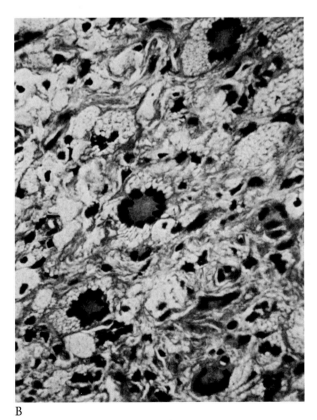

B

II. Predominantly lymphocytes

A. Lymphoma cutis (Fig. 18-6)

1. Epidermis usually normal
2. Papillary dermis spared (Grenz zone)
3. Dense nodular aggregates, patchy aggregates, or **diffuse dermal infiltration of lymphoid cells** throughout entire reticular dermis, often extending into subcutaneous fat
4. Nuclear atypia and atypical mitoses characteristic, though quantitatively variable
5. Cells often infiltrate between collagen fibers in a linear array
6. Nuclei packed tightly together appear distorted and "smudged"

See also Ch. 19, IV

Differential diagnosis:
Leukemia cutis
Lymphocytoma cutis
Lymphocytic infiltrate
Arthropod bite reaction
Mycosis fungoides
Langerhans cell histiocytosis
Lymphomatoid papulosis
Actinic reticuloid
Urticaria pigmentosa

Fig. **18-6.** Lymphoma cutis.
A. The dermis is filled with atypical
cells. The grenz zone near the
epidermis is characteristic of diffuse
B cell lymphomas.
B. Higher magnification shows densely
compacted cells with nuclear
hyperchromatism.

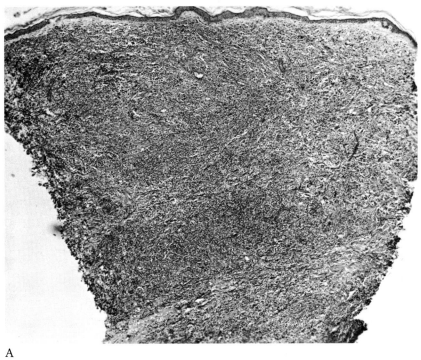

A

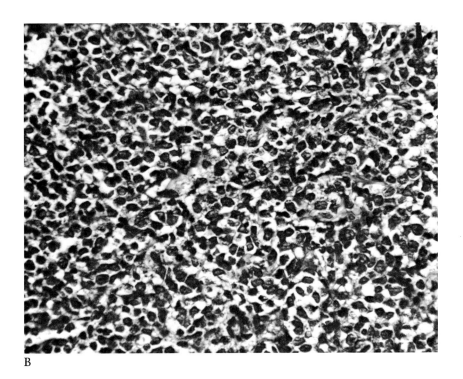

B

B. Leukemia cutis
(lymphocytic type)

1. Normal epidermis
2. Grenz zone of uninvolved papillary dermis
3. Diffuse or nodular aggregates of **immature leukocytes** extending throughout the reticular dermis, often into the subcutaneous tissue
4. Cells infiltrate between collagen bundles
5. Cells tightly packed together and sometimes appear "smudged"

The cells of cutaneous leukemia infiltrates usually have the morphology of the circulating leukemic cells; granulocytic leukemia cells may be distinguished from lymphocytic leukemia cells by the presence of chloracetate esterase–positive cytoplasmic granules (Fig.18-7)

Differential diagnosis: lymphoma cutis

III. Predominantly plasma cells

A. Plasmacytoma, primary lesions, and lesions associated with multiple myeloma

1. Normal or flattened epidermis
2. Dense infiltrate of atypical **plasma cells** in reticular and often papillary dermis
3. Atypical mitoses common

Round, homogeneous, eosinophilic PAS-positive Russell bodies may be present intracellularly and extracellularly

Differential diagnosis: lymphoma cutis

> *Plasma cells* conspicuous in
>
> Syphilis, all stages
> Rhinoscleroma
> Granuloma inguinale
> Chronic folliculitis
> Plasmacytoma
> Zoon's balanitis
> Syringocystadenoma papilliferum
> Inflammatory infiltrates on head and neck and periorificial areas
> Nodular amyloidosis
> Inflammation adjacent to neoplasm

IV. Predominantly mast cells

A. Urticaria pigmentosa
(Fig. 18-8)

1. Epidermis normal or flattened
2. Increased melanin in basal layer
3. Infiltrate of cuboidal **mast cells** fills papillary dermis and upper and mid-reticular dermis, occasionally extending into subcutaneous tissue

See also Ch. 11, II.O; Ch. 12, XIV, Ch. 13, IV

The cuboidal mast cell with distinct cell walls and round to oval, dense, basophilic nucleus has a "fried egg" appearance

Fig. **18-7.** *Involvement of the subcutis by chronic myelogenous leukemia. Numerous atypical megakaryocytes, immature myeloid cells, and rare neutrophils are present in this biopsy.*

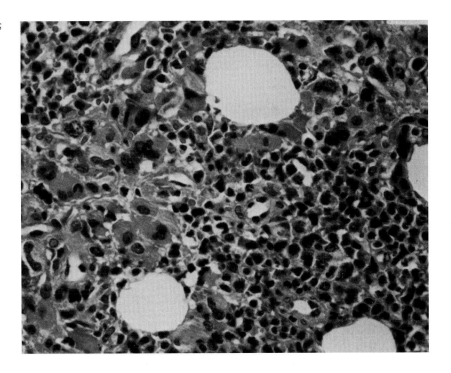

Fig. **18-8.** *Urticaria pigmentosa. The mast cell infiltrate is present in the mid and upper dermis. Mast cells may be mistaken for lymphocytes, but their nuclei stain less intensively and more uniformly than do those of lymphocytes. Mast cells also have more cytoplasm and better demarcated cytoplasmic borders than lymphocytes. Giemsa stains demonstrate metachromasia of mast cell granules.*

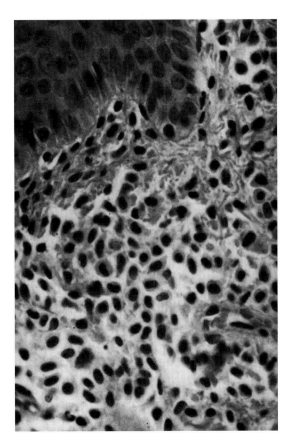

4. Variable number of **eosinophils** admixed with mast cells

Diagnostic cytoplasmic granules may be seen in H&E-stained sections or may be stained with Giemsa, toluidine blue, or chloracetate esterase stains

Differential diagnosis:
Dermal nevus
Leukemia cutis
Lymphoma cutis
Langerhans cell histiocytosis

Mastocytoma may be readily distinguished from Langerhans cell histiocytosis by its absence of exocytosis and ulceration

V. Predominantly neutrophils

A. Granuloma faciale (Fig. 18-9)

1. Normal epidermis
2. **Grenz zone** of uninvolved papillary or adventitial dermis separates epidermis and adnexal structures from infiltrate
3. Nodular and diffuse aggregates of lymphocytes and **eosinophils** (up to 90%) plus neutrophils, plasma cells, and mast cells
4. Infiltrate usually confined to upper and middle dermis but may extend to subcutaneous tissue
5. **Leukocytoclastic vasculitis** with endothelial cell swelling, neutrophils within vessel walls, and nuclear debris often observed
6. Fibrin deposition in and around vessels
7. Extravasation of erythrocytes
8. Hemosiderin-laden macrophages
9. Variable fibrosis

See also Ch. 16, II.E

While the infiltrate in granuloma faciale is truly of mixed composition, neutrophils and eosinophils generally predominate

B. Erythema elevatum diutinum

See Ch. 16, II.D

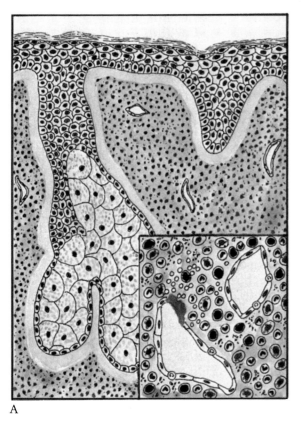

A

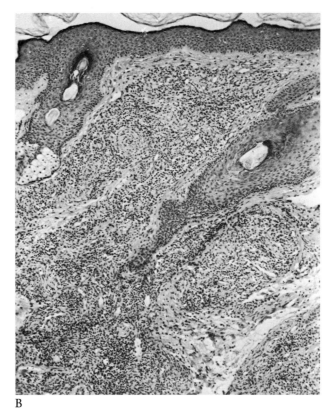

B

Fig. **18-9.** *Granuloma faciale.*
A. *The diffuse polymorphous infiltrate, including neutrophils, eosinophils, and lymphocytes, spares the upper papillary dermis (the grenz zone). Changes suggestive of vasculitis frequently are present. The inset illustrates the polymorphous nature of the infiltrate and vascular damage.*
B. *Photomicrograph for comparison. The low-power pattern of the grenz zone and numerous eosinophils is distinctive.*

C. Acute febrile neutrophilic dermatosis (Sweet's syndrome) (see Fig. 16-3)

1. Intercellular edema (spongiosis)
2. Migration of neutrophils into epidermis, sometimes forming microabscesses
3. **Edema of the papillary dermis, often severe**
4. **Dense diffuse and perivascular** infiltrate predominantly of neutrophils, infiltrate may extend into the subcutis
5. Nuclear fragments or "dust"
6. Vascular ectasia

Differential diagnosis:
Cellulitis
Pyoderma gangrenosum
Leukocytoclastic vasculitis

D. Cellulitis

1. Papillary dermal edema
2. Vascular ectasia
3. Perivascular and predominantly diffuse infiltrate composed of neutrophils, lymphocytes, occasional eosinophils, and plasma cells in deep dermis and subcutis
4. Extravasation of erythrocytes

Special stains for bacteria and mycobacteria may demonstrate organisms

The differential diagnosis varies in a spectrum from massive edema (e.g., angioedema) to massive suppurative infiltrates (e.g., Sweet's syndrome)

E. Leukemia cutis, granulocytic (Fig. 18-7)

1. Epidermal changes minimal
2. Grenz zone of uninvolved papillary dermis
3. Diffuse or perivascular infiltrate of **immature granulocytes** extending throughout the dermis and subcutis

Differential diagnosis: lymphoma cutis

Recognition of cells as granulocytic depends on degree of differentiation

VI. Predominantly eosinophils

A. Eosinophilic cellulitis (Wells' syndrome)

1. Normal epidermis
2. Edema of reticular dermis may be marked
3. Perivascular and diffuse infiltrate composed predominantly of eosinophils admixed with lymphocytes, histiocytic cells, and occasional giant multinucleate cells
4. Eosinophil granules scattered loosely in dermis
5. **Focal areas of altered collagen surrounded by eosinophils,** eosinophil granules, and histiocytic cells (so-called **flame figure**)
6. Infiltrate may extend through panniculus, fascia, and muscle

Flame figures have also been observed in:

Bullous pemphigoid
Eczema
Prurigo
Dermatophytosis
Arthropod bite reaction

VII. Mixed infiltrate

    A. Lymphoma cutis, polymorphous infiltrate

1. Hodgkin's disease	1. Epidermis usually normal
	2. Grenz zone of spared papillary dermis
	3. Diffuse or nodular infiltrate throughout the reticular dermis composed of:
	   a. **atypical mononuclear cells** admixed with histiocytic cells, lymphocytes, and variable numbers of neutrophils, eosinophils, plasma cells, and multinucleate giant cells
	   b. **Reed–Sternberg cells,** which are large cells with abundant cytoplasm, bilobed nuclei, and prominent nucleoli, giving an "owl's eye" appearance
		Differential diagnosis:
		   Lymphomatoid papulosis
		   Arthropod bite reaction
		   Mycosis fungoides
		
		See also Ch. 19, IV

2. Cutaneous T-cell lymphoma, including mycosis fungoides (see Fig. 5-6)	1. Epidermal changes variable and include psoriasiform hyperplasia, atrophy, or ulceration with or without Pautrier microabscesses
	2. Dense accumulations of **atypical mononuclear cells** characterized by convoluted or cerebriform, hyperchromatic large nuclei; these atypical cells may be admixed with lymphocytes, histiocytic cells, eosinophils, and plasma cells
		Cutaneous T-cell lymphoma, as a category, contains entities distinct from the traditional concept of mycosis fungoides. Identification of cellular phenotype and clinicopathologic correlation are required to distinguish confidently between the various forms.
		Tumor stage mycosis fungoides falls best within the broader concept of cutaneous T-cell lymphoma
		See also Ch. 5, III.B; Ch. 12, X
		
		Differential diagnosis:
		   Lymphomatoid papulosis
		   Actinic reticuloid
		   Hodgkin's disease
		   Langerhans cell histiocytosis

3. Large cell anaplastic lymphoma	1. Epidermis usually unremarkable 2. Rare cases with minimal epidermotropism 3. **Diffuse infiltrate of large, atypical lymphocytes** throughout dermis 4. Vesicular nuclei, pleomorphic nuclei 5. Abundant mitotic figures 6. Extensive individual cell necrosis 7. Variable numbers of eosinophils present	It can be impossible to distinguish primary large cell anaplastic lymphoma from secondary large cell anaplastic lymphoma, transformed mycosis fungoides or type C lymphomatoid papulosis. Clinical history is essential.

B. Chancroid (Fig. 18-10)

1. Epithelial hyperplasia adjacent to central ulceration
2. **Three relatively distinct zones** of inflammation present at base of ulcer
   a. *Superficial zone*: thin band of neutrophils admixed with extravasated erythrocytes, fibrin, and necrotic debris
   b. *Middle zone*: wide band of markedly edematous stroma containing many thin-walled, dilated, vertically oriented blood vessels with variable necrosis of vessel walls and variable inflammatory infiltrate
   c. *Deep zone*: dense perivascular and diffuse infiltrate composed predominantly of plasma cells and lymphocytes

Causative organism: *Haemophilus ducreyi*
Short, 1- to 2-μm, rodlike organisms in clusters or chains often demonstrable in superficial zone with either Giemsa (organisms blue) or Brown–Brenn (organisms red) stains

C. Primary syphilis

1. Erosion, ulceration, or epidermal hyperplasia with variable spongiosis and invasion by neutrophils
2. Dense, diffuse, and perivascular infiltrate composed of plasma cells, lymphocytes, and histiocytic cells
3. Neutrophils prominent only in infiltrate beneath ulceration
4. Marked vascular proliferation with endothelial cell swelling

Silver stains (see Ch. 3) demonstrate numerous spirochetes around vessels and occasionally within epithelium

D. Rhinoscleroma

1. Epithelial hyperplasia may be extreme
2. Dense infiltrate of many plasma cells, with histiocytic cells, lymphocytes, and neutrophils
3. Large (100–200 μm) vacuolated histiocytes called **Mikulicz cells** contain organisms
4. Round, eosinophilic, homogeneous extracellular and intracellular **Russell bodies** may be prominent
5. Fibrosis common in older lesions

Cutaneous involvement restricted to nose
Causative organism: *Klebsiella rhinoscleromatis*
2- to 3-μm, oval to round, rodshaped, encapsulated organisms within Mikulicz cells are best visualized with Warthin–Starry or Giemsa stains

Differential diagnosis:
Leishmaniasis
Histoplasmosis
Granuloma inguinale
Squamous cell carcinoma
Lepromatous leprosy
Syphilis

Fig. **18-10.** *Chancroid.*
A. *Penile ulcer with adjacent epithelium and underlying dermal zones characteristic of chancroid.*
B. *Zone A consists of neutrophils. Zone B consists of vascular proliferation. Zone C consists of plasma cells.*

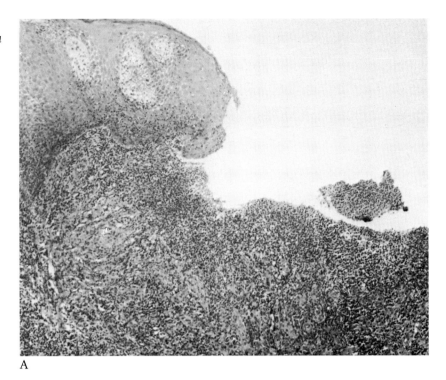

A

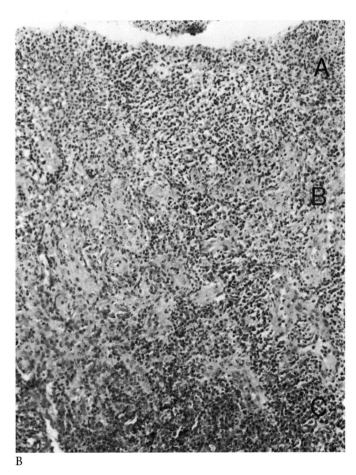

B

E. Histoplasmosis

1. Epidermis may be ulcerated
2. Diffuse dermal infiltrate composed of histiocytic cells and giant cells
3. Organisms present in histiocytic cells

Causative organism: *Histoplasma capsulatum*

Organisms may be visualized in H&E-stained sections but are better seen with PAS and methenamine silver stains. Organisms are present as spores measuring 2 to 5 μm

---

Obligate *intrahistiocytic organisms* occur in:

Granuloma inguinale
Leishmaniasis
Histoplasmosis
Rhinoscleroma

F. Leishmaniasis (Fig. 18-11)

1. Epidermis may be normal, flattened, hyperplastic, or ulcerated
2. Dense infiltrate composed primarily of histiocytic cells mixed with epithelioid cells, lymphocytes, plasma cells, and occasional giant cells
3. Edematous stroma with proliferation and ectasia of vessels
4. Variable fibrosis
5. Organisms more frequently found in deep dermis within histiocytic and epithelioid cells and free in tissue

Causative organisms:
Leishmania tropica
L. braziliensis
L. donovani

2 to 3 μm in diameter, round to oval organisms with thin cell wall, large nucleus, and rodshaped paranucleus (kinetoplast) are visible in sections stained with H&E; Giemsa stain accentuates nucleus and kinetoplast

Late lesions may show epithelioid cell granuloma and few organisms

Differential diagnosis:
Lepromatous leprosy
Xanthoma
Histoplasmosis
Cryptococcosis and other deep mycoses

Fig. **18-11.** *Leishmaniasis. The organisms measure 2 to 4 μm and are intracellular, within histiocytic cells.*

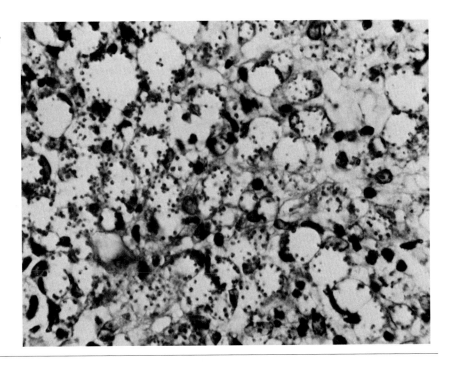

G. Granuloma inguinale

1. Epithelium adjacent to ulceration commonly hyperplastic with spongiosis and intraepithelial neutrophilic abscesses
2. Dense, dermal or submucosal infiltrate with **neutrophilic microabscesses surrounded by** plasma cells, histiocytic cells, and lymphocytes

Causative organism:
   Calymmatobacterium granulomatis

Intracytoplasmic inclusion (Donovan) bodies visible as either 1- to 2-μm, black, oval to rod-shaped structures with silver stains or as encapsulated bipolar "safety pin" bodies with Giemsa stain; these organisms are better visualized in smears or touch preps from biopsy material rather than tissue section

Differential diagnosis:
   Syphilis
   Squamous cell carcinoma

Obligate *intrahistiocytic organisms* occur in:

Granuloma inguinale (E)*
Leishmaniasis
Histoplasmosis
Rhinoscleroma (E)

---

*(E), encapsulated organisms.

Suggested Reading

Xanthomas

Altman, J., and Winkelmann, R. K. Diffuse normolipemic plane xanthoma: Generalized xanthelasma. *Arch. Dermatol.* 85:633, 1962.

Bulkley, B. H., Buja, L. M., Ferrans, V. J., et al. Tuberous xanthoma in homozygous type II hyperlipoproteinaemia: A histologic, histochemical, and electron microscopy study. *Arch. Pathol.* 99:293, 1975.

Cho, H. R., Lee, M. H., and Haw, C. R. Generalized tuberous xanthoma with type IV hyperlipoproteinemia. *Cutis* 59:315–318, 1997.

Cooper, P. H. Eruptive xanthoma: A microscopic simulant of granuloma annulare. *J. Cutan. Pathol.* 13:207–215, 1986.

Crowe, M. J., and Gross, D. J. Eruptive xanthoma. *Cutis* 50:31–32, 1992.

Ferrando, J., and Bombi, J. A. Ultrastructural aspects of normolipidemic xanthomatosis. *Arch. Dermatol. Res.* 266:143, 1979.

Filling-Katz, M. R., Miller, S. P., Merrick, H. F., Travis, W. D., Greeg, R. E., Tsokos, M., Comly, M., et al. Clinical, pathologic, and biochemical features of a cholesterol lipidosis accompanied by hyperlipidemia an xanthomas. *Neurology* 42:1768–1774, 1992.

Marcoval, J., Moreno, A., Bordas, X., Gallardo, F., and Peyri, J. Diffuse plane xanthoma: Clinicopathologic study of 8 cases. *J. Am. Acad. Dermatol.* 39:439–442, 1998.

Modiano, P., Gillet-Terver, M. N., Reichert, S., Francois-Griffaton, A., Beaumont, J. L., Weber, M., and Schmutz, J. L. Normolipemic plane xanthoma, monoclonal gammopathy, anti-lipoprotein activity, hypocomplementemia. *Ann. Dermatol. Venereol.* 122:507–508, 1995.

Parker, F. Xanthomas and hyperlipidemias. *J. Am. Acad. Dermatol.* 13:1, 1985.

Parker, F., Bagdade, J. D., Odland, G. F., and Bierman, E. L. Evidence for the chylomicron origin of lipids accumulation in diabetic eruptive xanthomas: A correlative lipid biochemical, histiochemical and electron microscopic study. *J. Clin. Invest.* 49:2172, 1970.

Parker, F., and Odland, G. F. Electron microscopic similarities between experimental xanthomas and human eruptive xanthomas. *J. Invest. Dermatol.* 52:136, 1969.

Zemel, H., Deeken, J., Asel, N., and Packer, J. The ultrastructural features of normolipemic plane xanthoma. *Arch. Pathol.* 89:111, 1970.

Leprosy

Azulay, R. D. Histopathology of skin lesions in leprosy. *Int. J. Lepr.* 39:244, 1971.

Liu, T-C., Yen, L-Z., Ye, G-Y., and Dung, G. L. Histology of indeterminate leprosy. *Int. J. Lepr.* 50:172, 1982.

Modlin, R. L., Hotman, F. M., Taylor, C. R., and Rea, T. H. T-lymphocyte subsets in the skin lesions of patients with leprosy. *J. Am. Acad. Dermatol.* 8:182, 1983.

Ridley, D. S. Histological classification and the immunological spectrum of leprosy. *Bull. W.H.O.* 51:451, 1974.

Ridley, D. S., and Joplin, W. H. Classification of leprosy according to immunity. A five-group system. *Int. J. Lepr.* 34:255, 1966.

Sehgal, V. N. *Clinical Leprosy* (3rd ed.). New Delhi: Jaypee Brothers, 1993.

Sehgal, V. N. Leprosy. *Dermatol. Clin.* 12:629–644, 1994.

Van Voorhis, W. C., Kaplan, G., Nunes Sarno, E., Horowitz, M. A., Steinman, R. M., Levis, W. R., Nogueira, N., et al. The cutaneous infiltrates of leprosy. Cellular characteristics and the predominant T-cell phenotypes. *N. Engl. J. Med.* 307:1593–1597, 1982.

Langerhans cell histiocytosis

Axiotis, C. A., Merino, M. J., and Duray, P. H. Langerhans cell histiocytosis of the female genital tract. *Cancer* 67:1650–1660, 1991.

Caputo, R., and Gianotti, F. Cytoplasmic markers ultrastructural features in histiocytic proliferations of the skin. *J. Ital. Dermatol. Venereol.* 115:107, 1980.

Caputo, R., Grimalut, R., Laterza, A., Bencini, P. L., and Veraldi, S. Mucocutaneous expressions of Langerhans cell histiocytosis in adults. *Eur. J. Dermatol.* 4:528–531, 1994.

Ceci, A., de Terlizzi, M., Coiella, R., Loiacono, G., Balducci, D., Surico, G., Castello, M., et al. Langerhans cell histiocytosis in childhood: Results from the Italian Cooperative AIEOP-CNR-H.X '83 study. *Med. Pediatr. Oncol.* 21:259–264, 1993.

Divaris, D. X. G., Ling, F. C. K., and Prentice, R. S. A. Congenital self-healing histiocytosis. Report of two cases with histochemical and ultrastructural studies. *Am. J. Dermatopathol.* 13:481–487, 1991.

Favara, B. E. Langerhans cell histiocytosis: Pathobiology and pathogenesis. *Semin. Oncol.* 18:3–7, 1991.

Komp, D. M. Langerhans cell histiocytosis. N. *Engl. J. Med.* 316:747–748, 1987.

Meehan, S., and Smoller, B. R. Langerhans cell histiocytosis of the genitalia in the elderly: A unique clinical pathologic presentation. *J. Cutan. Pathol.* 25:370–374, 1998.

Mierau, G. W., Favara, B. E., and Brenman, J. M. Electron microscopy in histiocytosis X. *Ultrastruct. Pathol.* 3:137, 1982.

Murphy, G. F., Harrist, T. J., Bhan, A. K., and Mihm, M. C., Jr. Distribution of cell surface antigens in histiocytosis X cells: Quantitative immunoelectron microscopy using monoclonal antibodies. *Lab. Invest.* 48:90, 1983.

Risdall, R. J., Dehner, L. P., Duray, P., et al. Histiocytosis X (Langerhans' cell histiocytosis): Prognostic role of histopathology. *Arch. Pathol. Lab. Med.* 107:59, 1983.

Zelger, B., Cerio, R., Orchard, G., Fritsch, P., and Wilson-Jones, E. Histologic and immunohistochemical study comparing xanthoma disseminatum and histiocytosis X. *Arch. Dermatol.* 128:1207–1212, 1992.

Xanthogranuloma

Flach, D. B., and Winkelmann, R. K. Juvenile xanthogranuloma with central nervous system lesions. *J. Am. Acad. Dermatol.* 14:405, 1986.

Guinnepain, M. T., and Puissant, A. Juvenile xanthogranuloma. *J. Ital. Dermatol. Venereol.* 115:101, 1980.

Helwig, E. B., and Hackney, V. C. Juvenile xanthogranuloma (nevoxanthoendothelioma). *Am. J. Pathol.* 30:625, 1954.

Rodriguez, J., and Ackerman, A. B. Xanthogranuloma in adults. *Arch. Dermatol.* 112:43, 1976.

Rotte, J. J., de Vaan, G. A., and Koopman, R. J. Juvenile xanthogranuloma and acute leukemia: A case report. *Med. Pediatr. Oncol.* 23:57–59, 1994.

Webster, S. B., Reister, H. C., and Harman, L. E. Juvenile xanthogranuloma with extracutaneous lesions. *Arch. Dermatol.* 93:71, 1966.

Zvulunov, A., Barak, Y., and Metzker, A. Juvenile xanthogranuloma, neurofibromatosis, and juvenile myelogenous leukemia. World statistical analysis. *Arch. Dermatol.* 131:904–908, 1995.

Reticulohistiocytosis

Barrow, M. V., and Holubar, K. Multicentric reticulohistiocytosis: A review of 33 patients. *Medicine* 48:287, 1969.

Goltz, R. W., and Laymon, C. W. Multicentric reticulohistiocytosis of the skin and synovia: Reticulohistiocytoma or ganglioneuroma. *Arch. Dermatol.* 69:717, 1954.

Heathcote, J. G., Guenther, L. C., and Wallace, A. C. Multicentric reticulohistiocytosis: A report of a case and a review of the pathology. *Pathology* 17:601, 1985.

Lesher, J. L., Jr., and Allen, B. S. Multicentric reticulohistiocytosis: A review of 33 patients. *Medicine* 48:287, 1969.

Nunnink, J. C., Krusinksi, P. A., and Yates, J. W. Multicentric reticulohistiocytosis and cancer: A case report and review of the literature. *Med. Pediatr. Oncol.* 13:273, 1985.

Perrin, C., Lacour, J. P., Michiels, J. F., Flory, P., Ziegler, G., and Ortonne, J. P. Multicentric reticulohistiocytosis. Immunohistochemical and ultrastructural study: A pathology of dendritic cell lineage. *Am. J. Dermatopathol.* 14:418–425, 1992.

Tani, M., Hori, K., Nakanishi, T., et al. Multicentric reticulohistiocytosis: Electron microscopic and ultracytochemical studies. *Arch. Dermatol.* 117:495, 1981.

Turner, R. R., Wood, G. S., Beckstead, H. J., et al. Histiocytic malignancies: Morphologic, immunologic, and enzymatic heterogeneity. *Am. J. Surg. Pathol.* 8:485, 1984.

Valencia, I. C., Colsky, A., and Berman, B. Multicentric reticulohistiocytosis associated with recurrent breast carcinoma. *J. Am. Acad. Dermatol.* 39:864–866, 1998.

Lymphoma Cutis

Agnarsson, B. A., and Kadin, M. E. Ki-1 positive large cell lymphoma: A morphologic and immunologic study of 19 cases. *Am. J. Surg. Pathol.* 21:264–274, 1988.

Chan, J. K. C., Ng, C. S., Hui, P. K., Leung, T. W., Los, E. S., Lau, W. H., and McGuire, L. J. Anaplastic large cell Ki-1 lymphoma. Delineation of two morphologic types. *Histopathology* 15:11–34, 1989.

Chan, J. K. C., Ng, C. S., Ngan, K. C., Hui, P. K., Lo, S. T., and Lau, W. H. Angiocentric T-cell lymphoma of the skin. *Am. J. Surg. Pathol.* 12:861–876, 1988.

Chott, A., Kaserer, K., Augustin, I., Vesely, M., Heniz, R., Oehlinger, W., Hanak, H., et al. Ki-1-positive large cell lymphoma. A clinicopathologic study of 41 cases. Am. J. Surg. Pathol. 14:439–448, 1990.

Crane, G. A., Variakojis, D., Rosen, S. T., Sands, A. M., and Roenigk, J. Cutaneous T-cell lymphoma in patients with human immunodeficiency virus infection. Arch. Dermatol. 127:989–994, 1991.

Dabski, K., Banks, P. M., and Winkelmann, R. K. Clinicopathologic spectrum of cutaneous manifestations in systemic follicular lymphoma. A study of 11 patients. Cancer 64:1480–1485, 1989.

Davis, T. H., Morton, C. C., Miller-Cassman, R., Balk, S. P., and Kadin, M. E. Hodgkin's disease, lymphomatoid papulosis, and cutaneous T-cell lymphoma derived from a common T-cell clone. N. Engl. J. Med. 326:1115–1122, 1992.

Evans, H. L., Winkelmann, R. K., and Banks, P. M. Differential diagnosis of malignant and benign cutaneous lymphoid infiltrates. Cancer 44:699, 1979.

Fisher, E. R., Park, E. J., and Wechsler, H. L. Histologic identification of malignant lymphoma cutis. Am. J. Clin. Pathol. 65:149, 1976.

Greer, J. P., Kinney, M. C., Collins, R. D., Salhany, K. E., Wolff, S. N., Hainsworth, J. D., Flexner, J. M., et al. Clinical features of 31 patients with Ki-1 anaplastic large cell lymphoma. J. Clin. Oncol. 9:539–547, 1991.

Lukes, R. J. The immunologic approach to the pathology of malignant lymphomas. Am. J. Clin. Pathol. 72:657, 1979.

Mehregan, D. A., Su, W. P. D., and Kurtin, P. J. Subcutaneous T-cell lymphoma: A clinical, histopathologic, and immunohistochemical study of six cases. J. Cutan. Pathol. 21:110–117, 1994.

Natkuranan, Y., Smoller, B. R., Zehnder, J. L., Dorfman, R. F., and Warnke, R. A. Aggressive cutaneous NK and NK-like T-cell lymphomas: Clinicopathologic, immunohistochemical, and molecular analyses of 12 cases. Am. J. Surg. Pathol. 23:571–581, 1999.

Perniciaro, C., Winkelmann, R. K., Daoud, M. S., and Su, W. P. D. Malignant angioendotheliomatosis is an angiotropic intravascular lymphoma. Immunohistochemical, ultrastructural, and molecular genetics studies. Am. J. Dermatopathol. 17:242–248, 1995.

Sander, C. A., Kind, P., Kaudewitz, P., Raffeld, M., and Jaffe, E. S. The revised European–American classification of lymphoid neoplasms (REAL): a new perspective for the classification of cutaneous lymphomas. J. Cutan. Pathol. 24:329–341, 1997.

Shimoyama, M., Minato, K., Saito, H., et al. Comparison of clinical, morphologic, and immunologic characteristics of adult T-cell leukemia-lymphoma and cutaneous T-cell leukemia: A clinicopathologic study of five cases. Blood 62:758, 1983.

Sleater, J. P., Segal, G. H., Scott, M. D., and Masih, A. S. Intravascular (angiotropic) large cell lymphoma: Determination of monoclonality by polymerase chain reaction on paraffin-embedded tissues. Mod. Pathol. 7:593–598, 1994.

Smith, J. L., and Butler, J. J. Skin involvement in Hodgkin's disease. Cancer 45:354, 1980.

Sterry, W., Korte, B., and Schubert, C. Pleomorphic T-cell lymphoma and large cell anaplastic lymphoma of the skin. Am. J. Dermatopathol. 11:112–123, 1989.

Su, I. J., Hseih, H. C., Lin, K. H., Uen, W. C., Kao, C. L., Chen, C. J., Cheng, A. L., et al. Aggressive peripheral T-cell lymphomas containing Epstein–Barr viral DNA: A clinicopathologic and molecular analysis. Blood 77:799–808, 1991.

Plasmacytoma

Alberts, D. S., and Lynch, P. Cutaneous plasmacytomas in myeloma. Arch. Dermatol. 114:1784, 1978.

Mikhail, G. R., Spindler, A. C., and Kelly, A. P. Malignant plasmacytoma cutis. Arch. Dermatol. 101:59, 1979.

Torne, R., Su, W. P. D., Winkelmann, R. K., Smolle, J., and Kerl, H. Clinicopathologic study of cutaneous plasmacytoma. Int. J. Dermatol. 29:562–566, 1990.

Wuepper, K. D., and MacKenzie, M. R. Cutaneous extramedullary plasmacytomas. Arch. Dermatol. 100:155, 1969.

Urticaria Pigmentosa

Burgoon, C. F., Graham, J. H., and McCaffree, D. L. Mast cell disease: A cutaneous variant with multisystem involvement. Arch. Dermatol. 98:590, 1968.

Monheit, G. D., Murad, T., and Conrad, M. Systemic mastocytosis and the mastocytosis syndrome. J. Cutan. Pathol. 6:42, 1979.

Eosinophilic Cellulitis

Spigel, G. T., and Winkelmann, R. K. Well's syndrome: Recurrent granulomatous dermatitis with eosinophilia. *Arch. Dermatol.* 115:611, 1979.

Stern, J. B., Sobel, H. J., and Rotchford, J. P. Well's syndrome: Is there collagen damage in the flame figures? *J. Cutan. Pathol.* 11:501, 1984.

Wells, G. C., and Smith, N. P. Eosinophilic cellulitis. *Br. J. Dermatol.* 100:101, 1979.

Hodgkin's Disease

Cerroni, L., Beham-Schmidt, C., and Kerl, H. Cutaneous Hodgkin's disease: An immunohistiocemical analysis. *J. Cutan. Pathol.* 22:229–235. 1995.

Morman, M. R., and Petrozzi, J. W. Cutaneous Hodgkin's disease. *Cutis* 26:483–484, 1980.

Shaw, M. T., and Jacobs, S. R. Cutaneous Hodgkin's disease in a patient with human immunodeficiency virus infection. *Cancer* 64:2585–2587, 1989.

Smith, J. L., and Butler, J. J. Skin involvement in Hodgkin's disease. *Cancer* 45:354, 1980.

Mycosis Fungoides

Degreef, H., Holvoet, C., Van Vloten, W. A., et al. Woringer–Kolopp disease: An epidermotropic variant of mycosis fungoides. *Cancer* 38:2154, 1976.

Jimbow, K., Chiba, M., and Horikoshi, T. Electron microscope identification of Langerhans cells in the dermal infiltrates of mycosis fungoides. *J. Invest Dermatol.* 78:102, 1982.

Lutzner, M., Edelson, R., Schein, P., et al. Cutaneous T-cell lymphomas: The Sezary syndrome, mycosis fungoides and related disorders. *Ann. Intern. Med.* 83:534, 1975.

McMillan, E. M., Wasik, R., and Everett, M. A. In situ demonstration of T cell subsets in atrophic parapsoriasis. *J. Am. Acad. Dermatol.* 6:32, 1982.

McNutt, N. S., and Crain, W. R. Quantitative electron microscopic comparison of lymphocyte nuclear contours in mycosis fungoides and in benign infiltrates in skin. *Cancer* 47:698, 1981.

Picker, L. J., Weiss, L. M., Medeires, L. J., et al. Immunophenotypic criteria for the diagnosis of non-Hodgkin's lymphoma. *Am. J. Pathol.* 128:181, 1987.

Smoller B. R., Bishop, K., Glusac, E. J., Kim, Y. H., and Hendrickson, M. R. Re-evaluation of histologic parameters in diagnosing mycosis fungoides. *Am. J. Surg. Pathol.* 19:1423–1430, 1995.

Waldorf, D. S., Ratner, A. C., and Van Scott, E. J. Cells in lesions of mycosis fungoides lymphoma following therapy: Changes in number and type. *Cancer* 21:264, 1968.

Weiss, L. M., Hu, E., Wood, G. S., et al. Clonal rearrangements of T-cell receptor genes in mycosis fungoides and dermatopathic lymphadenopathy. *N. Engl. J. Med.* 313:539, 1985.

Chancroid

Freinkel, A. L. Histological aspects of sexually transmitted genital lesions *Histopathology* 11:819, 1987.

Margolis, R. J., and Hood, A. F. Chancroid: Diagnosis and treatment. *J. Am. Acad. Dermatol.* 6:493, 1982.

Sheldon, W. H., and Weyman, A. Studies on chancroid. I. Observations on the histology with an evaluation of biopsy as a diagnostic procedure. *Am. J. Pathol.* 22:415, 1946.

Rhinoscleroma

Hyams, V. J. Rhinoscleroma. In C. H. Binford and D. H. Connor (Eds.), *Pathology of Tropical and Extraordinary Diseases,* Vol. I. Washington, D.C.: Armed Forces Institute of Pathology, 1976, pp. 187–189.

Tapia, A. Rhinoscleroma: A naso-oral dermatosis. *Cutis* 40:101, 1987.

Leishmaniasis

Grevelink, S. A., and Lerner, E. A. Leishmaniasis. *J. Am. Acad. Dermatol.* 34:257–272, 1996.

Kenner, J. R., Aronson, N. E., Bratthauer, G. L., Turnicky, R. P., Jackson, J. E., Tang, P. B., and Sau, P. Immunohistochemistry to identify *Leishmania* parasites in fixed tissues. *J. Cutan. Pathol.* 26:130–136, 1999.

Kurban, A. K., Malak, J. A., Farah, F. S., et al. Histopathology of cutaneous leishmaniasis. *Arch. Dermatol.* 93:396–401, 1966.

Sangueza, O. P., Sangueza, J. M., Stiller, M. J., and Sangueza, P. Mucocutaneous leishmaniasis: A clinicopathologic classification. *J. Am. Acad. Dermatol.* 28:927–932, 1993.

Granuloma Inguinale

Davis, C. M. Granuloma inguinale: A clinical, histological and ultrastructural study. JAMA 211:632, 1970.

Rosen, T., Tschen, J. A., Ransdell, W., et al. Granuloma inguinale. J. Am. Acad. Dermatol. 11:433, 1984.

Sehgal, V. N., Shyamprasad, A. L., and Bechar, P. E. The histopathological diagnosis of donovanosis. Br. J. Venereol. Dis. 60:45, 1984.

Chapter 19

Nodular Infiltrate

    I. Lymphocytoma cutis
   II. Arthropod bite reaction
  III. Angiolymphoid hyperplasia with eosinophilia
  IV. Lymphoma cutis, nodular pattern
      A. Monomorphous infiltrate (non-Hodgkin's lymphoma)
   V. Tertiary syphilis

Recognition of a nodular infiltrate implies a certain cohesiveness in the cellular patterning. The entities discussed in this chapter are grouped because of their predominant lymphoid component. Nodular infiltrates also arise with nonlymphoid tumors such as carcinoma, metastases, and benign neoplasms, including histiocytoid hemangioma. These conditions are described elsewhere. Distinguishing between lymphocytoma cutis and lymphoma cutis may be challenging and occasionally impossible.

The Reactive Process and the Disease	Histopathology	Comments
I. Lymphocytoma cutis (Fig. 19-1)	1. Normal or sometimes atrophic epidermis 2. Sparing of the upper dermis (Grenz zone) 3. Dense nodular aggregates of lymphocytes and histiocytic cells admixed with occasional eosinophils 4. Infiltrate present in the reticular dermis, occasionally in a perivascular or perifollicular array	Lymphadenitis benign cutis, an entity more commonly seen in Europe, is a form of lymphocytoma cutis related to infection with *Borrelia burgdorferi*
	5. **Germinal centers (lymphoid follicles)** often present	Lymphoid follicles are made up of a collection of large, pale lymphoblasts and macrophages containing nuclear debris (tingible bodies), surrounded by small, mature lymphocytes; the presence of lymphoid follicles may help differentiate lymphocytoma from lymphoma cutis

Lymphoid follicles may be seen in:

Lymphocytoma cutis
Insect bite reaction
Angiolymphoid hyperplasia with eosinophilia
Lymphoma cutis
Necrobiosis lipoidica
Lupus profundus
Necrobiotic xanthogranuloma

Differential diagnosis:
  Lymphoma cutis
  Arthropod bite reaction
  Angiolymphoid hyperplasia with eosinophilia

Fig. **19-1.** *Lymphocytoma cutis. This section contains nodular aggregates of lymphoid cells within the reticular dermis.*

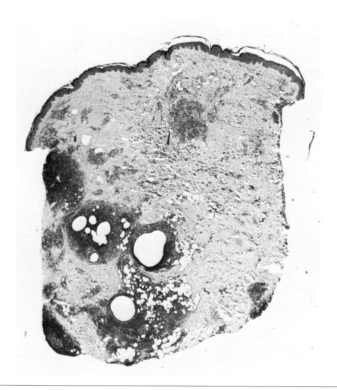

II. Arthropod bite reaction (see Fig. 16-2)

1. Hyperkeratosis and/or crust
2. Epidermal hyperplasia may be marked
3. Ulceration at site of puncta
4. Bandlike or nodular, polymorphous infiltrate composed of lymphocytes and many **eosinophils** with variable numbers of plasma cells and neutrophils
5. Occasional germinal center formation
6. Prominent endothelial cell swelling and vascular proliferation

See also Ch. 5, III.A; Ch. 12, IV; Ch. 13, I.F; Ch. 16, I.A.2

May be indistinguishable from lymphocytoma cutis

III. Angiolymphoid hyperplasia
with eosinophilia (Fig. 19-2)

1. Epidermis normal
2. Aggregates of lymphocytes with histiocytic cells and eosinophils; **eosinophils** and plasma cells scattered between collagen fibers throughout dermis
3. Lymphoid follicles may be present
4. Dermal hemorrhage and hemosiderin deposition common
5. Sheetlike cellular aggregates composed of histiocytic cells and/or endothelial cells
6. Numerous **prominent vessels,** occasionally branching and stellate
7. Plump endothelial cells protrude into vascular lumen ("hobnail" appearance)
8. Proliferation of delicate reticulin fibers and deposition of acid mucopolysaccharide around vessels

Fig. **19-2.** *Angiolymphoid hyperplasia with eosinophilia.*
A. There is a diffuse infiltrate of lymphoid cells and endothelial cells within the reticular dermis.
B. Higher magnification reveals a polymorphous lymphoid infiltrate and vessels with plump, "hobnail" nuclei.

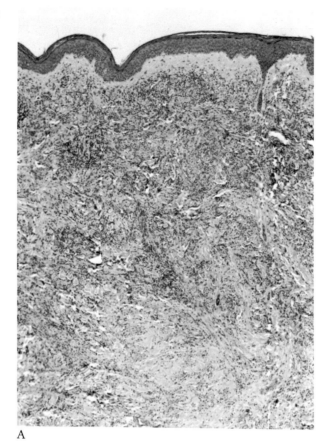

A

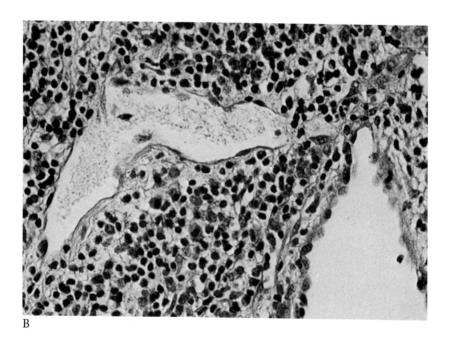

B

Fig. **19-3.** Lymphoma cutis. The
nodular quality of this B-cell lymphoma
is evident in the clustering of lymphoid
follicles that comprise this tumor nodule
(A). Atypical cells with nuclear
pleomorphism are seen at higher
magnification (B).

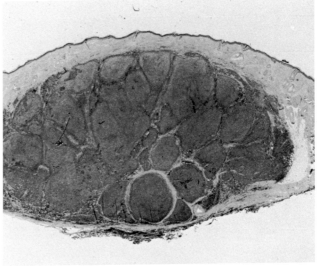

A

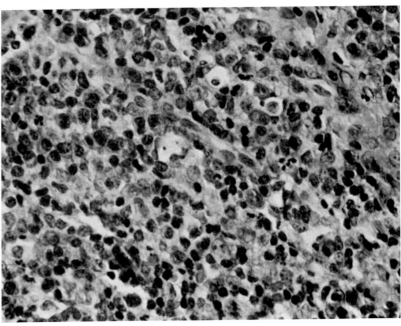

B

IV. Lymphoma cutis, nodular pattern (Fig. 19-3)

A. Monomorphous infiltrate (non-Hodgkin's lymphoma)

1. Epidermis usually normal
2. Papillary dermis spared (Grenz zone)
3. Dense nodular aggregates of lymphoid cells at any level of the reticular dermis or into subcutaneous fat
4. Nuclear atypia and atypical mitoses characteristic, though quantitatively variable
5. Cells often infiltrate between collagen fibers in a linear array
6. Nuclei, packed tightly together, appear distorted and "smudged"

The term *nodular* refers to two different histologic patterns:

1. Discrete aggregates within the dermis with little or no accompanying infiltrate
2. Diffuse infiltrate of cells in reticular dermis within which a distinct nodularity is evident.

Both patterns can be associated with the diagnosis of lymphoma cutis. The first pattern is relatively nonspecific, and the second pattern is consistent with a B-cell lymphoma.

Lymphocyte immunophenotypic characterization is very helpful in separating benign from malignant infiltrates and in classifying the lymphomas (Table 19-1)

Table **19-1.** *Features Helpful in Distinguishing Lymphocytoma from Lymphoma Cutis*

	Lymphocytoma	Lymphoma
Location of infiltrate	Predominantly upper dermis "top heavy"	Predominantly lower dermis and subcutis "bottom heavy"
Lymphoid follicles	Common	Uncommon (typical of some B-cell lymphomas)
Ulceration	Very uncommon	Occasionally seen
Cell composition	Polymorphous, including eosinophils and plasma cells	Often monomorphous; Hodgkin's disease and mycosis fungoides often have accompanying eosinophils
Cytologic features		
Nuclear atypia	Absent[a]	Hyperchromatism Pleomorphism frequent
Nucleoli	Inconspicuous	May be large and often multiple
Mitotic figures	Infrequent, not atypical[a]	Often numerous, may be atypical
Crush artifact	Uncommon	Common

[a] The cells within germinal centers of lymphoid follicles are often large and somewhat pleomorphic and exhibit mitotic figures.

Differential diagnosis:
  Lymphomatoid papulosis
  Cutaneous T-cell lymphoma
  Lymphocytoma cutis
  Arthropod bite reaction
  Mycosis fungoides
See also Ch. 18, VII.A

V. Tertiary syphilis

1. Epidermis normal, flattened, or ulcerated
2. Edema of papillary dermis with mild perivascular lymphohistiocytic and plasma cell infiltrate
3. Perivascular and periappendageal nodular infiltrate composed of aggregates of epithelioid and giant cells surrounded by lymphocytes, histiocytic cells, and plasma cells
4. Endothelial cell proliferation prominent and may produce narrowing and/or obliteration of vessel lumen

The overall dermal infiltrate may take on a nodular pattern

See also Ch. 16, II.L; Ch. 17, III.I

Suggested Reading

Lymphocytoma Cutis

Caro, W. A., and Helwig, E. B. Cutaneous lymphoid hyperplasia. *Cancer* 24:487, 1969.

Clark, W. H., Mihm, M. C., Jr., Reed, R. J., and Ainsworth, A. M. The lymphocytic infiltrates of the skin. *Hum. Pathol.* 5:25, 1974.

Evans, H. L., Winkelmann, R. K., and Banks, P. M. Differential diagnosis of malignant and benign cutaneous lymphoid infiltrates. *Cancer* 44:699, 1979.

Mach, K. W., and Wilgram, G. F. Characteristic histopathology of cutaneous lymphoplasia (lymphocytoma). *Arch. Dermatol.* 94:26, 1966.

Arthropod Bite Reaction

Fernandez, N., Torres, A., and Ackerman, A. B. Pathologic findings in human scabies. *Arch. Dermatol.* 113:320, 1977.

Goldman, L., Rockwell, E., and Richfield, D. F., III. Histopathological studies on cutaneous reactions to the bites of various arthropods. *Am. J. Trop. Med. Hyg.* 1:514, 1952.

Horen, W. P. Insect and scorpion sting. *JAMA* 221:894, 1972.

Larrivee, D. H., Benjamini, E., Feingold, B. F., et al. Histologic studies of guinea pig skin: Different stages of allergic reactivity to flea bites. *Exp. Parasitol.* 15:491, 1964.

Steffen, C. Clinical and histopathologic correlation of midge bites. *Arch. Dermatol.* 117:785, 1981.

Thomson, J., Cochran, T., Cochran, R., and McQueen, A. Histology simulating reticulosis in persistent nodular scabies. *Br. J. Dermatol.* 90:421, 1974.

Angiolymphoid Hyperplasia

Henry, P. G., and Burnett, J. W. Angiolymphoid hyperplasia with eosinophilia. *Arch. Dermatol.* 114:1168, 1978.

Olsen, T. G., and Helwig, E. B. Angiolymphoid hyperplasia with eosinophilia. A clinicopathologic study of 116 patients. *J. Am. Acad. Dermatol.* 12:781, 1985.

Lymphoma Cutis

Agnarsson, B. A., and Kadin, M. E. Ki-1 positive large cell lymphoma: A morphologic and immunologic study of 19 cases. *Am. J. Surg. Pathol.* 21:264–274, 1988.

Chan, J. K. C., Ng, C. S., Hui, P. K., Leung, T. W., Los, E. S., Lau, W. H., and McGuire, L. J. Anaplastic large cell Ki-1 lymphoma. Delineation of two morphologic types. *Histopathology* 15:11–34, 1989.

Chan, J. K. C., Ng, C. S., Ngan, K. C., Hui, P. K., Lo, S. T., and Lau, W. H. Angiocentric T-cell lymphoma of the skin. *Am. J. Surg. Pathol.* 12:861–876, 1988.

Chott, A., Kaserer, K., Augustin, T., Vesely, M., Heniz, R., Oehlinger, W., Hanak, H., et al., Ki-1-positive large cell lymphoma. A clinicopathologic study of 41 cases. *Am. J. Surg. Pathol.* 14:439–448, 1990.

Cozzutto, C., DeBernardi, B., Comelli, A., and Mori, P. Primary cutaneous lymphoma with a nodular pattern in infancy. *Cancer* 54:603, 1980.

Crane, G. A., Variakojis, D., Rosen, S. T., Sands, A. M., and Roenigk, J. Cutaneous T-cell lymphoma in patients with human immunodeficiency virus infection. *Arch. Dermatol.* 127:989–994, 1991.

Dabski, K., Banks, P. M., and Winkelmann, R. K. Clinicopathologic spectrum of cutaneous manifestations in systemic follicular lymphoma. A study of 11 patients. *Cancer* 64:1480–1485, 1989.

Davis, T. H., Morton, C. C., Miller-Cassman, R., Balk, S. P., and Kadin, M. E. Hodgkin's disease, lymphomatoid papulosis, and cutaneous T-cell lymphoma derived from a common T-cell clone. *N. Engl. J. Med.* 326:1115–1122, 1992.

Evans, H. L., Winkelmann, R. K., and Banks, P. M. Differential diagnosis of malignant and benign cutaneous lymphoid infiltrates. *Cancer* 44:699, 1979.

Greer, J. P., Kinney, M. C., Collins, R. D., Salhany, K. E., Wolff, S. N., Hainsworth, J. D., Flexner, J. M. et al. Clinical features of 31 patients with Ki-1 anaplastic large cell lymphoma. *J. Clin. Oncol.* 9:539–547, 1991.

Lukes, R. J. The immunologic approach to the pathology of malignant lymphomas. *Am. J. Clin. Pathol.* 72:657, 1979.

Mehregan, D. A., Su, W. P. D., and Kurtin, P. J. Subcutaneous T-cell lymphoma: A clinical, histopathologic, and immunohistochemical study of six cases. *J. Cutan. Pathol.* 21:110–117, 1994.

Natkuranan, Y., Smoller, B. R., Zehnder, J. L., Dorfman, R. F., and Warnke, R. A. Aggressive cutaneous NK and NK-like T-cell lymphomas: clinicopathologic, immunohistochemical, and molecular analyses of 12 cases. *Am. J. Surg. Pathol.* 23:571–581, 1999.

Perniciaro, C., Winkelmann, R. K., Daoud, M. S., and Su, W. P. D. Malignant angioendotheliomatosis is an angiotropic intravascular lymphoma. Immunohistochemical, ultrastructural, and molecular genetics studies. *Am. J. Dermatopathol.* 17:242–248, 1995.

Sander, C. A., Kind, P., Kaudewitz, P., Raffeld, M., and Jaffe, E. S. The revised European–American classification of lymphoid neoplasms (REAL): A new perspective for the classification of cutaneous lymphomas. *J. Cutan. Pathol.* 24:329–341, 1997.

Sleater, J. P., Segal, G. H., Scott, M. D., and Masih, A. S. Intravascular (angiotropic) large cell lymphoma: determination of monoclonality by polymerase chain reaction on paraffin-embedded tissues. *Mod. Pathol.* 7:593–598, 1994.

Smith, J. L., and Butler, J. J. Skin involvement in Hodgkin's disease. *Cancer* 45:354, 1980.

Sterry, W., Korte, B., and Schubert, C. Pleomorphic T-cell lymphoma and large cell anaplastic lymphoma of the skin. *Am. J. Dermatopathol.* 11:112–123, 1989.

Su, I. J., Hseih, H. C., Lin, K. H., Uen, W. C., Kao, C. L., Chen, C. J., Cheng, A. L., et al. Aggressive peripheral T-cell lymphomas containing Epstein–Barr viral DNA: A clinicopathologic and molecular analysis. *Blood* 77:799–808, 1991.

Wolk, B. H. Primary malignant lymphoma cutis. *Can. Med. Assoc. J.* 117:750, 1977.

Chapter **20**

Disorders of Collagen and Elastic Tissue

In all of the entities in this chapter, a significant alteration is found in collagen and/or elastic tissue. Certain diseases are easily recognized by either accompanying inflammation or epidermal changes. Certain diseases (e.g., noninflammatory anetoderma) display minimal or no findings in routinely stained sections. Special stains for collagen and elastic tissue are then very helpful, especially if it is possible to compare diseased and normal skin.

The Reactive Process and the Disease	Histopathology	Comments
I. Solar elastosis	1. Epidermal changes variable 2. Grenz zone of papillary dermis 3. Individual and clumped, **wavy, basophilic fibers** amid collagen of upper reticular dermis or admixed with **homogeneous gray-blue material** 4. Vessels in upper dermis often ectatic	Fibers and amorphous material stain positively with elastic tissue stain
II. Morphea		
A. Early stage (Fig. 20-1)	1. Epidermis normal 2. Closely packed, new collagen fibers in lower dermis that run parallel to long axis of epidermis; normal pattern of interlacing collagen bundles in lower dermis is lost 3. Moderately intense lymphocytic infiltrate at junction of reticular dermis and subcutis 4. Inflammation and widening of septa of subcutaneous fat by new collagen fibers 5. Rarely, plasma cells predominate in inflammatory infiltrate	Formalin-fixed skin biopsies typically exhibit a tapered or "cone" shape; thickened or sclerotic collagen produces a rectangular or square biopsy Differential diagnosis of a *"square" biopsy*: Normal skin of back Morphea/progressive systemic sclerosis Scar Chronic graft-versus-host reaction Radiodermatitis Connective tissue nevus Scleredema
B. Late stage	1. Epidermal atrophy 2. Bundles of dermal collagen fibers appear closely packed or **hyalinized** because of loss of interbundle space 3. Marked decrease in cellularity of dermis 4. Eccrine glands completely surrounded and **entrapped** by collagen with loss of adventitial fat 5. Inflammation present in subcutis; slight to absent elsewhere	Aggregates of inflammatory cells may be prominent in areas of fibrosis and may persist many years; the presence of inflammation favors the diagnosis of morphea over progressive systemic sclerosis Differential diagnosis: Scar Chronic graft-versus-host disease

Fig. **20-1.** *Morphea. Swelling of collagen bundles in the deep dermis is characteristic. Note also the trapped eccrine glands near the base of the field. The amount of inflammatory infiltrate is a variable feature in biopsies of this disorder.*

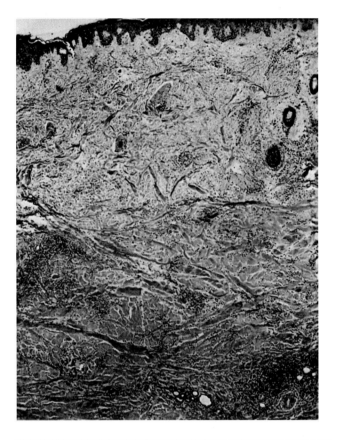

Fig. **20-2.** *Comparison of normal skin, scleroderma, and chronic radiodermatitis. Left, Normal skin: note the thickness of normal epidermis, the presence of pilosebaceous follicles and eccrine glands, and the appearance of normal collagen and perieccrine gland fat. Middle, Scleroderma: loss of pilosebaceous units, swollen and/or sclerotic collagen bundles, and "entrapped" eccrine glands are typical. Right, Chronic radiodermatitis: epidermal atrophy, hyalinized sclerotic collagen, vascular ectasia, loss of appendages, and bizarre "radiation fibroblasts" (inset) are characteristic.*

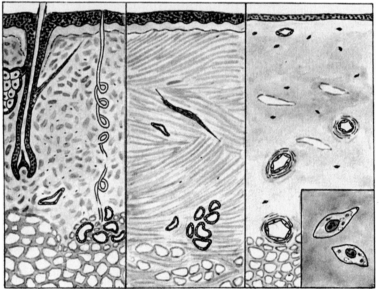

III. Progressive systemic sclerosis (scleroderma) (Figs. 20-1, 20-2)

Changes similar to those described for morphea except inflammation is usually minimal or absent

Systemic scleroderma in its early stages shows a mild inflammatory infiltrate

Late systemic scleroderma exhibits diminished vessels with frequent hyalinization of vessel walls and frequent luminal obliteration

IV. Sclerodermoid chronic graft-versus-host reaction

1. Basal vacuolization and dyskeratotic keratinocytes variably present
2. Dermal changes similar to those described for morphea except **sclerosis progresses from upper dermis downward**

V. Eosinophilic fasciitis

1. Inflammatory cell infiltrate in fascia, subcutis, and lower dermis, which is variable in intensity and composition
2. Eosinophils often present but not required for diagnosis
3. Plasma cells typically present
4. Dermal collagen changes variable but may be similar to morphea
5. Fascial collagen may be greatly increased and sclerotic

Peripheral eosinophilia may be observed

Changes similar to eosinophilic fasciitis are described in the eosinophilia–myalgia syndrome

VI. Radiodermatitis

    A. Acute stage

1. Frequent epidermal necrosis, even ulceration
2. **Prominent edema of dermis**
3. Fibroblasts in dermis often with **pyknotic nuclei**
4. Variable polymorphous inflammatory infiltrate throughout the dermis, especially in perivascular distribution
5. Swelling and occasional necrosis of endothelial cells

See also Ch. 11, I.E

    B. Chronic stage (Figs. 20-2, 20-3)

1. Hyperkeratosis and parakeratosis associated with epidermal hyperplasia and/or epidermal atrophy
2. Epidermal atypia with dyskeratosis
3. Variable ulceration
4. Increased melanin in basal layer
5. **Ectatic vessels** in upper dermis
6. Focal pigment incontinence with melanin free and within macrophages
7. Medium-sized arteries and veins exhibit fibrotic thickening of walls with frequent endothelial cell hyperplasia and luminal occlusion

Differential diagnosis:
    Lichen sclerosus et atrophicus
    Lupus erythematosus
    Scleroderma

Invasive squamous cell carcinoma may arise in areas of radio-dermatitis

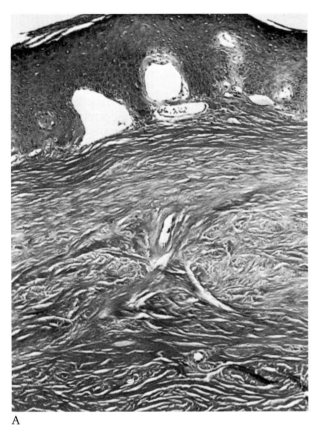

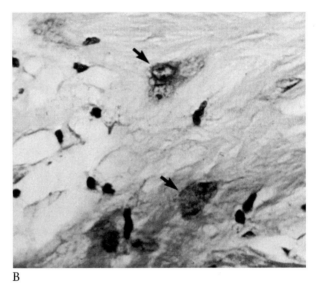

A   B

Fig. **20-3.** Chronic radiodermatitis. Superficial vascular ectasia with dense dermal fibrosis (A) and bizarre fibroblasts (B, arrows).

8. Hyalinized collagen **usually uniformly eosinophilic** from basement membrane zone to subcutaneous fat
9. Collagen fibers irregularly fragmented and often hyalinized
10. Fibroblasts exhibit irregular, large, variably pyknotic nuclei with variable shape; abundant cytoplasm of the so-called **radiation fibroblasts** is frequently vacuolated
11. Pilosebaceous units absent, eccrine glands preserved but atrophic

VII. Pseudoxanthoma elasticum (Fig. 20-4)

1. Epidermis normal
2. Grenz zone (normal papillary and reticular dermis)
3. **Swollen, fragmented, and irregularly clumped basophilic** (and sometimes eosinophilic) **fibers** in lower two-thirds of dermis
4. Foreign-body giant cells occasionally admixed with elastic fibers

Abnormal fibers stain both with elastic tissue and calcium stains (see Ch. 3)
Basophilia is due to calcium uptake by the fibers

Abnormal fibers may be eliminated transepidermally in perforating pseudoxanthoma elasticum, a disorder localized to the periumbilical skin of multiparous women

Fig. **20-4.** *Pseudoxanthoma elasticum. Elastic fiber alterations are noted in the mid-reticular dermis. Elastic fibers exhibit a characteristic frizzy appearance* (arrows). *Special stains* (*see* Ch. 3) *are recommended for optimal visualization of elastic fibers.*

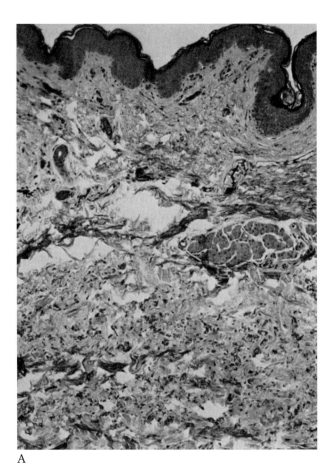

A

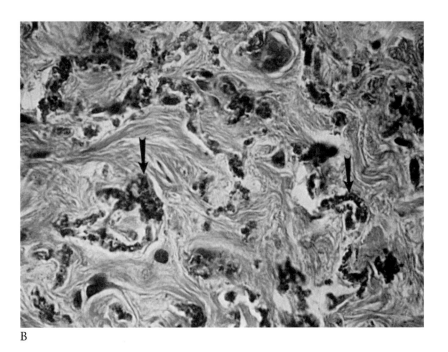

B

VIII. Ehlers–Danlos syndrome

No abnormal light microscopic findings

IX. Cutis laxa (Fig. 20-5)

1. **Reduced number of elastic fibers,** especially in papillary dermis
2. Elastic fibers exhibit granular degeneration

X. Anetoderma

    A. Inflammatory stage

1. Normal epidermis
2. Superficial perivascular infiltrate of lymphocytes and histiocytic cells
3. Nuclear debris occasionally present
4. Edema of papillary dermis

    B. Late stage

1. **Partial to complete loss of elastic fibers** in dermis with retention of elastica of vessels
2. **Apparent diminution in dermal thickness** when compared with normal skin

Differential diagnosis:
  Striae distensae
  Cutis laxa
  Connective-tissue nevus

Evaluation of elastic fiber abnormalities requires comparison of appropriately stained biopsies of normal and affected skin (see Ch. 3)

XI. Acrodermatitis chronica atrophicans (atrophic stage)

1. Profound atrophy of epidermis, dermis, and subcutis
2. Inflammatory infiltrate scant to absent
3. Atrophy of pilosebaceous units; preservation of eccrine glands

See also Ch. 8, IV; Ch. 12, VII

A borrelial spirochete may be found in affected tissue using silver stains

Fig. **20-5.**
A. *Cutis laxa. The elastic fibers exhibit attenuation and a granular, beaded appearance.*
B. *Control (adjacent normal) skin. The normal appearance of elastic fibers for comparison. (Both are van Gieson stained.)*

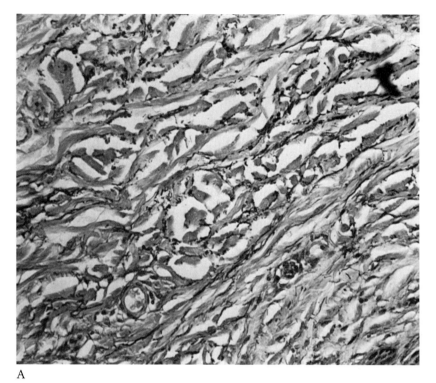

A

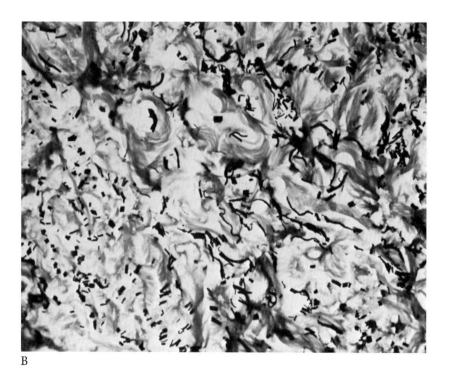

B

XII. Focal dermal hypoplasia (Goltz syndrome) (Fig. 20-6)

1. Normal epidermis
2. **Thinned or absent dermis**
3. Abnormally superficial location of adipose tissue
4. Edematous, widened papillary dermis may be present

Some clinical features include:
Erythematous linear patches
Perianal fat herniation
Lobster-claw deformity of hands

Superficially placed adipose tissue occurs in nevus lipomatosis superficialis

XIII. Aplasia cutis congenita

1. Absence of varying anatomic levels of the skin and subcutaneous tissue to include epidermis, dermis, subcutis, periosteum, and bone
2. If healed, changes of a scar remain

XIV. Perforating disorder of diabetes and renal failure (Fig. 20-7)

1. Epidermal invagination filled with keratin plug and basophilic debris
2. **Atrophy of epidermis at base of invagination associated with loss of granular layer**
3. Keratin plug, at times, in direct contact with epidermis

While the pathogenesis of this disorder probably relates to a focus of altered keratinization and is thus primarily epidermal in origin, the entity is considered here due to its connective tissue alteration

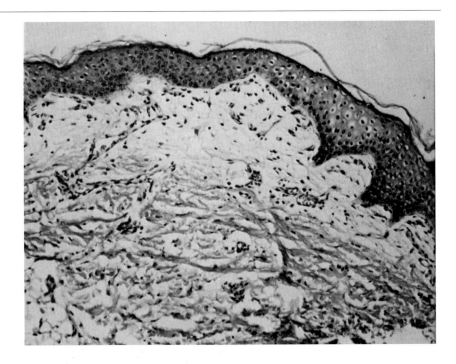

Fig. **20-6.** *Focal dermal hypoplasia. Edematous, wispy papillary dermis is seen in this tissue from a patient with Goltz syndrome.*

Fig. **20-7.** *Perforating disorder of diabetes and renal failure.*

A. *An epidermal invagination is plugged by parakeratotic and basophilic material. Notice the attenuation of the epidermis at the base of the plug.*

B. *Where the plug contacts the dermis, neutrophils and altered collagen bundles can be observed.*

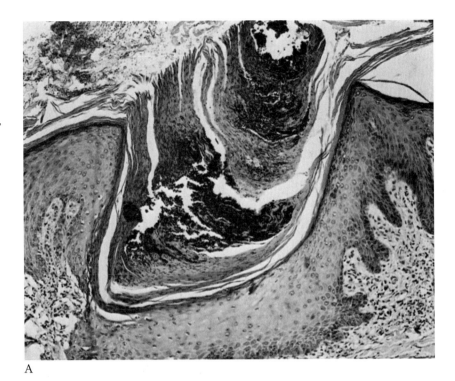

A

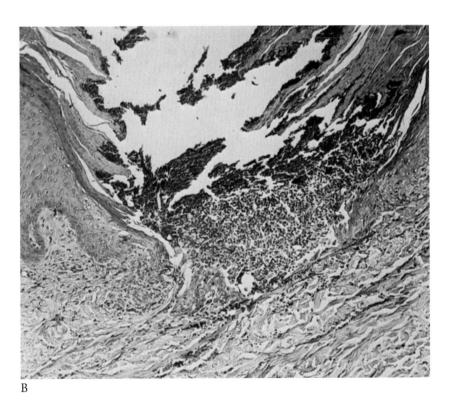

B

4. Altered connective tissue elements present within the epidermal invagination
5. Inflammatory cell infiltrate in dermis

> *Transepidermal elimination* may occur in:
>
> Perforating disorder of diabetes and renal failure
> Elastosis perforans serpiginosa
> Reactive perforating collagenosis
> Perforating folliculitis
> Pseudoxanthoma elasticum
> Nevocellular nevi and melanoma
> Granuloma annulare
> Calcinosis cutis
> Gouty tophus

XV. Elastosis perforans serpiginosa

1. Focally hyperplastic epidermis surrounds and engulfs degenerated elastic fibers and accompanying inflammatory infiltrate
2. Abnormal elastic tissue progressively extruded (transepidermal elimination)
3. Abnormal elastic tissue present in adjacent dermis

An elastic tissue stain defines the abnormal connective tissue elements

Pathophysiology: *Penicillamine, known to cause elastosis perforans serpiginosa, does so by chelating copper. Copper deficiency reduces elastin content in fibers via diminished lysyl oxidase acivity. A unique finding in this setting is the presence of lateral budding on elastic fibers using stains for elastic tissue.*

XVI. Reactive perforating collagenosis (Fig. 20-8)

1. Epidermal invagination filled with keratin, basophilic debris, and neutrophils
2. Collagen bundles, often oriented **vertically,** located in base of invagination and within debris

Elastic tissue is not altered. Trichrome stain shows that extruded connective tissue is collagen. The structure of the collagen is not greatly altered

XVII. Wrinkling due to middermal elastolysis

1. Unremarkable epidermis
2. Increased space between collagen bundles in superficial reticular dermis
3. Elastic tissue stains demonstrate preservation of elastic tissue fibers around hair follicles, but **elastolysis in interstitial reticular dermis**

Fig. **20-8.** *Perforating collagenosis. At the base of an invagination similar to that of Figure 20-7, collagen fibers appear to traverse the epidermis.*

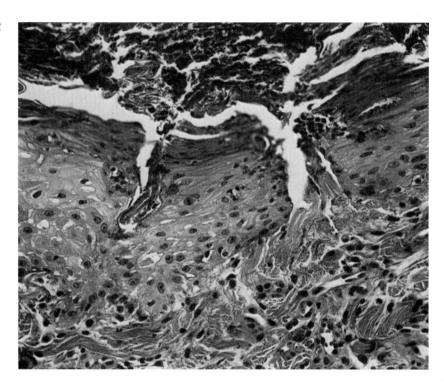

Suggested Reading

Morphea

Fleischmajer, R., and Nedwich, A. Generalized morphea. I. Histology of the dermis and subcutaneous tissue. *Arch. Dermatol.* 106:509, 1972.

O'Leary, P. A., Montgomery, H., and Ragsdale, W. E., Jr. Dermatohistopathology of various types of scleroderma. *Arch. Dermatol.* 75:78, 1957.

Peters, M. S., and Su, W. P. D. Eosinophils in lupus panniculitis and morphea profunda. *J. Cutan. Pathol.* 18:189–192, 1991.

Progressive Systemic Sclerosis (Scleroderma)

Barnett, A. J., Miller, M. H., and Littlejohn, G. O. A survival study of patients with scleroderma diagnosed over 30 years (1953–1983): The value of a simple cutaneous classification in the early stages of the disease. *J. Rheumatol.* 15:276–283, 1988.

Buckingham, R. B., Pince, R. K., and Rodnan, G. P. Progressive systemic sclerosis (PSS, scleroderma) dermal fibroblasts synthesize increased amounts of glycoaminoglycan. *J. Lab. Clin. Med.* 101:659, 1983.

Fleischmajer, R., Damiano, V., and Nedwich, A. Alteration of subcutaneous tissue in systemic scleroderma. *Arch. Dermatol.* 105:59, 1972.

Fleischmajer, R., Perlish, J. S., and Reeves, J. R. Cellular infiltrates in scleroderma skin. *Arthritis Rheum.* 20:975, 1977.

Livingston, J. Z., Scott, T. E., Wigley, F. M., Anhalt, G. J., Bias, W. B., McLean, R. H., and Hochberg, M. C. Systemic sclerosis (scleroderma): Clinical, genetic, and serologial subsets. *J. Rheumatol.* 14:512–518, 1987.

Piper, W. N., and Helwig, E. B. Progressive systemic sclerosis. *Arch. Dermatol.* 72:535, 1955.

Rodnan, G. P., Lipinski, E., and Luksick, J. Skin thickness and collagen content in progressive systemic sclerosis and localized scleroderma. *Arthritis Rheum.* 22:130, 1979.

Silver, R. M. Clinical aspects of systemic sclerosis (scleroderma). *Ann. Rheum. Dis.* 50:846–853, 1991.

Young, E. M., Jr., and Barr, R. J. Sclerosing dermatoses. *J. Cutan. Pathol.* 12:426, 1985.

Eosinophilic Fasciitis

Barnes, L., Rodnan, G. P., Medsger, T. A., and Short, D. Eosinophilic fasciitis: A pathologic study of twenty cases. *Am. J. Pathol.* 96:493–518, 1979.

Kahari, V.-M., Heino, J., Niskanen, L., Fraki, J., and Uitto, J. Eosinophilic fasciitis. *Arch. Dermatol.* 126:613–617, 1990.

Krauser, R. E., and Tuthill, R. J. Eosinophilic fasciitis. *Arch. Dermatol.* 113:1092, 1977.

Rodnan, G. P., DiBartolomeo, A. G., Medsger, T. A., Jr., et al. Eosinophilic fasciitis—report on seven cases of a newly recognized scleredema-like syndrome. *Arthritis Rheum.* 18:422, 1975.

Shulman, L. E. Diffuse fasciitis with hypergammaglobulinemia and eosinophilia: A new syndrome? *J. Rheumatol.* 1 (Suppl. 1):46, 1974.

Radiodermatitis

Fajardo, L. F., and Berthrong, M. Radiation injury in surgical pathology. Part III. Salivary glands, pancreas, and skin. *Am. J. Surg. Pathol.* 5:279, 1981.

Price, N. M. Radiation dermatitis following electron beam therapy. *Arch. Dermatol.* 114:63, 1978.

Pseudoxanthoma Elasticum

Christiano, A. M., Lebwohl, M. G., Boyd, C. D., and Uitoo, J. Workshop on Pseudoxanthoma elasticum: Molecular biology and pathology of the elastic fibers. Jefferson Medical College, Philadelphia, Pennsylvania, June 10, 1992. *J. Invest. Dermatol.* 99:660–663, 1992.

Goodman, R. M., Smith, E. W., Paton, D., et al. Pseudoxanthoma elasticum: A clinical and histopathological study. *Medicine* 42:297, 1963.

Hicks, J., Carpenter, C. L., and Reed, R. J. Periumbilical perforating pseudoxanthoma elasticum. *Arch. Dermatol.* 115:300, 1979.

Lund, H. Z., and Gilbert, C. F. Perforating pseudoxanthoma elasticum: Its distinction from elastosis perforans serpiginosa. *Arch. Pathol. Lab. Med.* 100:544, 1976.

Yoles, A., Phelps, R., and Lebwohl, M. Pseudoxanthoma elasticum and pregnancy. *Cutis* 58:161–164, 1996.

Ehlers–Danlos Syndrome

Holbrook, K. A., and Byers, P. H. Structural abnormalities in the dermal collagen and elastic matrix from the skin of patients with inherited connective tissue disorders. *J. Invest. Dermatol.* 9:7s, 1982.

Sulica, V. I., Cooper, P. H., Poper, F. M., et al. Cutaneous histologic features in Ehlers-Danlos syndrome. *Arch. Dermatol.* 115:40, 1979.

Wechsler, H. L., and Fisher, E. R., Ehlers–Danlos syndrome: Pathologic, histochemical and electron microscope observations. *Arch. Pathol.* 77:613, 1964.

Cutis Laxa

Sephel, G. C., Byers, P. H., Holbrook, K. A., et al. Heterogeneity of elasti expression in cutis laxa fibroblast strains. *J. Invest. Dermatol.* 93:147, 1989.

Goltz, R. W., Hult, A. M., Goldfarb, M., et al. Cutis laxa, *Arch. Dermatol.* 92:373, 1965.

Anetoderma

Feldman, S. Macular atrophy (Schweninger and Buzzi type). *Arch. Dermatol.* 85:209, 1962.

Kossard, S., Kronman, K. R., Dicken, C. H., et al. Inflammatory macular atrophy: Immunofluorescent and ultrastructural findings. *J. Am. Acad. Dermatol.* 1:325, 1979.

Varadi, D. P., and Saqueton, A. C. Perifollicular elastolysis. *Br. J. Dermatol.* 83:143, 1970.

Verhagen, A. R., and Woerdeman, M. J. Post-inflammatory elastolysis and cutis laxa. *Br. J. Dermatol.* 18:595, 1979.

Acrodermatitis Chronica Atrophicans (Atrophic Stage)

Burdorf, W. H. C., Worret, W. I., and Schultka, O. Acrodermatitis chronica atrophicans. *Int. J. Dermatol.* 18:595, 1979.

de Koning, J., Tazelaar, D. J., Hoogkamp-Kostanoje, J. A., and Elema, J. D. Acrodermatitis chronica atrophicans: A light and electron microscopic study. *J. Cutan. Pathol.* 22:23–32, 1995.

Montgomery, H., and Sullivan, R. R. Acrodermatitis atrophicans chronica. *Arch. Dermatol. Syphilol.* 51:32, 1945.

Patmas, M. A. Lyme disease: The evolution of erythema chronicum migrans into acrodermatitis chronica migrans. *Cutis* 52:169–170, 1993.

Focal Dermal Hypoplasia (Goltz Syndrome)

Goltz, R. W., Henderson, R. R., Hitch, J. M., et al. Focal dermal hypoplasia syndrome: A review of the literature and report of two cases. *Arch. Dermatol.* 101:1, 1970.

Gunduz, K., Gunalp, I., and Erden, I. Focal dermal hypoplasia (Goltz's syndrome). *Ophthalmic Genet.* 18:143–149, 1997.

Ishii, N., Baba, N., Kanaizuka, I., Nakajima, H., Ono, S., and Amemiya, F. Histopathological study of focal dermal hypoplasia (Goltz syndrome). *Clin. Exp. Dermatol.* 17:24–26, 1992.

Sato, M., Ishikawa, O., Yokoyama, Y., Kondo, A., and Miyachi, Y. Focal dermal hypoplasia (Goltz syndrome): a decreased accumulation of hyaluronic acid in three-dimensional culture. *Acta Derm. Venereol.* 76:365–367, 1996.

Uitto, J., Bauer, E. A., Santa Cruz, P. J., et al. Focal dermal hypoplasia: Abnormal growth characteristics of skin fibroblasts in culture. *J. Invest. Dermatol.* 75:170, 1982.

Aplasia Cutis Congenita

Frieden, I. Aplasia cutis congenita: A clinical review and proposal for classification. *J. Am. Acad. Dermatol.* 14:646, 1986.

Perforating Disorder of Diabetes and Renal Failure

Bank, D. E., Cohen, P. R., and Kohn, S. R. Reactive perforating collagenosis in a setting of double disaster: Acquired immunodeficiency syndrome and end-stage renal disease. *J. Am. Acad. Dermatol.* 21:371–374, 1989.

Carter, V. H., and Constantine, V. S. Kyrle's disease. I. Clinical findings in five cases and review of literature. *Arch. Dermatol.* 97:624, 1968.

Constantine, V. S., and Carter, V. H. Kyrle's disease. II. Histopathologic findings in five cases and review of the literature. *Arch. Dermatol.* 97:633, 1968.

Hood, A. F., Hardegen, G. L., Zarate, A. R., et al. Kyrle's disease in patients with chronic renal failure. *Arch. Dermatol.* 118:85, 1982.

Squier, C. A., Eady, R. A., and Hopps, R. M. The permeability of epidermis lacking normal membrane-coating granules: An ultrastructural tracer study of Kyrle–Flegel disease. *J. Invest. Dermatol.* 70:361, 1978.

Elastosis Perforans Serpiginosa

Faver, I. R., Daoud, M. S., and Su, W. P. D. Acquired reactive perforating collagenosis. Report of six cases and review of the literature. *J. Am. Acad. Dermatol.* 30:575–580, 1994.

Hashimoto, K., McEvoy, B., and Belcher, R. Ultrastructure of penicillamine-induced skin lesions. *J. Am. Acad. Dermatol.* 4:300, 1981.

Mehregan, A. H., Elastosis perforans serpiginosa: A review of the literature and report of 11 cases. *Arch. Dermatol.* 97:381, 1968.

O'Donnell, B., Kelly, P., Dervan, P., and Powell, F. C. Generalized elastosis perforans serpiginosa in Down's syndrome. *Clin. Exp. Dermatol.* 17:31–33, 1992.

Patterson, J. W. The perforating disorders. *J. Am. Acad. Dermatol.* 10:561–581, 1984.

Reactive Perforating Collagenosis

Fretzin, D. F., Beal, D. W., and Jao, W. Light and ultrastructural study of reactive perforating collagenosis. *Arch. Dermatol.* 116:1054, 1980.

Poliack, S. C., Lebwohl, M. G., Parris, A., et al. Reactive perforating collagenosis associated with diabetes mellitus. *N. Engl. J. Med.* 306:81, 1982.

Chapter 21

Diseases Recognized Histologically by Deposition of Material in the Dermis

I. Amyloidosis
   A. Systemic amyloidosis
      1. Primary
      2. Secondary
   B. Localized amyloidosis
      1. Nodular amyloidosis
II. Mucinoses
   A. Focal mucinosis; cutaneous myxoma
   B. Digital mucous cyst; myxoid cyst
   C. Mucous cyst of oral mucosa; mucocele
   D. Myxedema
   E. Pretibial myxedema
   F. Papular mucinosis
   G. Scleromyxedema
   H. Scleredema
III. Gouty tophus
IV. Calcinosis cutis (metastatic, dystrophic, idiopathic)
V. Ochronosis
VI. Hemochromatosis
VII. Tattoo
VIII. Argyria
IX. Lipoid proteinosis
X. Amiodarone hyperpigmentation
XI. Minocycline hyperpigmentation

The types of material deposited in the dermis that are described in this chapter are from vastly different sources. Overproduction of acid mucopolysaccharides by fibroblasts is the hallmark of the mucinoses. The substances deposited in amyloidosis and ochronosis are not made in significant amounts in normal cells. Some materials are completely exogenous, such as ink and graphite in a tattoo. The degree of inflammatory cell reaction is quite variable among these entities. Although not illustrated in this text, bovine collagen is now iatrogenically deposited in the dermis for cosmetic purposes.

The Reactive Process and the Disease	Histopathology	Comments
I. Amyloidosis		
A. Systemic amyloidosis (Fig. 21-1)		

1. Primary	1. Epidermal changes range from atrophy to hyperkeratosis and acanthosis
	2. Grenz zone (normal papillary dermis) may be present
	3. Pale **eosinophilic, homogeneous, acellular, sometimes fissured material** deposited in the dermis
	4. Deposition of amyloid usually in upper and mid-reticular dermis but may extend up to the epidermis or down to involve the subcutaneous fat
	5. Amyloid is often present within vessel walls
	6. Extravasation of erythrocytes common
	7. Deposition of amyloid around individual fat cells produces characteristic **"amyloid rings"**
		Frozen sections of unfixed skin stained with either Congo red or thioflavin-T optimally demonstrate amyloid deposition
		Amyloid deposits may be seen in arrector pili muscles and lamina propria of sweat ducts and glands
		Amyloid is derived from immunoglobulin light chains
		
		Differential diagnosis:
		  Colloid milium
		  Lipoid proteinosis
		  Solar elastosis
		  Scleroderma
		
		Electron microscopy is required to differentiate colloid milium from amyloid

2. Secondary	Amyloid sometimes observed around appendages and fat cells	Amyloid is derived from acute phase reactant in serum Biopsy of clinically normal skin or subcutaneous fat from abdomen may reveal amyloid deposition

Fig. **21-1.** *Systemic amyloidosis. Waxy, eosinophilic deposits are seen around blood vessels in the reticular dermis (arrow).*

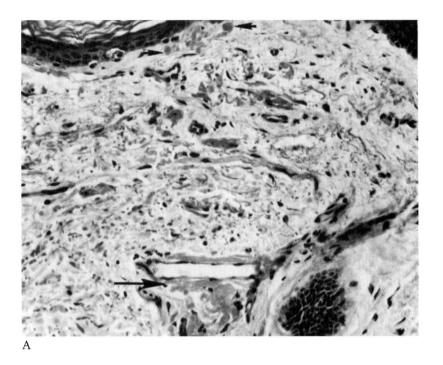

A

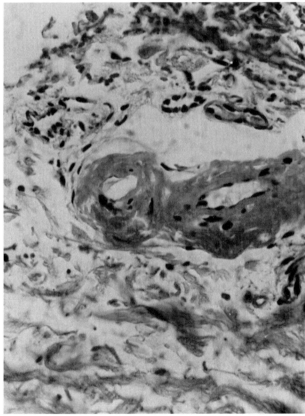

B

B. Localized amyloidosis

1. Nodular amyloidosis (Fig. 21-2)	1. Epidermis flattened and often atrophic 2. **Large masses of amyloid** deposited in papillary dermis, reticular dermis, and subcutaneous fat 3. Amyloid deposited in vessel walls and eccrine glands and around fat cells 4. Variable lymphocytic, plasma cell, and giant-cell infiltrate around amyloid deposits 5. Foci of calcification occasionally present	Amyloidosis is derived from immunoglobulin light chains Nodular amyloidosis cannot be distinguished histologically from systemic amyloidosis (see also I.A) Two other diseases—macular amyloidosis and lichen amyloidosis—are characterized by amyloid deposition limited to the papillary dermis (see also Ch. 14, I). Amyloid is derived from keratin protein. Amyloid P is a normal constituent in the skin surrounding elastic fibers
II. Mucinoses		This group of disorders is characterized by the dermal deposition of mucin (usually the acid mucopolysaccharide, hyaluronic acid), which can be seen as faint, wispy basophilic threads and granules with H&E-stained sections; it is better demonstrated with colloidal iron, alcian blue, or toluidine blue stains.
A. Focal mucinosis; cutaneous myxoma	1. Epidermis normal to flattened 2. **Mucin deposition displaces and replaces collagen fibers of reticular dermis** 3. Proliferation of fibroblasts in areas of mucin deposition 4. Small cystic spaces may occur	

B. Digital mucous cyst; myxoid cyst	1. Elevated, dome-shaped lesion with flattened epidermis
	2. Variable mucin deposition:
	  a. Between collagen fibers
	  b. Within fissures or cleftlike spaces in the dermis
	  c. Within large cystic spaces which may fill entire dermis
	3. Compressed rim of collagen gives impression of encapsulation
	4. Proliferation of fibroblasts in and around areas of mucin deposition
		Early lesions may resemble focal mucinosis

Fig. **21-2.** Nodular amyloidosis. Nodular aggregates of waxy eosinophilic globules replace normal dermal components.

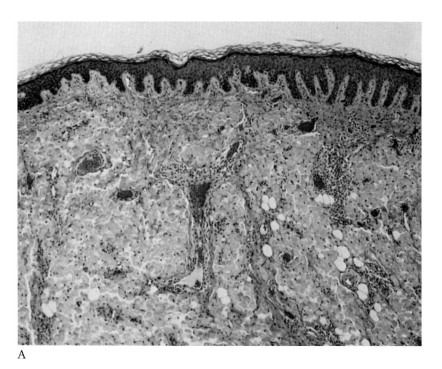

A

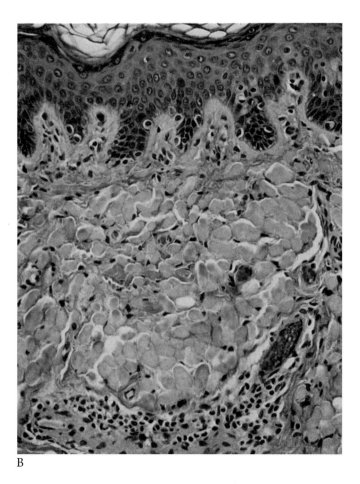

B

C. Mucous cyst of oral mucosa; mucocele

1. Thinned epithelium
2. Well-circumscribed accumulation of amorphous eosinophilic material admixed with histiocytic cells and neutrophils within the submucosa

The material in mucous cysts of the oral mucosa is sialomucin, which contains acid and neutral mucopolysaccharides; sialomucin will stain with PAS as well as alcian blue and colloidal iron

D. Myxedema

1. Variable hyperkeratosis, follicular plugging with keratin, and follicular atrophy
2. **Mucin deposited in small amounts about venules and appendages as well as in the reticular dermis;** this feature may be quite mild and subtle
3. Slight swelling and separation of collagen fibers

Increased mucin deposition in the papillary and upper reticular dermis may be seen in dermatomyositis and lupus erythematosus

E. Pretibial myxedema (Fig. 21-3)

1. Hyperkeratosis, keratin plugs in follicular openings
2. Grenz zone of normal papillary dermis
3. **Bandlike deposition of mucin throughout upper reticular dermis**
4. Displacement and replacement of collagen fibers by mucin
5. Fibroblast proliferation
6. Increased number of mast cells
7. Mucin frequently deposited between fat cells in subcutaneous tissue

F. Papular mucinosis

1. Flattened epidermis
2. Mucin deposition and fibroblast proliferation largely confined to papillary and upper reticular dermis
3. Increased number of mast cells

Serum protein immunoelectrophoresis may demonstrate the presence of paraprotein, usually IgG with lambda light chains

Differential diagnosis: granuloma annulare

G. Scleromyxedema

1. Flattened epidermis
2. Widespread deposition of **mucin with fibroblast proliferation** extending throughout papillary reticular dermis

Fig. **21-3.** *Pretibial myxedema.*
A. *The lightly stained band in the upper reticular dermis indicates the area of acid mucopolysaccharide deposition.*
B. *The higher magnification shows the loosely cellular nature of the myxedematous zone, as well as a dilated lymphatic channel.*

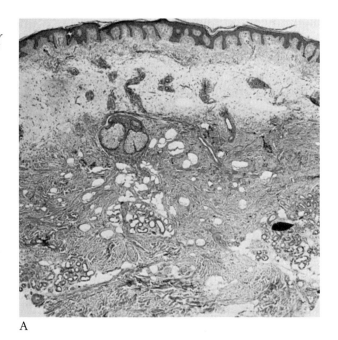

A

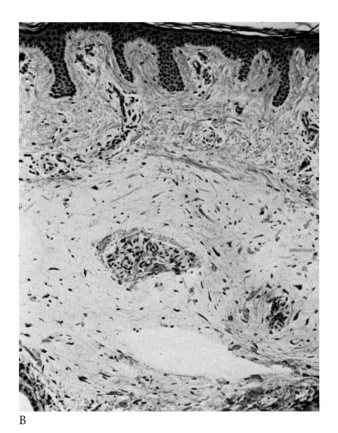

B

H. Scleredema

1. Normal epidermis
2. Markedly thickened dermis with broad collagen bundles in lower dermis
3. "Entrapment" of appendages
4. Mucin may be demonstrable between collagen fibers and fat cells in early lesions
5. No fibroblast proliferation

Differential diagnosis:
    Scleroderma
    Normal skin

Condition often occurs on the upper back, which normally displays thickened dermis

Histologic changes may be very subtle and diagnosis difficult to establish

III. Gouty tophus (Fig. 21-4)

1. Normal or ulcerated epidermis
2. Variously sized deposits of amorphous amphophilic material with characteristic **parallel, needle-shaped clefts** present in dermis and subcutaneous tissue
3. Lymphohistiocytic and **giant-cell infiltrate around urate deposits**
4. Calcification of urate deposits may occur

If tissue is fixed in 100% ethanol instead of formalin, needle-shaped urate crystals may be better visualized

Fig. **21-4.** Gouty tophus.
A. The urate deposits form the dome-shaped lesion and compress normal dermis.
B. Higher magnification shows the amorphous material surrounded by a foreign-body-type giant-cell reaction.

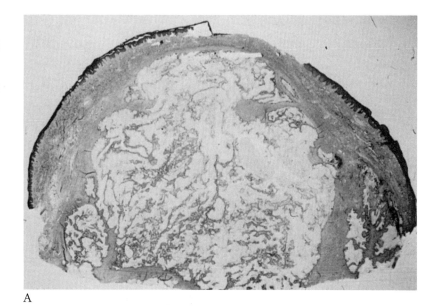

A

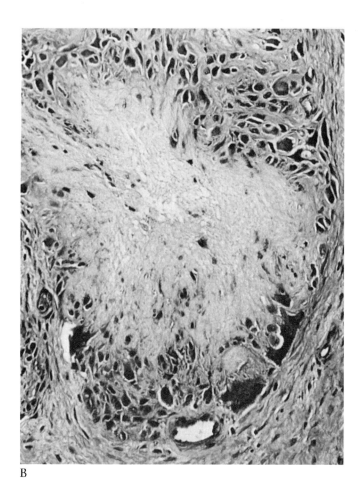

B

IV. Calcinosis cutis (metastatic, dystrophic, idiopathic) (Fig. 21-5)

1. Epidermis normal or occasionally ulcerated
2. Small to massive deposition of **dark blue particles** in dermis and subcutaneous tissue
3. Foreign-body giant-cell reaction sometimes present adjacent to calcium deposits

Special stains such as von Kossa's or alizarin red stain may be helpful in confirming the presence of calcium

---

Dystrophic calcification occurs in the following entities:

Basal cell carcinoma
Pilomatrixoma
Trichilemmal cyst
Acne
Lupus profundus
Dermatomyositis
Scleroderma

V. Ochronosis (Fig. 21-6)

Pathophysiology: *Ochronosis refers to pigment deposition in connective tissue. Endogenous production occurs due to autosomal recessive absence of homogentisic acid oxidase (alkaptonuria). Exogenous causes include hydroquinone application and quinacrine ingestion.*

1. Normal epidermis
2. Intracellular and extracellular deposition of yellow to **light brown granules and globules composed of homogentisic acid**
3. Particles often seen within endothelial cells and secretory cells of eccrine gland
4. **Large deposits within collagen, and elastic fibers may assume bizarre, irregular shapes**
5. Giant multinucleate cells occasionally present

Homogentisic acid crystals stain black with cresyl violet or methylene blue

VI. Hemochromatosis

1. **Increased melanin** in basal layer
2. Intracellular and extracellular deposition of **golden brown, irregularly shaped** hemosiderin granules
3. Granules commonly found in and around basement membrane of eccrine units and around blood vessels

Hemosiderin deposition can be demonstrated with the Prussian blue stain

Differential diagnosis:
Venous stasis
Progressive pigmented purpura

Fig. **21-5.** *Calcinosis cutis. Basophilic islands of calcium are present within a fibrotic and compressed dermis.*

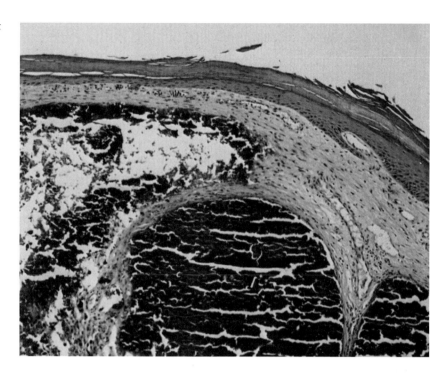

Fig. **21-6.** *Ochronosis. Glassy amorphous material (arrows) is present in the dermis. In routine stains, these islands stain yellowish brown.*

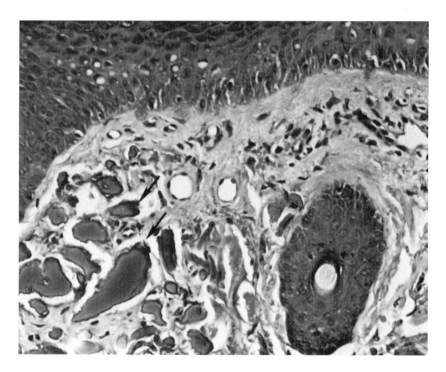

VII. Tattoo (Fig. 21-7)

1. Epidermis usually normal
2. Dark pigment granules dispersed in the upper and middle reticular dermis, both **free and within macrophages**
3. Most tattoo pigments appear black with routine microscopy but occasionally a reddish hue (cinnabar) or bluish hue (cobalt) is apparent

Rarely, eczematous or granulomatous reactions to the injected material may occur

VIII. Argyria (Fig. 21-8)

1. Increased melanin may be present in basal cells
2. Uniform, small, round, brown-black refractile granules deposited intracellularly and extracellularly in papillary and reticular dermis
3. **Granules characteristically deposited in basement membrane of vessels and eccrine glands** and within endothelial cells

Dark-field examination demonstrates particles of heavy metals and emphasizes the uniformity in the size of the silver granules; uniform size of granules helps differentiate argyria from ochronosis, tattoo, hemosiderin, and other heavy-metal deposition

IX. Lipoid proteinosis

1. Hyperkeratosis and papillomatosis
2. **Homogeneous eosinophilic hyaline material present in papillary dermis**
3. In reticular dermis the material surrounds and deposits in vessel walls, eccrine glands, and arrector pili muscles
4. Elastosis frequently present peripheral to hyaline deposition
5. Increased number of mast cells

The hyaline material contains abundant type IV collagen and has the following staining properties:
PAS-positive, diastase-resistant
Alcian blue positive at pH of 3
Slightly positive with Congo red and variably positive with other lipid stains

Fig. **21-7.** Tattoo. Black pigment within and outside dermal histiocytic cells is characteristic.

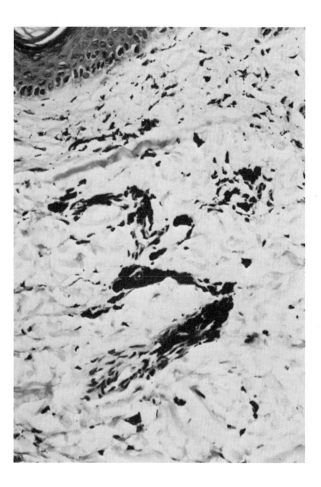

Fig. **21-8.** Argyria. Deposition of dark, almost refractile granules in the basement membrane zone of these eccrine glands is characteristic of argyria. Deposition of granules about other skin appendages and upon elastic fibers as well as hypermelanosis also occurs in this disorder.

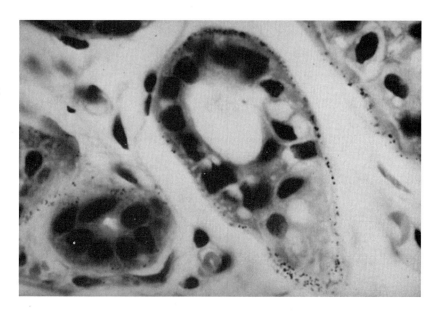

X. Amiodarone hyper-
pigmentation

1. Unremarkable epidermis
2. Superficial perivascular
   lymphocytic infiltrate
3. Yellow-brown granules within
   macrophages and free in dermis

The pigment granules stain
positively uniformly with
periodic acid–Schiff stains and
variably with Ziehl–Neelsen and
Fontana–Masson stains

Differential diagnosis of
conditions causing
pigment-laden macrophages
in dermis:

Amiodarone
Argyria
Bismuth
Busulfan
Chyrsiasis
Desipramine
Doxyrubicin
Hemosiderin
Lead
Mercury
Minocycline
Postinflammatory
  hyperpigmentation
Regression

XI. Minocycline hyperpigmentation

1. Unremarkable epidermis
2. Superficial perivascular
   lymphocytic infiltrate
3. Black pigment in dermal
   macrophages

The pigment granules stain with
iron stains

Suggested Reading

Amyloidosis

Breathnach, S. M. The cutaneous amyloidoses: Pathogenesis and therapy. *Arch. Dermatol.* 121:470, 1985.

Breathnach, S. M. Amyloid and amyloidosis. *J. Am. Acad. Dermatol.* 18:1–16, 1988.

Habermann, M. C., and Montenegro, M. R. Primary cutaneous amyloidosis: Clinical, laboratorial and histopathological study in 25 cases. *Dermatologica* 160:240, 1980.

Hashimoto, K. Diseases of amyloid, colloid, and hyalin. *J. Cutan. Pathol.* 12:322, 1985.

Kobayashi, H., and Hashimoto, K. Amyloidogenesis in organ-limited cutaneous amyloidosis: An antigenic identity between epidermal keratin and skin amyloid. *J. Invest. Dermatol.* 80:66, 1983.

Kyle, R. A., and Gertz, M. A. Primary systemic amyloidosis: Clinical and laboratory features in 474 cases. *Semin. Hematol.* 32:45–59, 1995.

Robert, C., Aractingi, S., Prost, C., Verola, O., Blanchet-Bardon, C., Blanc, F., et al., Bullous amyloidosis. *Medicine* 24:124–138, 1994.

Westermark, P. Amyloidosis of the skin: A comparison between localized and systemic amyloidosis. *Acta Derm. Venereol. (Stockh.)* 80:341–345, 1979.

Mucinoses

Cohn, B. A., Wheeler, C. E., Jr., and Briggaman, R. A. Scleredema adultorum of Buschke and diabetes mellitus. *Arch. Dermatol.* 101:27, 1970.

Dineen, A. M., and Dicken, C. H. Scleromyxedema. *J. Am. Acad. Dermatol.* 33:37–43, 1995.

Farmer, E. R., Hambrick, G. W., and Shulman, L. E. Papular mucinosis: A clinicopathologic study of four patients. *Arch. Dermatol.* 118:9, 1982.

Farrell, A. M., Branfoot, A. C., Moss, J., Papadaki, L., Woodrow, D. F., and Bunker, C. B. Scleredema diabeticorum of Buschke confined to the thighs. *Br. J. Dermatol.* 134:1113–1115, 1996.

Gabriel, S. E., Perry, H. O., Oleson, G. B., and Bowles, C. A. Scleromyxedema: A sclerodermal-like disorder with systemic manifestations. *Medicine (Baltimore)* 67:58–65, 1988.

Johnson, W. C., Graham, J. H., and Helwig, E. B. Cutaneous myxoid cyst: A clinicopathological and histochemical study. *JAMA* 191:15, 1965.

Lynch, P. J., Maize, J. C., and Sisson, J. C. Pretibial myxedema and nonthyrotoxic thyroid disease. *Arch. Dermatol.* 107:107, 1973.

Miyagawa, S., Dohi, K., Tsuruta, S., and Shirai, T. Scleredema of Buschke associated with rheumatoid arthritis and Sjorgren's syndrome. *Br. J. Dermatol.* 121:517–520, 1989.

Reed, R. J., Clark, W. H., and Mihm, M. C. The cutaneous mucinoses. *Hum. Pathol.* 4:201, 1973.

Rudner, E. J., Mehregan, A., and Pinkus, H. Scleromyxedema: A variant of lichen myxedematosus. *Arch. Dermatol.* 93:3, 1966.

Truban, A. P., and Roenizk, H. H. The cutaneous mucinoses. *J. Am. Acad. Dermatol.* 14:1, 1986.

Venencie, P. Y., Powell, F. C., Su, W. P. D., and Perry, H. O. Scleredema: A review of thirty-three cases. *J. Am. Acad. Dermatol.* 11:128–134, 1984.

Yaron, M., Yaron, I., Yust, I., and Brenner, S. Lichen myxedematosus (scleromyxedema) serum stimulates hyaluronic acid and prostaglandin E production by human fibroblasts. *J. Rheumatol.* 12:171–175, 1985.

Gout

Lichtenstein, L., Scott, H. W., and Levin, M. H. Pathologic changes in gout. *Am. J. Pathol.* 32:871, 1956.

Calcinosis Cutis

Kolton, B., and Pedersen, J. Calcinosis cutis and renal failure. *Arch. Dermatol.* 110:256, 1974.

Steward, V. L., Herling, P., and Dalinka, M. Calcification in soft tissue. *J.A.M.A.* 250:78, 1983.

Whiting, D. A., Simson, I. W., Kalimeyer, J. C., et al. Unusual cutaneous lesions in tumoral calcinosis. *Arch. Dermatol.* 102:465, 1970.

Ochronosis

Egorin, M. J., Trump, D. L., and Wainwright, C. W. Quinacrine ochronosis and rheumatoid arthritis. *JAMA* 236:385, 1976.

Lichtenstein, L., and Kaplan, L. Hereditary ochronosis. *Am. J. Pathol.* 30:99, 1954.

O'Brien, W. M., La Du, B. N., and Bunim, J. J. Biochemical, pathologic and clinical aspects of alcaptonuria ochronosis and ochronotic arthropathy: Review of world literature (1584–1962). *Am. J. Med.* 34:813, 1963.

Hemochromatosis

Cawley, E. P., Hsu, Y. T., Wood, B. T., et al. Hemochromatosis and the skin. *Arch. Dermatol.* 100:1, 1969.

Chevrant-Breton, J., Simon, M., Bourel, M., and Ferrand, B. Cutaneous manifestations of idiopathic hemochromatosis, study of 100 cases. *Arch. Dermatol.* 113:161, 1977.

Milder, M. S., Cook, J. D., Stray, S., and Finch, C. A. Idiopathic hemochromatosis, an interim report. *Medicine (Baltimore)* 59:34–49, 1980.

Perdrup, A., and Poulsen, H. Hemochromatosis and vitiligo. *Arch. Dermatol.* 90:34, 1964.

Tattoo

Goldstein, A. P. Histologic reactions in tattoos. *J. Dermatol. Surg. Oncol.* 5:896, 1979.

Rostenberg, A., Jr., Brown, R. A., and Caro, M. R. Discussion of tattoo reactions with report of a case showing a reaction to a green color. *Arch. Dermatol. Syphilol.* 62:540, 1950.

Taaffe, A., Knight, A. G., and Marks, R. Lichenoid tattoo hypersensitivity. *Br. Med. J.* 1:616, 1978.

Argyria

Hill, W. R., and Montgomery, H. Argyria (with special reference to the cutaneous histopathology). *Arch. Dermatol. Syphilol.* 44:588, 1941.

Mehta, A. C., Dawson-Butterworth, K., and Woodhouse, M. A. Argyria. Electron microscopic study of a case. *Br. J. Dermatol.* 78:175, 1966.

Pariser, R. J. Generalized argyria. Clinicopathologic features and histochemical studies. *Arch. Dermatol.* 114:373, 1978.

Lipoid Proteinosis

Caro, I. Lipoid proteinosis. *Int. J. Dermatol.* 17:388, 1978.

Harper, J. I., Duance, V. C., Sims, T. J., and Light, N. D. Lipoid proteinosis: An inherited disorder of collagen metabolism? *Br. J. Dermatol.* 113:145–151, 1985.

Moy, L. S., Moy, R. L., and Matscroka, L. Y. Lipoid proteinosis: Ultrastructural and biochemical studies. *J. Am. Acad. Dermatol.* 16:1193, 1987.

Muda, A. O., Paradisi, M., Angelo, C., Mostaccioli, S., Atzori, F., Puddu, P., and Faraggiana, T. Lipoid proteinosis: Clinical, histologic, and ultrastructural investigations. *Cutis* 56:220–224, 1995.

Van Der Walt, J. J., and Heyl, T. Lipoid proteinosis and erythropoietic protoporphyria: A histological and histochemical study. *Arch. Dermatol.* 104:501, 1971.

Chapter **22**

Hyperplasias and Neoplasms

I. Fibrohistiocytic
  A. Skin tag; fibroepithelial polyp; acrochordon; soft fibroma
  B. Nevus lipomatosis superficialis
  C. Acquired digital fibrokeratoma
  D. Supernumerary digit
  E. Angiofibroma
  F. Accessory tragus
  G. Scar; hypertrophic scar; keloid
  H. Connective-tissue nevus
  I. Elastofibroma dorsi
  J. Fibromatosis
  K. Recurrent infantile digital fibromatosis
  L. Dermatofibroma/fibrous histiocytoma
  M. Dermatofibrosarcoma protuberans (DFSP)
  N. Atypical fibroxanthoma (AFX); malignant fibrous histiocytoma (MFH)
  O. Fibrosarcoma
  P. Dermatomyofibroma
  Q. Solitary fibrous tumor

II. Vascular
  A. Stasis dermatitis
  B. Lobular capillary hemangioma
    1. Capillary hemangioma
    2. Pyogenic granuloma
    3. Angiokeratoma
    4. Bacillary angiomatosis
    5. Histiocytoid (epithelioid) hemangioma
  C. Intravascular papillary endothelial hyperplasia (IPEH) (Masson's pseudo-angiosarcoma)
  D. Cavernous hemangioma
  E. Lymphangioma circumscripta
  F. Kaposi's sarcoma
  G. Glomus tumor
  H. Glomangioma (multiple glomus tumors)
  I. Hemangiopericytoma
  J. Angiosarcoma
  K. Acquired tufted angioma
  L. Targeted hemosiderotic hemangioma
  M. Retiform hemangioendothelialioma
  N. Spindle cell hemangioendothelioma

III. Neural
  A. Neurofibroma
  B. Palisaded encapsulated neuroma (true neuroma)
  C. Traumatic or amputation neuroma
  D. Neurilemmoma; schwannoma
  E. Malignant schwannoma
  F. Granular cell tumor
  G. Neuroendocrine carcinoma (Merkel cell tumor)

IV. Smooth muscle
  A. Leiomyoma
  B. Leiomyosarcoma

V. Miscellaneous
  A. Metastatic carcinoma
  B. Metastatic melanoma
  C. Epithelioid sarcoma

Many entities described in this chapter are common; many are rare. In most soft tissue tumors, the diagnosis is predicated on histologic finding and correlation with clinical features, particularly age of the patient and the body site of the tumor.

The Reactive Process and the Disease	Histopathology	Comments
I. Fibrohistiocytic		
A. Skin tag; fibroepithelial polyp; acrochordon; soft fibroma (Fig. 22-1)	1. Polypoid structure with variable hyperplasia and hyperkeratosis of epidermal surface 2. Central core composed of **fibrovascular or fibrofatty tissue without adnexal structures**	Some skin tags display seborrheic keratosis-like epidermal hyperplasia Differential diagnosis: Fibrous papule Neurofibroma Dermal nevus, pedunculated
B. Nevus lipomatosis superficialis	Polypoid structure with **mature adipose tissue** extending into the upper and papillary dermis	Characteristically located on the buttock or posterior thigh
C. Acquired digital fibrokeratoma (Fig. 22-2)	1. Dome-shaped papule with hyperkeratosis and acanthoses 2. **Dense fibrotic dermis;** collagen fibers arrayed vertically 3. Appendages absent	Characteristically located on the digits, palms, and soles
D. Supernumerary digit	1. Fibroepithelial polyp with **nerves** 2. Bone, cartilage, and appendages may also be present	Located on the ulnar side of hand
E. Angiofibroma	1. **Fibrovascular hyperplasia** of the upper dermis 2. May be histologically indistinguishable from a fibrous papule; usually the concentric perifollicular fibrosis and bizarre cells in the dermis (present in a fibrous papule) are absent	Differential diagnosis: Fibrous papule Scar Regressed nevus Connective-tissue nevus

Fig. **22-1.** *Fibroepithelial polyp. Note the lack of appendages in this polyp.*

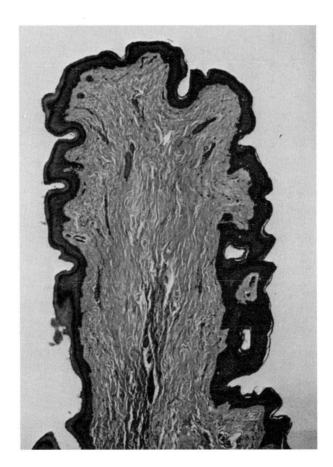

Fig. **22-2.** *Acquired digital fibro-keratoma. A papule is seen with acanthosis, thick collagen, and absent appendages.*

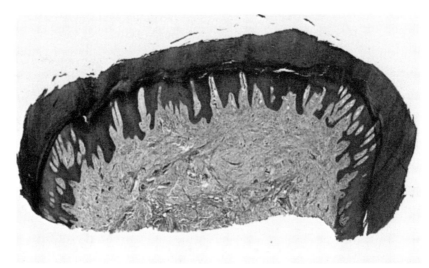

F. Accessory tragus (Fig. 22-3)	Polypoid structure with flattened epidermis, vellus hairs, cartilage centrally, and fibrofatty stroma	Located in preauricular area

G. Scar; hypertrophic scar; keloid (Fig. 22-4)	1. Epidermis normal or flattened
	2. Fibroblast proliferation
	3. Collagen proliferation variable
	   a. Scar: Dense collagen fibers usually **arrayed parallel** to epidermis
	   b. Hypertrophic scar: **Irregularly arranged** collagen fibers of variable shapes and sizes
	   c. Keloid: Smudged, **hyalinized, thickened collagen fibers** admixed with dense collagen bundles
	4. Variable inflammatory infiltrate	

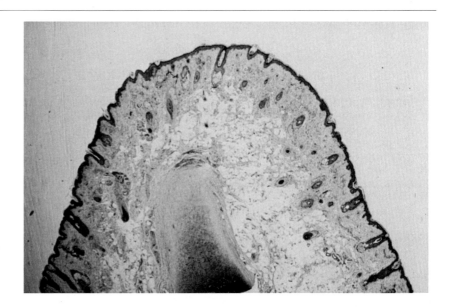

Fig. **22-3.** *Accessory tragus. This papule contains a central core of cartilage with overlying fibroadipose tissue and epidermis.*

Fig. **22-4.**
A. *Keloid. These large, eosinophilic collagen bundles with a glassy, hyalinized appearance are characteristic.*
B. *Hypertrophic scar. The dense fibrous tissue frequently runs parallel to the surface in scars. The histologic patterns of keloid and hypertrophic scar often are mixed within a biopsy.*

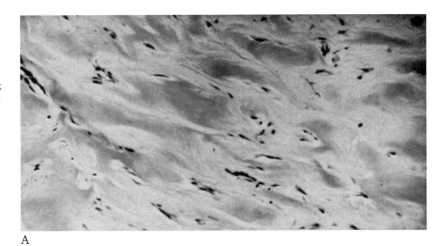

A

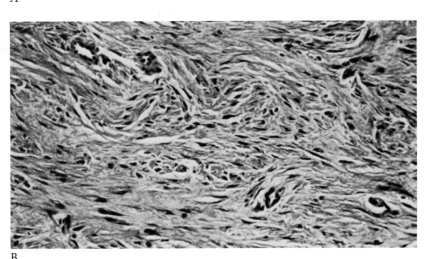

B

H. Connective-tissue nevus (Fig. 22-5)

Reticular dermis widened by increased collagen with normal, increased, or decreased number of elastic fibers

This lesion is essentially a hamartoma of connective tissue

I. Elastofibroma dorsi

1. Increase in number and size of collagen *and* elastic fibers
2. Elastic fibers cut in cross-section show a **serrated margin**

Elastic stains highlight proliferation and abnormalities of elastic fibers

J. Fibromatosis

1. Dense cellular proliferation of fibroblasts with abundant collagen arranged in interlacing bundles
2. Rare to moderate mitoses present
3. Tumor tends to be **infiltrative,** especially into septa of subcutaneous fat, nerves, and skeletal muscle
4. Mucoid alteration and calcification may be observed

Forms of fibromatoses include:
Palmar fibromatosis (Dupuytren's)
Plantar fibromatosis
Desmoid tumor

Desmoid tumors arise from "muscular" aponeurosis and are commonly associated with pregnancy and Gardner's syndrome
Pleomorphism and atypical mitoses are not present in fibromatoses

Differential diagnosis:
Scar
Nodular fasciitis
Dermatofibrosarcoma protuberans
Fibrosarcoma

K. Recurrent infantile digital fibromatosis

1. Proliferation of myofibroblasts
2. Distinctive eosinophilic acellular **hyaline bodies** within cytoplasm of spindled cells

The hyalin bodies can be seen on H&E-stained sections but are accentuated by PTAH and trichrome stains

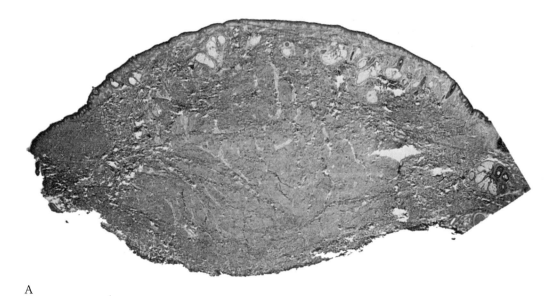

A

Fig. **22-5.** Connective-tissue nevus.
A. The nodular appearance of this dermal hamartomatous growth is evident in this low-power micrograph.
B. Collagen bundles appear smaller and vessels more numerous and thick-walled than usual. Alterations in collagen and elastic tissue vary in type and degree in this disorder.

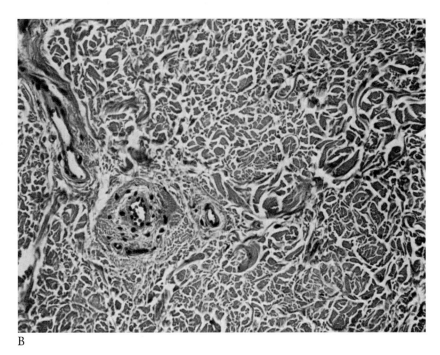

B

L. Dermatofibroma/fibrous histiocytoma (Fig. 22-6)

1. Overlying epidermis commonly (80%) shows elongated rete ridges and increased melanin in basal layer (so-called **dirty fingers**)

If many histiocytic cells are present, the lesion can be called a *histiocytoma*; if numerous vessels are present, the lesion can be called a *sclerosing hemangioma*; and if many comma-shaped spindle cells are present, the lesion can be called a *dermatofibroma*

2. Lesion composed of variable **mixture of spindle cells and histiocytic cells**

Cellular dermatofibroma may be difficult to distinguish from a dermatofibrosarcoma protuberans

3. Cellularity varies; spindle cells often interspersed between collagen bundles
4. Spindle cells commonly arranged in whorled, cartwheel patterns
5. **Border infiltrative** and ill-defined
6. **Collagen bundles entrapped** by proliferating cells

Polarizable normal collagen is present in dermatofibroma

7. Multinucleate giant cells, frequently Touton type, may be present

Features favoring the diagnosis of dermatofibroma include:

8. Tumor may involve deep dermis and rarely subcutaneous fat

  Vascular and lipophagic elements
  Ill-defined infiltrative border

9. Hemosiderin commonly present within histiocytic cells

  Hemosiderin deposition
  Polarizable collagen within tumor
  Tumor cells express factor XIIIa

Differential diagnosis:
  Dermatofibrosarcoma protuberans
  Scar
  Kaposi's sarcoma
  Cellular blue nevus
  Neurofibroma
  Fibromatosis
  Xanthoma
  Leiomyoma

Fig. **22-6.** Dermatofibroma (fibrous histiocytoma). The cellular area within the dermis is usually capped by epidermal hyperplasia (A) The dermis exhibits a spindle cell proliferation with a cart-wheel or storiform pattern (B) or a dense proliferation of comma-like cells, sometimes admixed with foam cells (C). The former pattern is called fibrous histiocytoma and the latter, dermatofibroma, but the terms are used interchangeably.

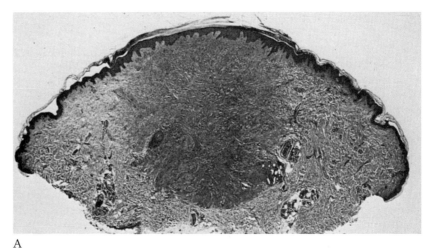

A

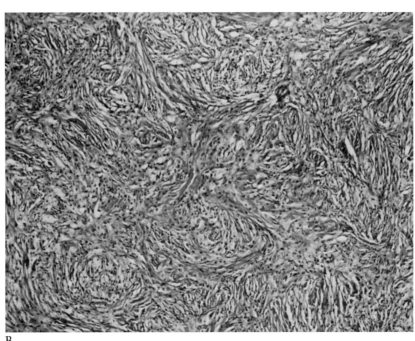

B

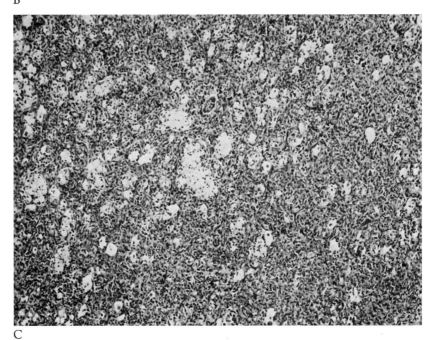

C

M. Dermatofibrosarcoma
protuberans (DFSP)
(Fig. 22-7)

1. Epidermis normal, atrophic, or ulcerated
2. **Expansile lesion present in dermis and subcutaneous tissue; may involve fascia**
3. Proliferation of spindle cells may be arranged in a cartwheel pattern
4. Slight to moderate nuclear atypia
5. Mitoses frequently present
6. Giant cells and foam cells rare
7. Intercalating infiltrative pattern in subcutaneous tissue

Differential diagnosis:
Dermatofibroma
Fibromatosis
Fibrosarcoma

Tumor cells express CD34

Normal dermal collagen replaced by dermatofibrosarcoma protuberans; polaroscopy is negative
Incisional biopsy is required for definitive diagnosis

A Bednar tumor is a melanin containing DFSP, often in a young person

Fig. **22-7.** *Dermatofibrosarcoma protuberans.*
A. *In the mid and deep reticular dermis is a dense proliferation of spindled cells replacing normal dermal architecture. A focus of hemorrhage (arrow) is present in the upper dermis.*
B. *The storiform architecture is evident in this photomicrograph.*

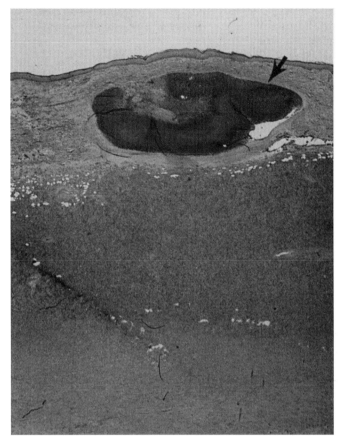

A

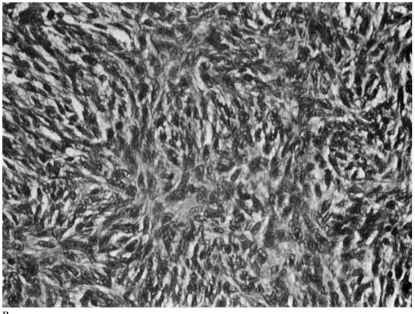

B

N. Atypical fibroxanthoma (AFX); malignant fibrous histiocytoma (MFH) (Fig. 22-8)

1. **Nodular proliferation of pleomorphic and spindle-shaped cells**
2. **Bizarre giant cells**
3. Mitoses frequent; often atypical
4. Foam cells variably present
5. Ulceration common in atypical fibroxanthoma
6. Zones of tumor necrosis common in malignant fibrous histiocytoma; some MFH have prominent mucinous degeneration and/or bizarre giant cells

Differential diagnosis of AFX:
Spindle-cell squamous carcinoma
Melanoma

Differential diagnosis of MFH:
Metastatic melanoma
Proliferative myositis
Nodular fasciitis
Other sarcomas or metastatic poorly differentiated neoplasms

Cellular features are similar in both tumors; however, AFX is superficially located, while MFH is more deeply situated

Fig. **22-8.** *Malignant fibrous histiocytoma.*
A. *The neoplasm fills the dermis and is present in the interlobular septae of the subcutis (arrow).*

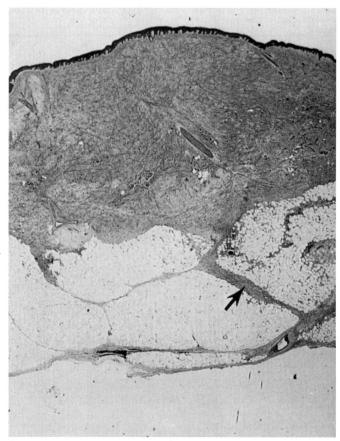

A

B. *Atypical cell with hyperchromatic irregular nucleus is seen (arrow) among the spindled cells.*
C. *Osteoclast-like multinucleated giant cells (arrows) may be seen.*

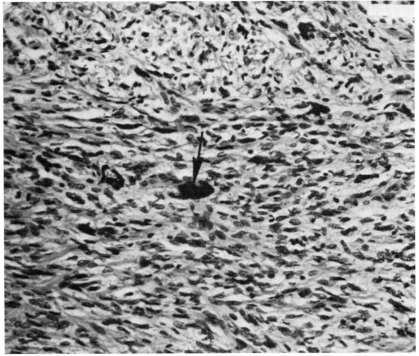

B

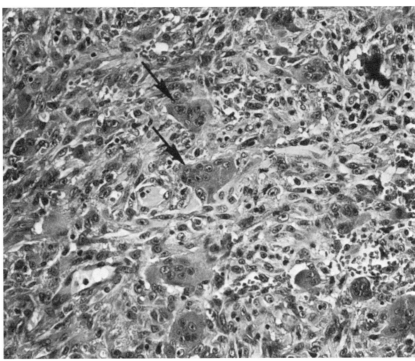

C

O. Fibrosarcoma

1. Densely cellular tumor composed of spindle cells
2. Nuclei are pleomorphic and may be arranged in a **herringbone pattern**
3. Mitoses usually numerous; **atypical mitoses often seen**
4. Tumor arises from fascia or deep subcutis; may arise in previously irradiated reticular dermis

Differential diagnosis:
Dermatofibrosarcoma protuberans
Malignant melanoma, desmoplastic type
Fibromatosis
Malignant schwannoma
Spindle-cell squamous carcinoma
Leiomyosarcoma
Malignant fibrous histiocytoma

P. Dermatomyofibroma (Fig. 22-9) .

1. Well-circumscribed, horizontally oriented, plaquelike pattern in reticular dermis variably extending into subcutis
2. Proliferation of uniform spindle-shaped cells in interlacing fascicles
3. Thin collagen bundles separate the fascicles
4. Mitotic figures rare

Smooth-muscle actin labels the spindle-shaped cells, helping to distinguish this entity from dermatofibroma

Differential diagnosis:
Dermatofibroma
Dermatomyosarcoma protuberans
Leiomyoma
Leimyosarcoma

Fig. **22-9.** *Dermatomyofibroma.*
A, B. A *proliferation of spindle cells in the reticular arranged in long intersecting fascicles.*

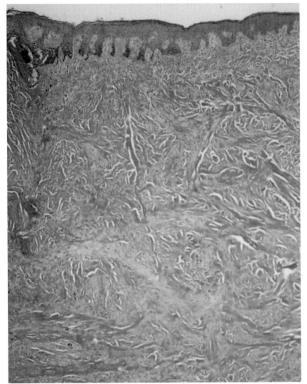

A

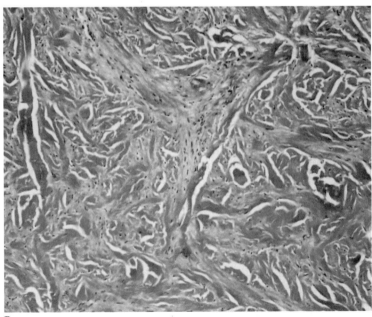

B

Q. Solitary fibrous tumor
(Fig. 22-10)

1. Normal to atrophic epidermis
2. Well-circumscribed nodule centered in reticular dermis
3. Proliferation of uniform spindle-shaped cells with little cytoplasm
4. Mitoses and nuclear pleomorphism rare
5. Increased vascularity, often accentuated at periphery of proliferation
6. Areas of myxoid change and others with hemangiopericytoma-like pattern variably present

Spindle-shaped cells in solitary fibrous tumors express CD34

Fig. **22-10.** *Solitary fibrous tumor.*
A, B. *Circumscribed nodule in the reticular dermis composed of a proliferation of spindle cells.*

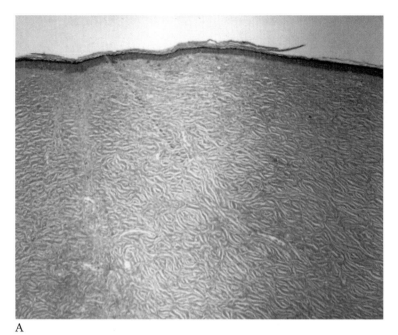

A

B

II. Vascular

A. Stasis dermatitis (Fig. 22-11)	1. Hyperkeratotic, flattened to atrophic epidermis, occasionally with spongiosis	See also Ch. 16, I.B.7

2. **Focal proliferation of capillaries** throughout papillary and reticular dermis
3. **Thickened vessel walls**
4. Dermal **fibrosis**
5. **Hemorrhage and hemosiderin deposition common**
6. Variable mononuclear cell infiltrate

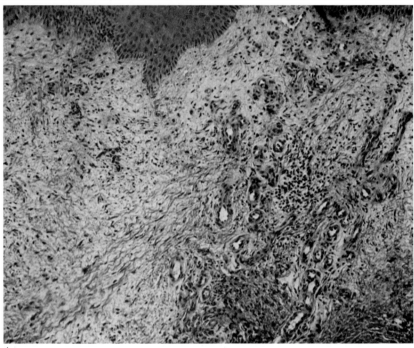

Fig. **22-11.** *Statis dermatitis. Dermal fibrosis and thick-walled vessels (A, B) with numerous hemosiderin-laden microphages (arrow, C) are typical.*

A

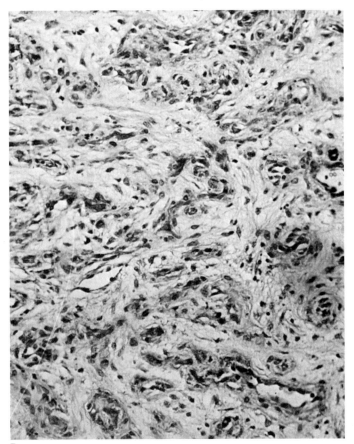

B

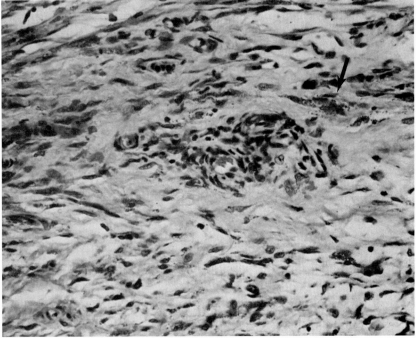

C

B. Lobular capillary
hemangioma

   1. Capillary hemangioma (Fig. 22-12)

1. Overlying epidermis normal or
flattened
2. Dermal proliferation of **capillary-sized endothelial
cell-lined** vessels

The concept of *lobular capillary
hemangioma* unifies several
patterns of benign vascular
neoplasia based upon the
architecture of the lesion and
the size of proliferating vessels.
These vessels may be situated at
upper cutaneous levels
(angiokeratoma) or more deeply
(tufted capillary hemangioma,
intravascular pyogenic
granuloma)

Fig. **22-12.** *Hemangioma. Two
patterns of hemangioma in the skin.*

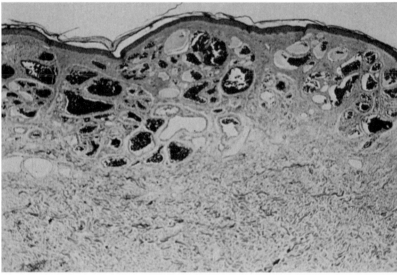

A

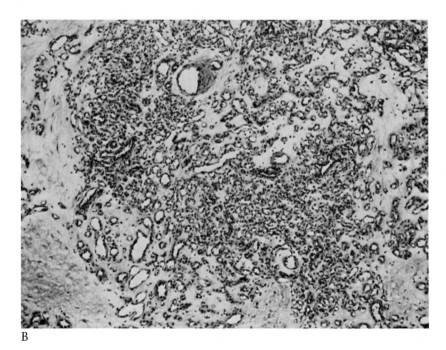

B

2. Pyogenic granuloma (Fig. 22-13)

1. Thin, often ulcerated epidermis, which may form a **lateral collarette**
2. Proliferation of capillaries with variable endothelial swelling and variable ectasia
3. **Acute inflammation** and **stromal edema** commonly associated with epidermal ulceration

Lesions are often elevated above the surface of the normal adjacent skin and may even be pedunculated

3. Angiokeratoma

1. Exophytic structure composed of **hyperkeratosis** overlying **epidermal hyperplasia** and **closely apposed, dilated, thin-walled capillary spaces**
2. Blood and sometimes thrombus fills the capillaries
3. Proliferation of capillary-sized vessels situated beneath ectatic spaces; reticular dermis normal
4. Dermal collagen appears normal

Differential diagnosis:
Lymphangioma circumscriptum
Chronic radiodermatitis

Fig. **22-13.** *Pyogenic granuloma. A lobular proliferation of endothelial cells is present. Notice the collarette of epidermis (arrow).*

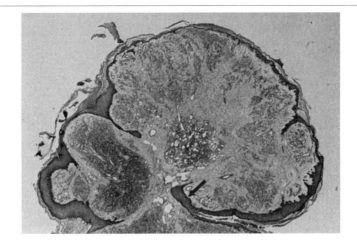

4. Bacillary angiomatosis (Fig. 22-14)

1. Well-circumscribed proliferation of capillary-sized vessels in upper and mid-dermis
2. Prominent endothelial cells with luminal obliteration
3. Slitlike vascular spaces not observed
4. Scattered inflammatory cells, predominantly neutrophils
5. Foci of dermal necrosis may be present

Bartonella-like organisms may be observed with silver stains

Fig. **22-14.** *Bacillary angiomatosis.*
A. *An ulcerated papule is present with a lobular proliferation of endothelial cells within the dermis.*

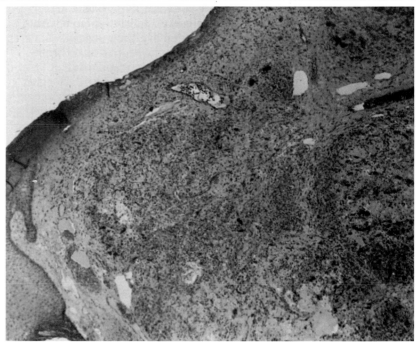

A

B. A *nodule of epithelioid endothelial cells with a hemorrhage* (arrow) is seen. A *polymorphous inflammatory cell infiltrate accompanies the vascular element.*
C. Warthin–Starry stain reveals clumps of coccobacillary organisms.

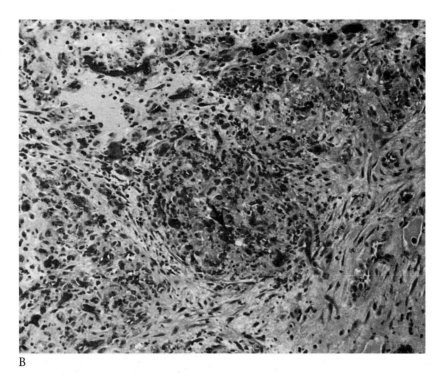

B

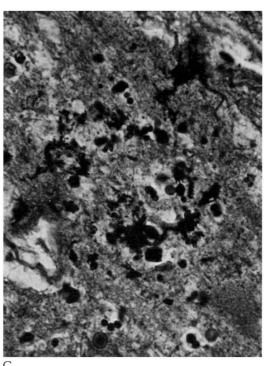

C

5. Histiocytoid (epithelioid) hemangioma (Fig. 22-15)	1. **Dermal nodule of endothelial cells** with oval, pale nuclei, inconspicuous nucleoli, and abundant eosinophilic cytoplasm 2. Vascular lumens variably evident 3. Mitotic figures rare 4. Inflammatory cells infiltrate endothelial proliferation 5. Lymphocytes common, eosinophils typically but not invariably present 6. Lymphoid follicles generally absent	Histiocytoid hemangioma is distinguished from angiolymphoid hyperplasia with eosinophilia by its more prominent endothelial cell component and less prominent inflammatory component. The two entities may be related Immunohistochemical analysis for type IV collagen highlights the vessels. Detection of factor VIII–related antigen confirms endothelial cells
C. Intravascular papillary endothelial hyperplasia (IPEH) (Masson's pseudo-angiosarcoma)	1. **Nodular aggregate within blood vessel** consisting of eosinophilic papillary fronds with fibrin core 2. Hypertrophy of endothelial cells, often spindle-shaped wavy fronds 3. Marked extravasation of erythrocytes 4. Residual thrombus as evidenced by amorphous hyalinized material merging with vascular wall	Papillary pattern simulates angiosarcoma and is differentiated by fibrous core and cellular benignity IPEH is a reactive pattern subsequent to thrombus; history of preceding trauma common
D. Cavernous hemangioma	Reticular, dermal, and/or subcutaneous proliferation of large, irregular, blood-filled vascular spaces lined by a single layer of endothelial cells surrounded by fibrous tissue	Cavernous hemangiomas are often associated with capillary hemangiomas

Fig. **22-15.** Histiocytoid
hemangioma.
A. A diffuse infiltrate replaces normal
   dermal architecture.
B. The tumor is composed of plump
   endothelial cells with oval, pale
   nuclei and small nucleoli (arrows),
   as well as numerous interspersed
   lymphocytes. Few vascular channels
   are identified (arrow-head).

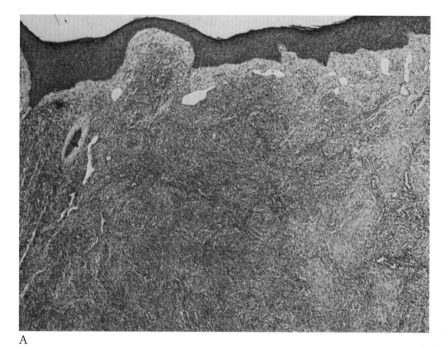

A

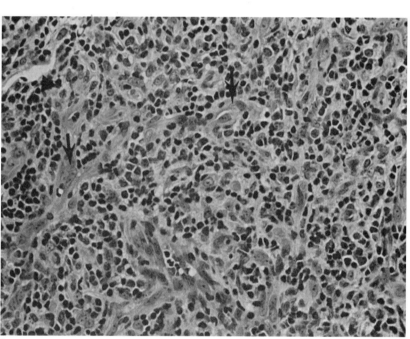

B

E. Lymphangioma
circumscripta
(Fig. 22-16)

1. Epidermis appears thin,
   normal, or hyperplastic
2. Numerous **dilated lymphatic
   channels are present in the
   upper dermis**, usually in close
   approximation to the epidermis
3. Lymphatic channels in this area
   of the dermis have extremely
   thin walls lined by a single layer
   of endothelial cells; valves also
   may be observed
4. Lymph is present within the
   channels, often admixed with
   erythrocytes
5. Communication with deep,
   thick-walled vessels is common
   but may not be apparent on
   histologic section

Differential diagnosis:
   Angiokeratoma
   Chronic radiodermatitis

Fig. **22-16.** *Lymphangioma circumscription. Numerous thinwalled, dilated lymphatic channels with valves are located high in the dermis (A), apparently pushing up the epidermis (B).*

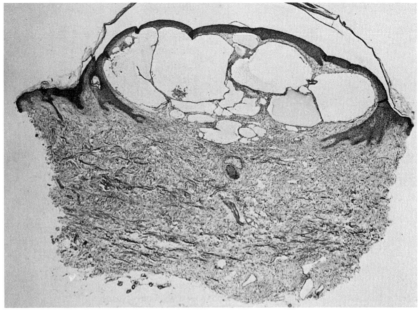

A

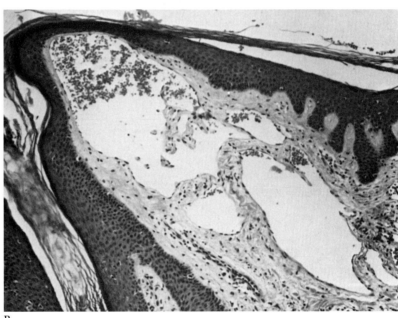

B

F. Kaposi's sarcoma
(Fig. 22-17)

Patch stage:
1. Epidermis normal
2. Low power reveals subtle, **diffuse hypercellularity** in the reticular dermis
3. Higher magnification shows **irregular spaces between collagen fibers** containing scattered erythrocytes
4. Small **foci of spindle cells** more notable in a periappendageal array

Normal capillary-sized vessel may be surrounded by spindle cells, vascular slits, and extravasated erythrocytes (so-called promontory sign)

Differential diagnosis:
Normal skin
Dermatofibroma, early

Plaque stage:
1. Epidermis normal
2. Low power. **Irregular vascular spaces** separating collagen; multifocal cellular aggregates including inflammatory cells visible
3. Higher power
   a. Spaces lined by prominent hyperchromatic endothelial cells with rare mitotic figures
   b. Cellular aggregates are composed of spindle cells, some containing eosinophilic hyaline globules and phagocytosed erythrocytes

Differential diagnosis:
Dermatofibroma
Stasis
Angiosarcoma, well-differentiated

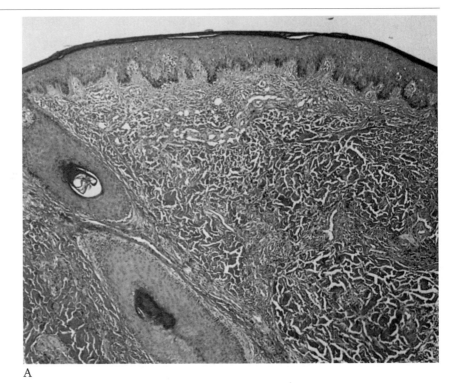

Fig. **22-17.** *Kaposi's sarcoma.*
A. *Patch stage Kaposi's sarcoma. At low magnification, there is a subtle hypercellularity in the dermis with "cracking" of the collagen.*

A

B, C. *Tumor nodule of Kaposi's sarcoma. Hyperchromatic atypical cells line a cleft within the collagen (arrows). Nuclear debris is also seen amid the collagen.*

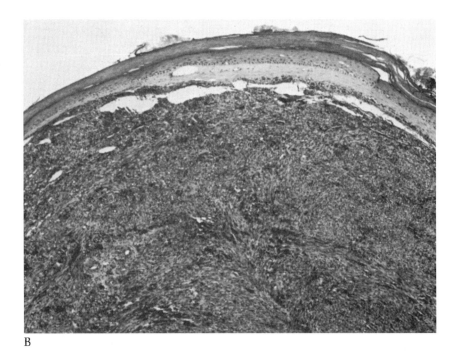

B

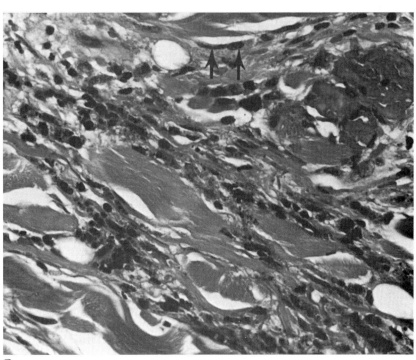

C

c. **Endothelial cell-lined vascular slits** contain stacked erythrocytes ("rouleaux")
d. Extravasation of erythrocytes and hemosiderin deposition
e. **Plasma cells** scattered amid spindle cells

Tumor stage:
1. Low power: well-defined exophytic nodule composed of spindle cells
2. High power
   a. Whorls of spindle cells with densely packed nuclei and interposed erythrocytes
   b. Some cells contain eosinophilic hyaline globules and phagocytosed erythrocytes
   c. Mitoses frequent
   d. Reticular dermis adjacent to nodule often shows ectatic vessels and aggregates of histiocytic cells

Differential diagnosis:
Other spindle-cell neoplasms, including spindle-cell melanoma

G. Glomus tumor (Fig. 22-18)

1. Small, endothelial cell-lined vessels surrounded by dense proliferation of glomus cells
2. **Glomus cells** are distinctive, large, cuboidal, or polygonal cells with clear or faintly eosinophilic cytoplasm, distinct cell walls, and large, round basophilic nuclei
3. Areas of mucoid degeneration often present
4. Fibrous capsule present

Glomus tumors usually present as solitary, painful lesions on the digits

Glomus cells are modified smooth muscle and are part of the normal glomus apparatus

H. Glomangioma (multiple glomus tumors)

1. Circumscribed but not encapsulated tumors
2. Many large, blood-filled, endothelial-cell–lined vascular channels
3. Variable numbers of glomus cells surround vascular channels

The presence of glomus cells around the vessels differentiates a glomangioma from a hemangioma

I. Hemangiopericytoma

1. Epidermis normal
2. Dense dermal proliferation of spindle-shaped or oval cells surrounding numerous vessels
3. **Branching of vascular channels** characteristic (so-called antler configuration)
4. Spindle cells may exhibit pleomorphism

Reticulum stain demarcates endothelial cells and vessel wall from proliferating pericytes

Presumed cell origin for this tumor is the pericyte

Differential diagnosis:
Glomus tumor

Fig. **22-18.** Glomus tumor. Numerous cells with bland, homogeneous nuclei surround these vascular spaces. (See also Fig. 1-5, glomus cells.)

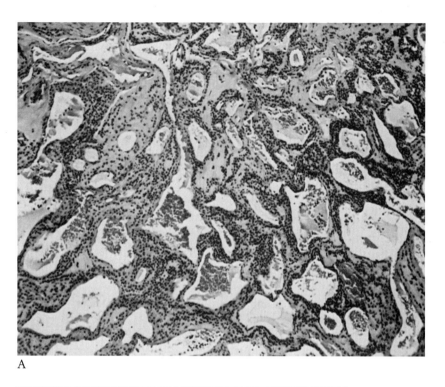

A

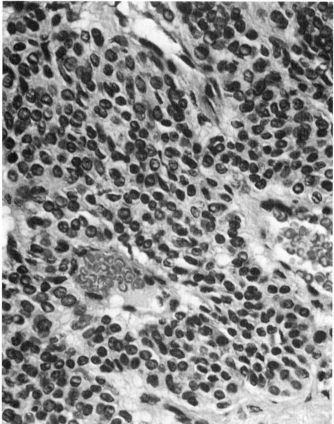

B

J. Angiosarcoma
(Fig. 22-19)

1. Extensive **infiltration of dermis by pleomorphic cells**, forming **large, irregular spaces**, which often contain erythrocytes
2. Cells exhibit large nuclei with variable hyperchromatism and striking dusky eosinophilic cytoplasm
3. Mitoses frequent
4. Pleomorphic cells form buds without stromal core that jut into lumen or may appear free floating in the lumen
5. Infiltration of muscle characteristic

Vessels surrounding tumor often show atypical hyperchromatic nuclei

Differential diagnosis:
Kaposi's sarcoma

Fig. **22-19.** Angiosarcoma.
A. A tumor nodule of angiosarcoma is present in the dermis.
B. Loosely aggregated sheets of malignant endothelial cells fill and partially occlude vessels in the dermis. This pattern of proliferation is typical of angiosarcoma and is often quite subtle. Inset: Nuclear pleomorphism and prominent nucleoli are noted.

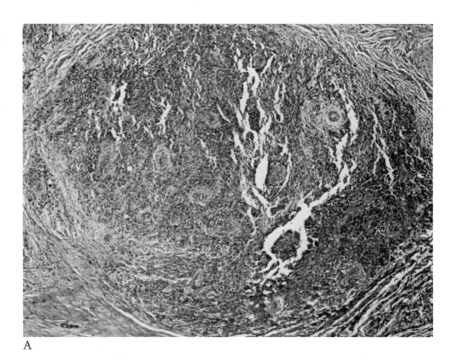

A

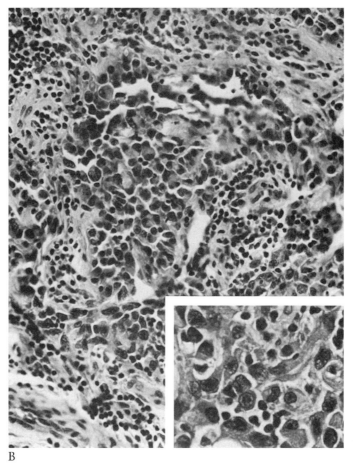

B

K. Acquired tufted angioma

1. Dilated, bloodless vessels with projections of vascular tufts in papillary dermis
2. Focal collections of clustered capillaries throughout primarily in deep reticular dermis
3. Increased numbers of spindle-shaped cells surrounding the tufts of capillaries
4. Vessels lined by enlarged endothelial cells
5. No cytologic atypia, but mitoses frequent
6. Increased numbers of eccrine glands

L. Targetoid hemosiderotic hemangioma

1. Epidermal hyperplasia
2. Ectatic dermal blood vessels lined by prominent "hobnail" endothelial cells
3. Dissecting vascular spaces extend deeply throughout reticular dermis
4. Extravasated erythrocytes and hemosiderin deposition
5. Prominent lymphangiecatasias at periphery

Endothelial cells tend to stain with CD31, but less commonly with CD34, suggesting a possible lymphatic origin for this neoplasm

M. Retiform hemangio-endothelioma

1. Poorly circumscribed proliferation of thin-walled vessels in a retiform pattern
2. Widespread dissection of arborizing vessels between collagen bundles
3. Extends deep into reticular dermis ablating cutaneous appendages
4. Variable confluent sheets of tumor cells
5. Monomorphic hobnail endothelial cells prominent
6. Minimal cytologic atypia or mitoses
7. Prominent lymphocytic infiltrate at periphery

Retiform hemangioendothelioma is a low-grade angiosarcoma with a high rate of local recurrence, but low metastatic potential

N. Spindle cell hemangio-endothelioma

1. Well-circumscribed nodule centered in reticular dermis
2. Alternating areas of thin-walled dilated cavernous vascular spaces and solid areas
3. Solid areas composed of spindle-shaped cells and epithelioid endothelial cells
4. Intracytoplasmic vacuoles variably present
5. Mitoses rare
6. Organized thrombi invariably present, most commonly in cavernous spaces

Spindle cell hemangio-endotheliomas are generally believed to be reactive processes and not true neoplasms and may be associated with Maffucci's syndrome

III. Neural

A. Neurofibroma
(Fig. 22-20)

1. Discrete but nonencapsulated dermal mass composed of a cellular proliferation within a fine eosinophilic stroma
2. **Thin, wavy, faintly eosinophilic fibers** lying in loosely textured strands
3. Slender, oval to spindle-shaped, **wavy nuclei**
4. Focal areas of myxoid change occasionally present
5. Increased number of mast cells often present
6. Few myelinated nerve fibers present, no demonstrable nerve bundles

Differential diagnosis:
"Neurotized" nevus
Neurilemmoma

Plexiform neurofibroma, a marker of neurofibromatosis, characteristically contains large, irregularly shaped nerve bundles in the lower dermis and subcutis. The nerve trunks show hypercellularity and often mucinous change

B. Palisaded encapsulated neuroma (true neuroma)

Well-defined aggregates of nerve trunks within papillary and reticular dermis

In contrast to the name, there is no real palisading and no encapsulation

Typically occurs as a small papule on the face

Multiple mucosal neuromas show similar histologic features

C. Traumatic or amputation neuroma

1. Large, irregular bundles of peripheral nerves associated with considerable connective-tissue proliferation
2. Organization into bundles is a distinctive feature

Fig. **22-20.** Neurofibroma. The elongated spindle cells have small nuclei that appear to loop and curl. The cells appear smaller than those of leiomyoma. Mucinous and edematous areas (not shown here) are common.

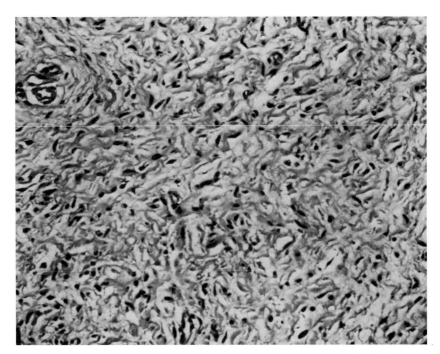

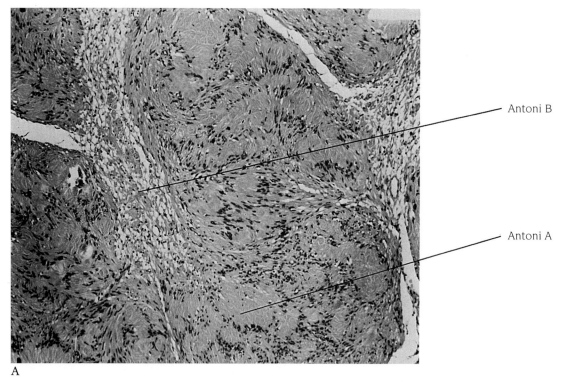

Antoni B

Antoni A

A

Fig. **22-21.** *Neurilemmoma.*
A. *When well-developed, this spindle
cell tumor exhibits Antoni A and B
patterns. Antoni A refers to areas of
loose, edematous connective tissue;
Antoni B to foci of nuclear
palisading.*

D. Neurilemmoma;
schwannoma
(Fig. 22-21)

1. Circumscribed encapsulated
spindle cell (Schwann cell)
proliferation within a delicate
fibrillar eosinophilic matrix
2. Antoni A (with Verocay bodies)
and Antoni B areas characteristic
3. Tumor arises within perineurium and lies adjacent to nerve
trunks
4. Mast cells may be present

Cells with closely apposed nuclei
in parallel array are called
Antoni A areas; rows of
palisaded nuclei that are
parallel but separated by an
acellular matrix are called
Verocay bodies; mucinous
edematous stroma with
scattered cells is called
Antoni B area

E. Malignant schwannoma

1. Nodular aggregate of highly
plemorphic spindle cells with
numerous mitotic figures,
sometimes showing Verocay
body formation
2. Evidence of residual plexiform
neurofibroma may be present
peripherally

Differential diagnosis:
Neutrotropic melanoma

B, C. *Two nuclear palisades enclosing a relatively anuclear central area are called a Verocay body.*

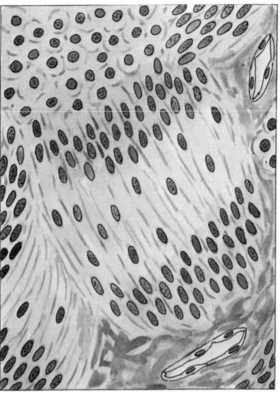

B

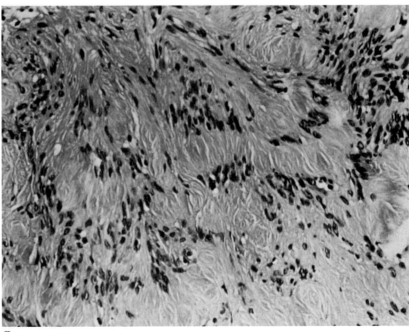

C

F. Granular cell tumor
(Fig. 22-22)

1. Epidermal hyperplasia, often marked, with increased melanin in basal layer
2. Distinctive, large, polygonal tumor cells with abundant, **pale eosinophilic granular cytoplasm,** usually distinct cytoplasmic membrane
3. Nuclei small, dark, and centrally placed
4. Cells may be arranged in sheets or cords or individually dispersed between collagen or muscle fibers
5. Discrete round eosinophilic globules are characteristically present in cytoplasm (pustuloovoid bodies)

The cytoplasmic granules are PAS-positive and diastase-resistant and also stain with colloidal iron and PTAH

Differential diagnosis:
Xanthoma
Lepromatous leprosy

Granular cell tumors occur commonly in the tongue; the prominent epithelial hyperplasia is sometimes mistaken for squamous cell carcinoma

Tumor cells are derived from Schwann cells and stain positively with S-100 protein

Fig. **22-22.** *Granular cell tumor. Polygonal cells with eosinophilic granular cytoplasm and small, dark nuclei are present within the dermis, infiltrating among collagen bundles.*

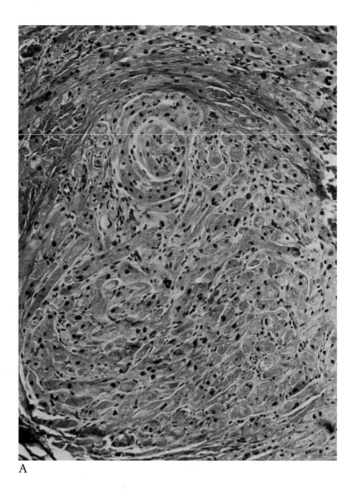

A

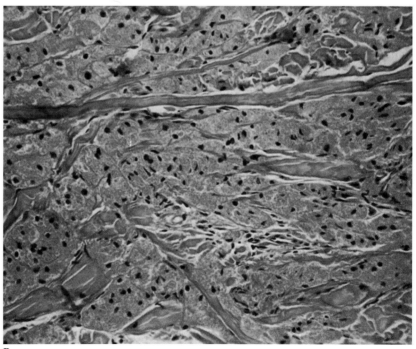

B

G. Neuroendocrine carcinoma (Merkel cell tumor) (Fig. 22-23)

1. Low power
   Large dermal aggregates of uniform cells with hyperchromatic nuclei and multifocal obvious zones of necrosis
2. High power
   a. Cells in sheets and trabecular array
   b. Nuclei are hyperchromatic; cytoplasms appear to form syncytia
   c. Mitoses are frequent
   d. Necrotic zones show shadowy rims of tumor cells

Differential diagnosis:
   Lymphoma
   Metastatic small cell carcinoma (including oat cell carcinoma and carcinoid)

Immunoperoxidase studies:
   Neuron-specific enolase positive
   Cytokeratin-20 paranuclear staining is uncharacteristically seen
   Chromagranin, if positive, is helpful

Electron microscopy:
   Membrane-bound dense core granules characteristic

Immunoperoxidase and electron microscopic findings do not differentiate Merkel cell tumor from metastatic tumors with neuroendocrine granules

Fig. **22-23.** *Neuroendocrine carcinoma.*
A. *There is a dense proliferation of basaloid cells within the dermis.*
B. *Higher magnification reveals a monomorphous infiltrate of atypical cells with large nuclei and syncytial cytoplasm.*

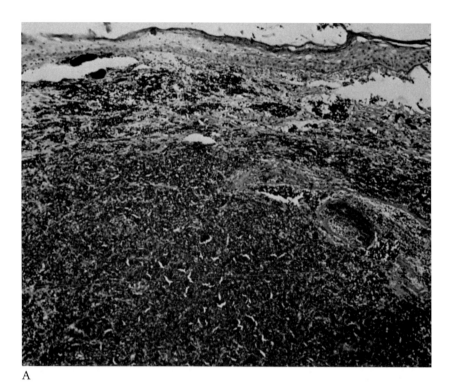

A

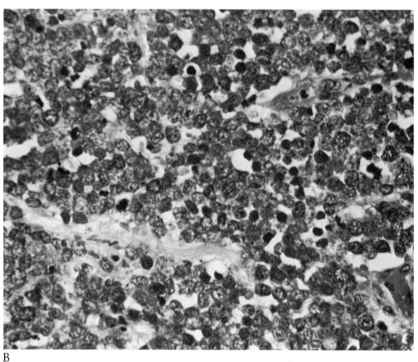

B

IV. Smooth muscle

A. Leiomyoma (Fig. 22-24)

1. Bundles of spindle-shaped cells with abundant cytoplasm and **oval, cigar-shaped nuclei**
2. In cross section, nuclei appear round and in the center of the cell with perinuclear vacuolization

Dermal leiomyomas commonly arise from the arrector pili or dartos muscle (piloleiomyoma) or vessel walls; subcutaneous leiomyomas typically arise from a vessel wall (angioleiomyoma)

Differential diagnosis:
Neurofibroma
Neurilemmoma

Special stains help confirm the diagnosis: with the trichrome stain, smooth muscle appears pink to red and collagen appears blue-green; using the van Gieson stain, muscle and nerves appear yellow and collagen appears red. Cells stain with antibodies to smooth muscle actin

Fig. **22-24.** *Leiomyoma. This spindle cell tumor has abundant eosinophilic cytoplasm and cigar-shaped nuclei. Compared with neurofibroma, these cells are larger, the cytoplasm is more abundant, and the shape of these cells is larger and less contorted.*

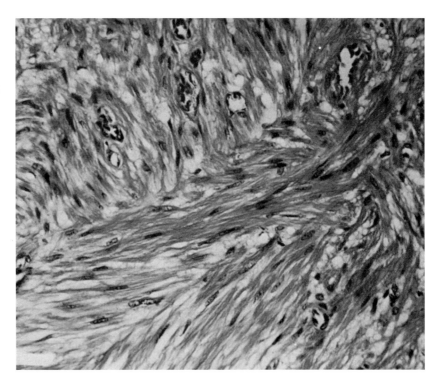

B. Leiomyosarcoma
(Fig. 22-25)

1. Nodule of pleomorphic spindle cells in fascicles containing oval to cigar-shaped nuclei
2. Clear separation of nuclei from cell membrane best observed in cross-section where nucleus lies centrally in cell
3. Striking **nuclear pleomorphism** associated with **numerous mitoses**
4. Tumor necrosis common in large lesion

Verocay bodies may occur in any spindle cell tumor and are most commonly associated with tumors of neurogenic origin but have occurred in leiomyosarcoma, malignant fibrous histiocytoma, and melanoma, among others

Fig. **22-25.** Leiomyosarcoma.
A. Fascicles of pleomorphic spindle cells with atypical nuclei are seen.
B. A higher magnification displays a mitotic figure and marked nuclear atypia (arrow).

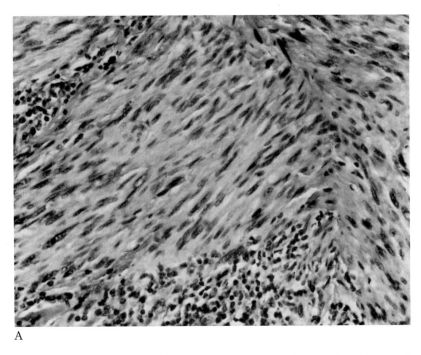

A

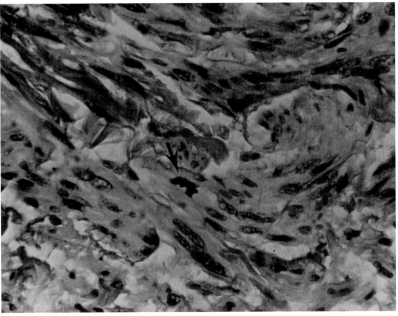

B

V. Miscellaneous

A. Metastatic carcinoma (Fig. 22-26)

1. Malignant tumor cells with hyperchromatic, large nuclei infiltrate and displaced collagen bundles
2. Some tumors are associated with a fibroblastic (desmoplastic) response
3. Metastases frequently exhibit histologic similarities to the primary tumor

Immunoperoxidase studies may help identify primary tumor, for example, prostate-specific antigen

Fig. **22-26.** Metastatic adenocarcinoma. Carcinoma cells are situated in the upper dermis. Note the glandular differentiation in B (arrow).

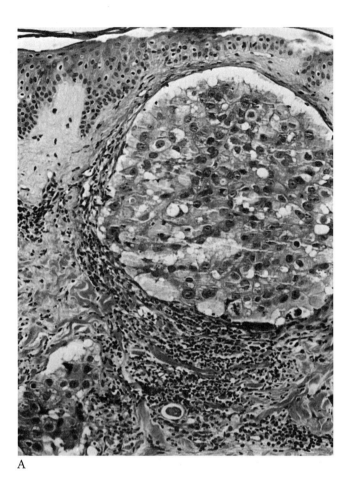

A

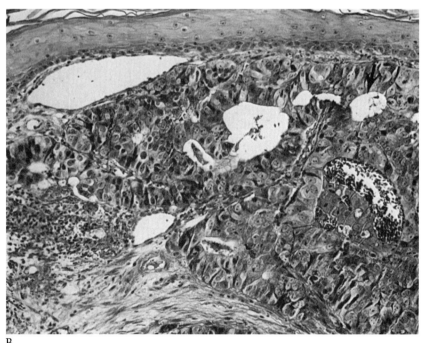

B

B. Metastatic melanoma (Fig. 22-27)

Metastases lack the polypoid architecture of primary melanoma; also given their origin outside the epidermis, they do not often involve it to a great extent, and epidermal collarettes seldom form. The inflammation, fibrosis, ulceration, and vascular changes often seen in primary lesions of malignant melanoma are uncommon in metastases. However, vascular invasion is much more common in metastases, again masking their likely origin.

Immunoperoxidase studies using S-100 and HMB 45 antibodies are useful

C. Epithelioid sarcoma

1. Nodular, deforming aggregates of epithelioid and spindle-shaped cells with eosinophilic cytoplasm surround necrotic zones in which shadowy outline and tumor cells can be identified.
2. Variable nuclear pleomorphism with frequent, prominent, and often atypical mitoses
3. Spindle-shaped and epithelioid cells associated with a variably hyalinized stroma

Differential diagnosis:
Palisading granulomas
Infectious granulomas with fibrosis

Areas of necrosis may exhibit calcification

A unique feature of this tumor is cellular staining for cytokeratin and vimentin using immunohistochemistry

Fig. **22-27.** Metastatic melanoma. The tumor nodule is situated in the reticular dermis and is composed of a loose syncytium of cells with pleomorphic nuclei and atypical mitotic figures.

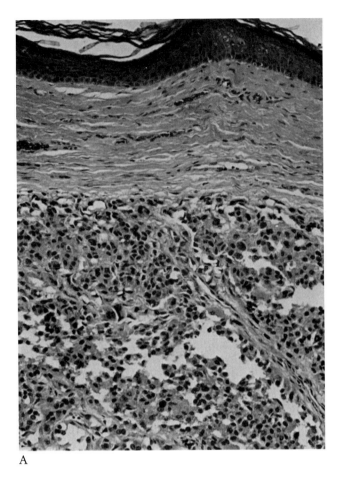

A

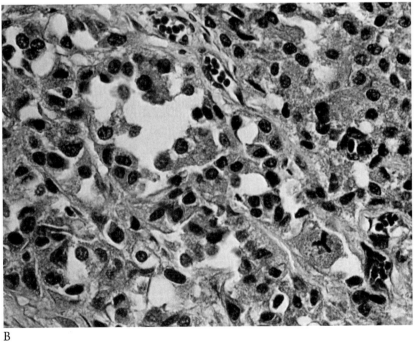

B

Suggested Reading
Fibrohistiocytic

Nevus Lipomatosis Superficialis
Dotz, W., and Prioleau, P. G. Nevus lipomatosis cutaneous superficialis. A light and electron microscope study. *Arch. Dermatol.* 120:376, 1984.

Reymond, J. L., Stoebner, P., and Ambeard, P. Nevus lipomatous cutaneous superficialis: An electron microscopic study of four cases. *J. Cutan. Pathol.* 7:295, 1980.

Acquired Digital Fibrokeratoma
Bart, R. S., Andrade, R., Kopf, A. W., et al. Acquired digital fibrokeratomas. *Arch. Dermatol.* 97:120, 1968.

Supernumerary Digit
Shapiro, L., Juhlin, E. A., and Brownstein, M. H. Rudimentary polydactyly: An amputation neuroma. *Arch. Dermatol.* 108:223, 1973.

Angiofibroma
Meigel, W. N., and Ackerman, A. B. Fibrous papule of the face. *Am. J. Dermatopathol.* 1:329, 1979.

Accessory Tragus
Brownstein, M. H., Wanger, N., and Helwig, E. B. Accessory tragi. *Arch. Dermatol.* 104:625, 1971.

Hypertrophic Scar and Keloid
Linares, H. A., Kischer, C. W., Dobrkovsky, M., et al. The histiotypic organization of the hypertrophic scar in humans. *J. Invest. Dermatol.* 59:323, 1972.

Linares, H. A., and Larson, D. L. Early differential diagnosis between hypertrophic and nonhypertrophic healing. *J. Invest. Dermatol.* 62:514, 1974.

Connective-Tissue Nevus
Racque, C. J., and Wood, M. G. Connective-tissue nevus. *Arch. Dermatol.* 102:390, 1970.

Schorr, W. F., Optiz, J. M., and Reyes, C. N. The connective tissue nevus-osteopoikilosis syndrome. *Arch. Dermatol.* 106:208, 1972.

Fibromatosis
Aviles, E., Arlen, M., and Miller, T. Plantar fibromatosis. *Surgery* 69:117, 1971.

Recurrent Infantile Digital Fibromatosis
Mehregan, A. H., Nabai, H., and Matthews, J. E. Recurring digital fibrous tumor of childhood. *Arch. Dermatol.* 106:375, 1972.

Dermatofibroma
Goette, D. K., and Helwig, E. B. Basal cell carcinomas and basal cell carcinomalike changes overlying dermatofibromas. *Arch. Dermatol.* 111:589, 1975.

Gonzales, B. Benign fibrous histiocytomas of the skin: An immunohistochemical analysis of 30 cases. *Pathol. Res. Pract.* 180:486, 1985.

Dermatofibrosarcoma Protuberans
Barr, R. J., Young, E. M., and King, D. F. Non-polarizable collagen in dermatofibrosarcoma protuberans: A useful diagnostic aid. *J. Cutan. Pathol.* 13:339, 1986.

Burkhardt, B. R., Soule, E. H., Winkelmann, R. K., et al. Dermatofibrosarcoma protuberans: Study of 58 cases. *Am. J. Surg.* 111:638, 1986.

Atypical Fibroxanthoma and Malignant Fibrous Histiocytoma
Fretzin, D. F., and Helwig, E. B. Atypical fibroxanthoma of the skin: A clinicopathologic study of 140 cases. *Cancer* 31:1541, 1973.

Weiss, S. W., and Enzuiger, F. M. Malignant fibrous histiocytoma: An analysis of 200 cases. *Cancer* 41:2250, 1978.

Fibrosarcoma
Pritchard, D. J., Soule, E. H., Taylor, W. F., et al. Fibrosarcoma, a clinicopathologic and statistical study of 199 tumors of the soft tissues of the extremities and trunk. *Cancer* 33:888, 1974.

Vascular

Lobular Capillary Hemangioma

Mills, S. E., Cooper, P. H., and Fechner, R. E. Lobular capillary hemangioma: The underlying lesion of pyogenic granuloma: A study of 73 cases from the oral and nasal mucous membranes. *Am. J. Surg. Pathol.* 4:471, 1980.

Bacillary Angiomatosis

Cockerall, C. J., and LeBoit, P. E. Bacillary angiomatosis: A newly characterized, pseudoneoplastic, infectious, cutaneous vascular disorder. *J. Am. Acad. Dermatol.* 22:501, 1990.

Knobler, E. H., Silvers, D. N., Fine, K. C., et al. Unique vascular skin lesions associated with human immunodeficiency virus. *JAMA* 260:524, 1988.

LeBoit, P. E. Bacillary angiomatosis. *Mod. Pathol.* 8:218–222, 1995.

Relman, D. A., Loutit, J. S., Schmidt, T. M., et al. The agent of bacillary angiomatosis: An approach to the identification of uncultured pathogens. *N. Engl. J. Med.* 323:1573, 1990.

Tappero, J. W., Koehler, J. E., Berger, T. G., Cockerell, C. J., Lee, T. H., Busch, M. P., Stites, D. P., et al. Bacillary angiomatosis and bacillary splenitis in immunocompetent adults. *Ann. Intern. Med.* 118:363–365, 1993.

Webster, G. F., Cockerell, C. J., and Friedman-Kien, A. E. The clinical spectrum of bacillary angiomatosis. *Br. J. Dermatol.* 126:535–541, 1992.

Intravascular Papillary Endothelial Hyperplasia

Hashimoto, H., Diamaru, Y., and Enjoji, M. Intravascular papillary endothelial hyperplasia: A clinicopathologic study of 91 cases. *Am. J. Dermatopathol.* 5:539, 1983.

Kaposi's Sarcoma

Blumenfeld, W., Egbert, B. M., and Sagebiel, R. W. Differential diagnosis of Kaposi's sarcoma. *Arch. Pathol. Lab. Med.* 109:123, 1985.

Chang, Y., Cesarman, E., Pessin, M. S., Lee, F., Culpepper, J., Knowles, D. M., and Moore, P. S. Identification of herpesvirus-like DNA sequences in AIDS-associated Kaposi's sarcoma. *Science* 266:1865–1869, 1994.

Chang, Y., and Moore, P. S. Kaposi's sarcoma (KS)-associated herpesvirus and its role in KS. *Infect. Agents Dis.* 5:215–222, 1996.

Francis, N. D., Parkin, J. M., Weber, J., et al. Kaposi's sarcoma in acquired immune deficiency syndrome (AIDS). *J. Clin. Pathol.* 39:469, 1986.

Fukunaga, M., and Silverberg, S. G. Hyaline globules in Kaposi's sarcoma: A light microscopic and immunohistochemical study. *Mod. Pathol.* 4:187–190, 1991.

McNutt, N. S., Fletcher, V., and Conant, M. A. Early lesions of Kaposi's sarcoma in homosexual men: An ultrastructural comparison with other vascular proliferations in skin. *Am. J. Pathol.* 111:62, 1983.

Moskowitz, L. B., Hensley, G. T., Gould, E. W., and Weiss, S. D. Frequency and anatomic distribution of lymphadenopathic Kaposi's sarcoma in the acquired immunodeficiency syndrome: An autopsy series. *Hum. Pathol.* 16:447–456, 1985.

Niedt, G. W., Myskowski, P. L., Urmacher, C., Niedzwiecki, D., Chapman, D., and Safai, B. Histology of early lesions of AIDS-associated Kaposi's sarcoma. *Mod. Pathol.* 3:64–70, 1990.

Tappero, J. W., Conant, M. A., Wolfe, S. F., and Berger, T. G. Kaposi's sarcoma. Epidemiology, pathogenesis, histology, clinical spectrum, staging criteria and therapy. *J. Am. Acad. Dermatol.* 28:371–395, 1993.

Glomus Tumor

Harris, M. Ultrastructure of a glomus tumor. *J. Clin. Pathol.* 24:520, 1971.

Miettinen, M., Lehto, V-P., and Virtanen, I. Glomus tumor cells: Evaluation of smooth muscle and endothelial cell properties. *Virchows. Arch.* (B). 43:139, 1983.

Hemangiopericytoma

Enzinger, F. M., and Smith, B. H. Hemangiopericytoma: An analysis of 106 cases. *Hum. Pathol.* 7:61, 1976.

Angiosarcoma

Cooper, P. H. Angiosarcomas of the skin. *Semin. Diagn. Pathol.* 4:2, 1987.

Hodgkinson, D. J., Soule, E. H., and Woods, J. E. Cutaneous angiosarcoma of the head and neck. *Cancer* 44:1106, 1979.

Maddox, J. C., and Evans, H. L. Angiosarcoma of skin and soft tissue: A study of forty-four cases. *Cancer* 48:1907, 1981.

Neural

Neurofibroma

Brasfield, R. D., and Das Gupta, T. K. Von Recklinghausen's disease: A clinico-pathological study. *Ann. Surg.* 175:86, 1972.

Crowe, F. W., Schull, J., and Neel, J. V. *A Clinical, Pathological and Genetic Study of Multiple Neurofibromatosis.* Springfield, IL: Thomas, 1956.

Megahed, M. Histopathologic variants of neurofibroma. *Am. J. Dermatopathol.* 16:486–495, 1994.

Neurofibromatosis: Consensus statement. National Institutes of Health Consensus Development Conference. *Arch. Neurol.* 45:575–578, 1988.

Reed, R. J. Cutaneous manifestations of neural crest disorders (neurocristo-pathies). *Int. J. Dermatol.* 16:807, 1977.

Riccardi, V. M. Cutaneous manifestations of neurofibromatosis: Cellular interaction, pigmentation and mast cells. *Birth Defects* 17:129–145, 1981.

Sorensen, S. A., Mulvihill, J. J., and Nielsen, A. Long term follow-up of von Recklinghausen neurofibromatosis: Survival and malignant neoplasms. *N. Engl. J. Med.* 314:1010, 1986.

Palisaded Encapsulated Neuroma

Reed, R. J., Fine, R. M., and Meltzer, H. D. Palisaded encapsulated neuromas of the skin. *Arch. Dermatol.* 106:865, 1972.

Neurilemmoma

Das Guptas, T. K., Brasfield, R. D., Strong, E. W., et al. Benign solitary schwannomas (neurilemmomas). *Cancer* 24:335, 1969.

Fletcher, C. D. M., and Davies, S. E. Benign plexiform (multinodular) schwannoma: A rare tumor unassociated with neurofibromatosis. *Histopathology* 10:971–980, 1986.

Val-Bernal, J. F., Figols, J., and Vazquez-Barquero, A. Cutaneous plexiform schwannoma associated with neurofibromatosis type 2. *Cancer* 76:1181–1186, 1995.

Woodruff, J. M., Godwin, T. A., Erlandson, R. A., Susin, M., and Martini, N. Cellular schwannoma: A variety of schwannoma sometimes mistaken for a malignant tumor. *Am. J. Surg. Pathol.* 5:733–744, 1981.

Malignant Schwannoma

Roth, M. J., Medeiros, J., Kapur, S., Wexler, L. H., Mims, S., Horowitz, M. E., and Tsokos, M. Malignant schwannoma with melanocytic and neuroepithelial differentiation in an infant with congenital giant melanocytic nevus: A complex neurocristopathy. *Hum. Pathol.* 24:1371–1375, 1993.

Taxy, J. B., Battifora, H., Trujillo, Y., et al. Electron microscopy in the diagnosis of malignant schwannoma. *Cancer* 48:1381, 1981.

Granular Cell Tumor

Armin, A., Connelly, E. M., and Rowden, G. An immunoperoxidase investigation of S-100 protein in granular cell myoblastomas: Evidence for Schwann cell derivation. *Am. J. Clin. Pathol.* 79:37, 1983.

Lack, E. E., Worsham, G. F., Callihan, M. D., et al. Granular cell tumor: A clinicopathologic study of 110 patients. *J. Surg. Oncol.* 13:301, 1980.

Smooth Muscle

Neuroendocrine Carcinoma

Warner, T. F. C. S., Uno, H., Hafez, R., et al. Merkel cells and Merkel cell tumors. Ultrastructure, immunocytochemistry, and review of the literature. *Cancer* 52:238, 1983.

Leiomyoma

Bures, J. C., Barnes, L., and Mercer, D. A comparative study of smooth muscle tumors utilizing light and electron microscopy, immunocytochemical staining and enzymatic assay. *Cancer* 48:2420, 1981.

Leiomyosarcoma

Headington, J. T., Beals, T. F., and Niederhuber, J. E. Primary leiomyosarcoma of the shin: A report and critical appraisal. *J. Cutan. Pathol.* 4:308, 1977.

Stout, A. P., and Hill, W. T. Leiomyosarcoma of the superficial soft tissues. *Cancer* 11(4):844, 1958.

Miscellaneous

Metastatic Carcinoma

Aguilar, A., Schoendorff, C., Lopez Redondo, M. J., Ambrojo, P., Requena, L., and Sanchez Yus, E. Epidermotropic metastases from internal carcinomas. *Am. J. Dermatopathol.* 13:452–458, 1991.

Brownstein, M. H., and Helwig, E. B. Patterns of cutaneous metastasis. *Arch. Dermatol.* 105:862, 1972.

Lookingbill, D. P., Spangler, N., and Helm, K. F. Cutaneous metastases in patients with metastatic carcinoma: A retrospective study of 4020 patients. *J. Am. Acad. Dermatol.* 29:228–236, 1993.

Reingold, I. M. Cutaneous metastases from internal carcinoma. *Cancer* 19:162–168, 1966.

Spencer, P. S., and Helma, T. N. Skin metastases in cancer patients. *Cutis* 39:119–121, 1987.

Zeligman, I., and Schwilm, A. Umbilical metastasis from carcinoma of the colon. *Arch. Dermatol.* 110:911, 1974.

Epithelioid Sarcoma

Wick, M. R., and Manivel, J. C. Epithelioid sarcoma and isolated necrobiotic granuloma: A comparative immunocytochemical study. *J. Cutan. Pathol.* 13:253, 1986.

Chapter **23**

Cysts in the Dermis

Careful examination of the cyst wall, in terms of epithelium cell type and associated appendages, is the key to proper identification.

The Reactive Process and the Disease	Histopathology	Comments
I. Epidermal inclusion cyst; milium (Figs. 23-1, 23-2)	1. Cyst wall lined with normal epidermis, including a **granular layer** 2. Cyst contains eosinophilic, often laminated, keratinous material 3. Rupture of cyst results in inflammatory infiltrate with multinucleate foreign-body giant cells	See Table 23-1 for a comparison of histologic features of dermal cysts Very small epidermal inclusion cysts are called *milia* The presence of a granular cell layer and visible intercellular bridges are features that distinguish an epidermal inclusion cyst from a pilar cyst
II. Pilar cyst (Figs. 23-1, 23-3)	1. Cyst wall composed of eosinophilic keratinocytes, which do not form a granular layer 2. Cell borders indistinct; **no visible intercellular bridges** 3. Cyst contains amorphous eosinophilic material and parakeratotic nuclear remnants 4. Focal calcification of cyst contents may occur	Pilar and epidermal inclusion cysts are indistinguishable clinically
III. Steatocystoma (Fig. 23-4)	1. Folded, or convoluted, cyst wall composed of keratinocytes with peripheral palisading basal cells and no apparent intracellular bridges 2. Amorphous eosinophilic corrugated keratin layer centrally 3. Cyst may contain hair and amorphous granular material 4. Characteristically, **sebaceus gland lobules** are present adjacent to or within the cyst wall	
IV. Dermoid cyst	1. **Cyst wall lined by epidermis with mature appendages** (hair follicles, sebaceous glands, and rarely apocrine glands) 2. Cyst cavity usually contains hair	These lesions, which occur most commonly on the face, often are present at birth

Fig. **23-1.** *Comparison of epidermal inclusion and pilar cysts. In the former, cells flatten as they mature and form a granular layer with recognizable squames (left). In the pilar cyst, the more rounded cells mature without a granular layer and form a solid-appearing keratin product (right).*

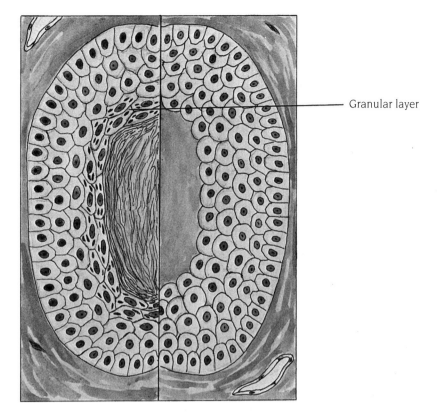

——————— Granular layer

Table **23-1.** *Histologic Features Differentiating Cysts in the Dermis*

	Epidermal Inclusion Cyst	Pilar Cyst	Steatocys-toma	Dermoid Cyst	Hidrocys-toma	Vellus Hair Cyst	Ganglion	Cutaneous Ciliated Cyst
Cyst wall	Normal epidermis; granular layer present	Peripherally palisading eosinophilic cells with no visible intercellular bridges; no granular layer present	Convoluted or wavy wall composed of basophilic cells without visible intercellular bridges; eosinophilic cuticle centrally	Normal epidermis	Cuboidal (eccrine) or columnar (apocrine) cells; decapitation secretion of columnar cells observed	Normal epidermis	Dense, fibrous connective tissue	Pseudostrati-fied co-lumnar epithelium
Cyst contents	Laminated, eosinophilic keratinous material	Homogeneous, eosinophilic, amorphous material	Hairs may be present	May contain hair	Granular, amorphous, pale, eosino-philic material	Laminated, eosinophilic, keratinous material; numerous small vellus hairs	Myxoid, slightly basophilic, amorphous material	Eosinophilic amorphous material
Appendages adjacent to or within	None	None	Sebaceous glands adjacent to or within cyst wall	Mature pilose-baceous units attach to cyst wall and open into lumen	None	Hair follicle occasionally attached to cyst wall	None	None
Other		Focal calcifica-tion of cyst contents common		Subcutaneous location	Outer layer of myoepithe-lial cells			Cilia on the inner surface of cyst lining

Fig. **23-2.** *Epidermal inclusion cyst.*

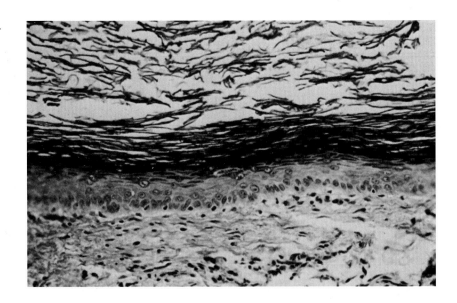

Fig. **23-3.** *Pilar cyst.*

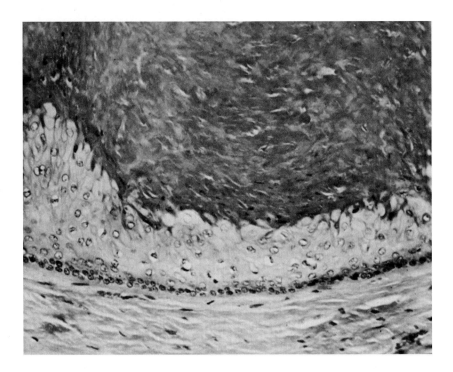

Fig. **23-4.** Steatocystoma. The folded
wall of the cyst is lined by stratified
squamous epithelium, and sebaceous
glands open into the lumen.

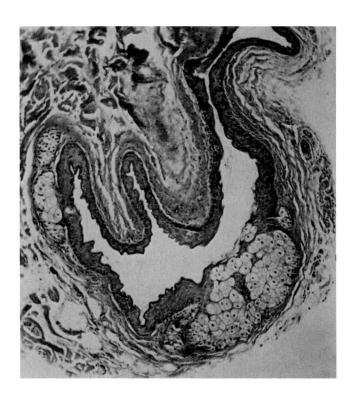

V. Hidrocystoma

    A. Eccrine (Fig. 23-5)

1. Unilocular or multilocular intradermal cyst
2. Cyst wall composed of one or two layers of **cuboidal or flattened, eccrine epithelial cells**

    B. Apocrine

1. Large cystic spaces within the dermis
2. Papillary projections into lumen
3. Cyst wall composed of one or more layers of **columnar cells,** which exhibit "decapitation" secretion
4. Myoepithelial cells are located peripheral to the columnar cells
5. Loose stroma around cyst often contains extravasated erythrocytes

This lesion often presents clinically as a slowly enlarging gray or bluish, soft cystic nodule on the scalp or face

Fig. **23-5.** A, B. *Hidrocystoma, probably eccrine.*

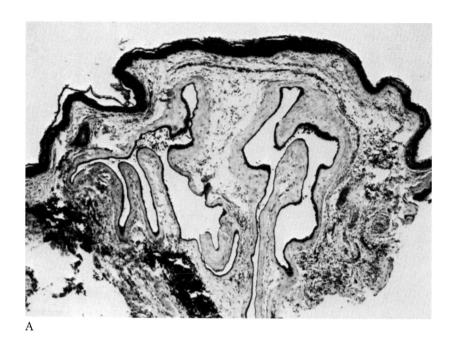

A

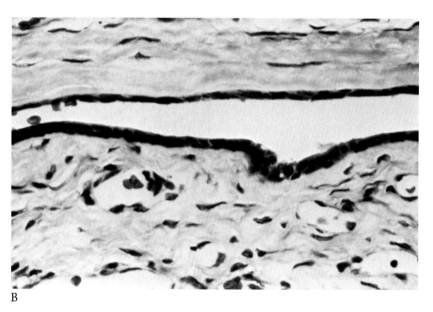

B

VI. Vellus hair cyst (Fig. 23-6)

1. Small cyst in middle dermis lined with normal epidermis
2. Cyst contains eosinophilic, laminated keratinous material and **numerous small vellus hairs**
3. Hair follicle occasionally attached to cyst wall

The presence of multiple small hairs within the cyst differentiates this lesion from an epidermal inclusion cyst

VII. Ganglion (synovial) cyst (Fig. 23-7)

1. Cystic space or spaces filled with **myxoid material** and surrounded by fibrous wall
2. Located in proximity to synovium, joint capsule, or other dense collagenous tissue

VIII. Digital myxoid cyst

    A. Digital mucous cyst; myxoid cyst

1. Elevated, dome-shaped lesion with flattened epidermis
2. Variable mucin deposition:
   a. Between collagen fibers
   b. Within fissures or cleftlike spaces in the dermis
   c. Within large cystic spaces, which may fill entire dermis
3. Proliferation of fibroblasts in and around areas of mucin deposition

Early lesions may resemble focal mucinosis

Fig. **23-6.** *Vellus hair cyst. The appearance is similar to that of epidermal inclusion cyst, but the lumen contains numerous vellus hairs.*

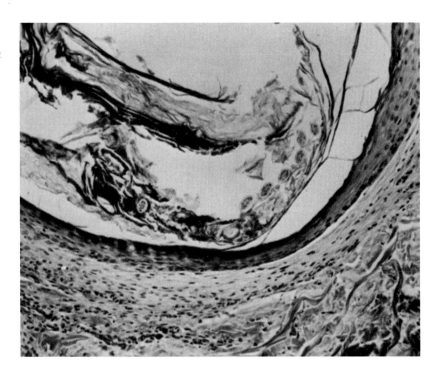

Fig. **23-7.** *Ganglion cyst. Mucoid material is present within a multilocular cyst, the walls of which are composed of fibrous tissue, probably related to joint capsule or tendon.*

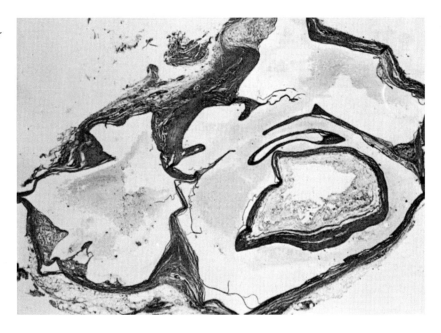

IX. Cutaneous ciliated cyst
(Fig. 23-8)

1. Unilocular or multilocular
2. **Pseudostratified, ciliated columnar epithelium**
3. Mucous glands and smooth muscle absent

Fig. **23-8.** *Cutaneous ciliated cyst. The cells lining this cyst are pseudostratified and ciliated (arrow, B).*

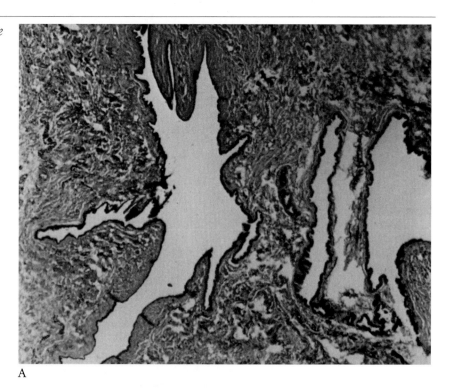

A

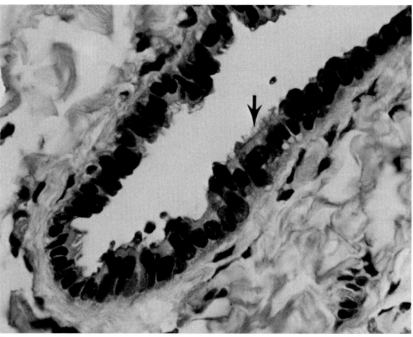

B

Suggested Reading

Epidermal Inclusion and Pilar Cysts

Cooper, P. H., and Fechner, R. E. Pilomatricoma-like changes in the epidermal cysts of Gardner's syndrome. *J. Am. Acad. Dermatol.* 8:639–644, 1983.

McGavran, M. H., and Binnington, B. Keratinous cysts of the skin: Identification and differentiation of pilar cysts from epidermal cysts. *Arch. Dermatol.* 94:499, 1966.

Rahbari, H. Epidermoid cysts with seborrheic verruca-like cyst walls. *Arch. Dermatol.* 118:326, 1982.

Steatocystoma

Brownstein, M. H. Steatocystoma simplex: A solitary steatocystoma. *Arch. Dermatol.* 118:409, 1982.

Marley, W. M., Buntin, D. M., and Chesney, T. M. Steatocystoma multiplex limited to the scalp. *Arch. Dermatol.* 117:673, 1981.

Schiff, B. L., Kern, A. B., and Ronchese, F. Steatocystoma multiplex. *Arch. Dermatol.* 77:516, 1958.

Dermoid Cyst

Brownstein, M. H., and Helwig, E. B. Subcutaneous dermoid cysts. *Arch. Dermatol.* 107:237, 1973.

Hidrocystoma

Smith, J. D., and Chernosky, M. E. Hidrocystomas. *Arch. Dermatol.* 108:676, 1973.

Smith, J. D., and Chernosky, M. E. Apocrine hydrocystoma (cystadenoma). *Arch. Dermatol.* 109:700, 1974.

Vellus Hair Cyst

Esterly, N. B., Fretzin, D. F., and Pinkus, H. Eruptive vellous hair cysts. *Arch. Dermatol.* 113:500, 1977.

Lee, S., and Kim, J-G. Eruptive vellus hair cyst: Clinical and histologic finding. *Arch. Dermatol.* 115:744, 1979.

Stiefler, R. E., and Bergfeld, W. F. Eruptive vellus hair cysts: An inherited disorder. *J. Am. Acad. Dermatol.* 3:425, 1980.

Cutaneous Ciliated Cyst

Farmer, E. R., and Helwig, E. B. Cutaneous ciliated cysts. *Arch. Dermatol.* 114:70, 1978.

True, L., and Golitz, L. E. Ciliated plantar cyst. *Arch. Dermatol.* 116:1066, 1980.

Part **V**

Appendages

Chapter 24

Disorders of the
Pilosebaceous Unit

I. Hyperkeratosis and inflammatory reactions
   A. Keratosis pilaris
   B. Pityriasis rubra pilaris
   C. Follicular eczema
   D. Folliculitis
      1. Acute superficial
      2. Acute deep
      3. Chronic deep
   E. Pityrosporon folliculitis
   F. Eosinophilic folliculitis
   G. Perforating folliculitis
   H. Majocchi's granuloma
   I. Invasive dermatophytosis
II. Alopecia, nonscarring
   A. Follicular mucinosis
   B. Alopecia areata
   C. Androgenic alopecia
   D. Traction alopecia and trichotillomania
   E. Telogen effluvium
III. Alopecia, scarring
   A. Lupus erythematosus
   B. Lichen planopilaris
   C. Pseudopelade of Brocq
   D. Alopecia neoplastica
IV. Hyperplasia and neoplasms
   A. Nevus sebaceous
      1. Childhood
      2. Adult
   B. Sebaceous hyperplasia
   C. Sebaceous adenoma
   D. Sebaceous epithelioma
   E. Sebaceoma
   F. Sebaceous carcinoma
   G. Trichofolliculoma
   H. Pilar tumor of the scalp (proliferating trichilemmal cyst)
   I. Trichilemmoma
   J. Trichoepithelioma
   K. Pilomatrixoma (calcifying epithelioma of Malherbe)
   L. Trichoblastoma

The inflammatory and neoplastic disorders discussed in this chapter are wide ranging and require careful study to gain the familiarity necessary to recognize the individual entities. The article by Drs. Headington, Mitchell, and Swanson referenced at the end of the chapter is especially recommended for readers interested in the histology and histopathology of the hair follicle.

The Reactive Process and the Disease	Histopathology	Comments
I. Hyperkeratosis and inflammatory reactions		
A. Keratosis pilaris	1. Dilated follicle 2. Keratinaceous concretion within follicular orifice 3. Variable perifollicular lymphocytic inflammation	
B. Pityriasis rubra pilaris (PRP)	1. Hyperkeratosis and spotty parakeratosis 2. Perifollicular psoriasiform hyperplasia 3. Focal "shoulder" parakeratosis sometimes present at follicular opening 4. Mild perivasculitis and perifollicular lymphocytic infiltrate	Parakeratoses in PRP may be in **vertical** columns, in **horizontal** sheets between orthokeratotic stratum corneum, or in **shoulder** alignment about follicular orifices The histology of PRP may be indistinguishable from that of psoriasis or chronic eczematous dermatitis See also Ch. 5, I.F

C. Follicular eczema

1. **Spongiosis** prominent, sometimes exclusively in follicular epithelium
2. Migration of lymphocytes into follicle

Differential diagnosis: Follicular mucinosa

D. Folliculitis

   1. Acute superficial

1. Subcorneal pustule present at follicular orifice
2. Perifollicular neutrophilic infiltration usually present

Special stains for bacteria frequently demonstrate organisms; sterile folliculitis also occurs

   2. Acute deep

Perifollicular abscess associated with destruction of follicle wall and sebaceous gland

Rosacea and acne vulgaris may have acute superficial and acute deep folliculitis as well as a chronic folliculitis. Rosacea may also show a granulomatous folliculitis (See Ch. 17, II.B)

   3. Chronic deep

1. Intrafollicular abscess frequently present
2. Perifollicular infiltrate of neutrophils, lymphocytes, macrophages, plasma cells, and foreign-body giant cells
3. Variable fibrosis, sometimes even keloid formation

This type of folliculitis commonly affects the beard area (folliculitis barbae) and/or scalp (folliculitis decalvans, folliculitis keloidalis nuchae)

E. Pityrosporon folliculitis
(Fig. 24-1)

1. Perifollicular lymphocytic infiltrate with a few neutrophils
2. **Dilated follicle,** sometimes with rupture, containing **numerous yeast consistent with pityrosporon organisms**
3. Focal granulomatous inflammation at the point of follicular rupture

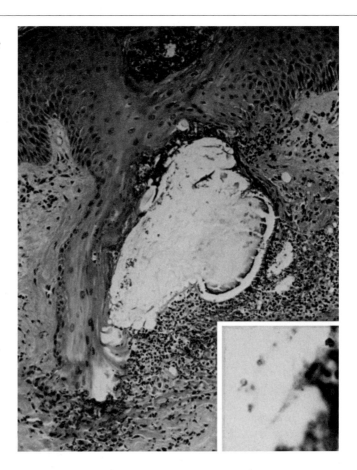

Fig. **24-1.** *Pityrosporon folliculitis. A dilated and ruptured follicle is seen. The follicle orifice contains yeast consistent with* Pityrosporon *organisms (inset).*

F. Eosinophilic folliculitis (Ofujii's disease) (Fig. 24-2)

Early lesion:
1. Parafollicular and interstitial **eosinophils with prominent eosinophil degranulation**
2. **Infiltration of follicular wall** and sebaceous glands by eosinophils with degranulation
3. Intercellular edema of follicle and sebaceous gland
4. Scattered lymphocytes about follicle

Late lesion:
1. Massive intrafollicular luminal and epithelial aggregation of eosinophils
2. Numerous eosinophils admixed with lymphocytes is perifollicular array
3. Interstitial eosinophils with marked degranulation present

Early lesions may clinically resemble follicular eczema

Clue to diagnosis is prominent eosinophil degranulation

Eosinophilic folliculitis is most frequently seen in patients with AIDS

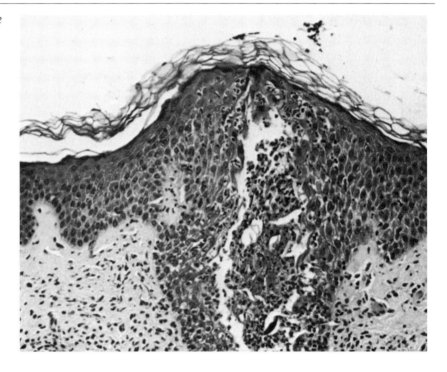

Fig. **24-2.** *Eosinophilic folliculitis. The granulocytes infiltrating this follicle are eosinophils.*

G. Perforating folliculitis

1. Dilated hair follicle filled with keratin, parakeratotic cells and sometimes degenerated collagen, and brightly eosinophilic elastic fibers
2. A curled-up hair is often present within the mass of material described above
3. Perforation of follicular epithelium occurs in the lateral aspect of the upper one-third of the follicle where brightly eosinophilic fibers bridge the wall

Differential diagnosis:
    Kyrle's disease
    Elastosis perforans
        serpiginosa
    Reactive perforating
        collagenosis

H. Majocchi's granuloma (Fig. 24-3)

1. Hyperkeratosis and variable epidermal hyperplasia
2. Dense, perifollicular and intrafollicular, lymphocytic and eosinophilic infiltrate
3. Giant cells occasionally present, especially if follicle has ruptured
4. Septate hyphae present within hair, follicle, and/or perifollicular infiltrate and often in overlying stratum corneum

Organisms best visualized with special stains (see Ch. 3)

Fig. **24-3.** *Majocchi's granuloma.*
A. *An acutely inflamed pilosebaceous follicle has ruptured, spilling its inflammatory contents, including hyphal forms, into the dermis (A), which elicits a further inflammatory response.*
B. *The hair and keratinaceous material contain numerous hyphal forms.*

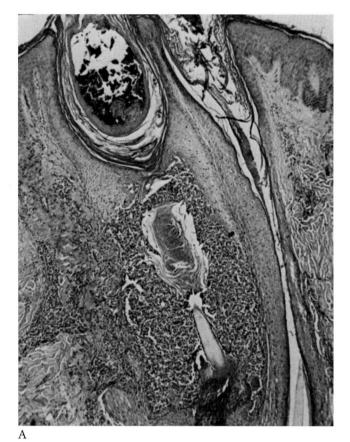

A

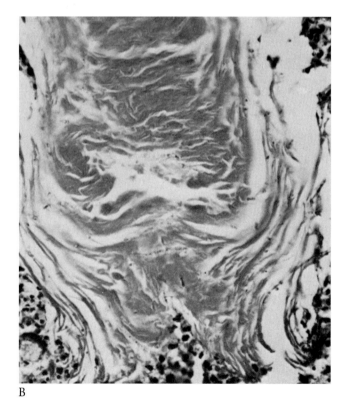

B

I. Invasive dermatophytosis (Fig. 24-4)

1. Hyperkeratosis and variable epidermal hyperplasia
2. Dense, perifollicular and intrafollicular, lymphocytic and eosinophilic infiltrate
3. Giant cells occasionally present, especially if follicle has ruptured
4. Septate hyphae present within hair, follicle, and/or perifollicular infiltrate and often in overlying stratum corneum
5. Septate hyphae present in reticular dermis and/or fat associated with variable granulomatous response

This entity occurs in association with immunosuppressed states

II. Alopecia, nonscarring

A. Follicular mucinosis (Fig. 24-5)

Pathophysiology: *Up to 50% of mononuclear cells within the follicular epithelium are CD1a-positive dendritic cells, i.e., Langerhans cells*

1. **Acid mucopolysaccharide** (AMP) deposition between epithelial cells results in a reticulate appearance to portions of the **hair follicle and sebaceus glands**
2. Extent of inflammation variable; infiltrate composed of lymphocytes and occasional eosinophils

AMP demonstrated with colloidal iron, Giemsa, or alcian blue stains

Follicular mucinosis has been associated with:

Letterer–Siwe disease in children
Angiolymphoid hyperplasia with eosinophilia
Cutaneous T-cell lymphoma, mycosis fungoides variant

Fig. **24-4.** Endothrix infection. Chains of fungal organisms are present within a hair shaft. Significant inflammation is absent.

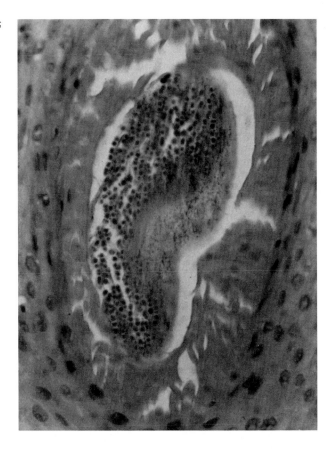

Fig. **24-5.** Follicular mucinosis. This pilosebaceous unit exhibits mucinous degeneration. Alcian blue stains (to demonstrate the presence of acid mucopolysaccharides) are positive and help to exclude the diagnosis of follicular eczema.

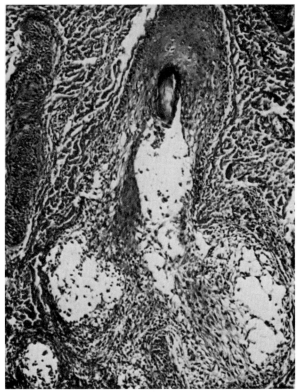

B. Alopecia areata
(Fig. 24-6)

Acute phase:
1. Peribulbar lymphocytic infiltrate ("swarm of bees")
2. Increased numbers of catagen and telogen follicles
3. Variable perivascular infiltrate

Chronic:
4. Diminished inflammation
5. Greatly increased number of telogen/vellus follicles
6. Dystrophic hair shafts
7. Eventual loss of follicles
8. Fibrous tracts (stela) extend downward from telogen follicles

Histologic findings in alopecia areata are quite variable depending on the site of biopsy within the lesion and current activity of disease

C. Androgenic alopecia

1. Shift of normal anagen: telogen ratio (approximately 9:1) to increased telogen/vellus follicles
2. Miniaturization of follicle and hair shaft sizes
3. Variable perivascular and perifollicular inflammation

The diagnosis of androgenic alopecia is best made in horizontally sectioned tissue

Fig. **24-6.** *Alopecia areata.*
A. *The lymphocytic infiltrate involving the lower portion of the hair follicle ("swarm of bees") is characteristic.*

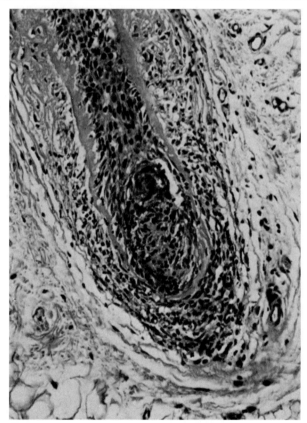

A

B. This scalp biopsy was cut in horizontal sections. The peribulbar infiltrate surrounds a stela (arrow) or fibrous sheath left by the upward migration of a telogen follicle.

C. A follicular unit is shown, consisting of two miniaturized follicles and associated sebaceous glands. A dystrophic shaft is present in one follicle (arrow). A follicle in telogen (arrowhead) is also present, characterized by a brightly eosinophilic rim outlining the hair shaft.

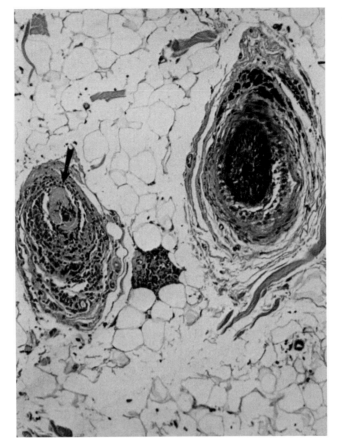

B

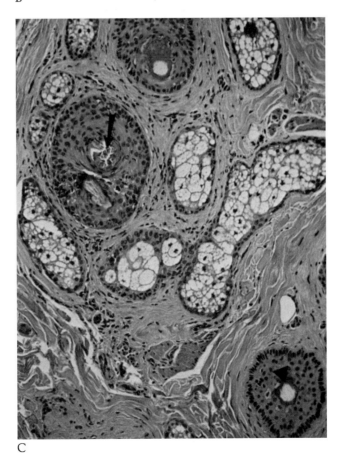

C

<table>
<tr>
<td>D. Traction alopecia and trichotillomania</td>
<td>
1. Variable perifollicular inflammation; may be granulomatous in presence of follicular rupture
2. Increased catagen and telogen follicles
3. Dilated follicles containing pigment casts
4. Fragmented hair shafts (trichomalacia)
5. Perifollicular hemorrhage
6. Perifollicular fibrosis (late stage)
</td>
<td></td>
</tr>
<tr>
<td>E. Telogen effluvium</td>
<td>
1. Great increase in number of telogen follicles
2. Numerous fibrous tracts (stela)
3. Significant inflammation absent
</td>
<td></td>
</tr>
</table>

III. Alopecia, scarring

<table>
<tr>
<td>A. Lupus erythematosus (Fig. 24-7)</td>
<td>
1. Striking perifollicular inflammation with exocytosis of lymphocytes is present
</td>
<td>See also Ch. 8, VI; Ch. 11, II.D; Ch. 12, III; Ch. 13, I.C; Ch. 16, I.B.I; Ch. 26, I.B</td>
</tr>
<tr>
<td>B. Lichen planopilaris</td>
<td>
1. Follicular plug
2. Follicular hypergranulosis
3. Around lower one-third of follicle, there is a bandlike, "hugging" lymphocytic infiltrate
4. Characteristic changes of lichen planus may affect interfollicular epidermis
5. Dermal fibrosis and absence of hair follicles and sebaceus glands characteristic of end-stage lesions
</td>
<td></td>
</tr>
</table>

Fig. **24-7.** *Lupus erythematosus, horizontal sections.*
A. *The inflammatory infiltrate hugs follicular epithelium with interface changes consisting of exocytosis, basal vacuolization, and dyskeratosis (arrow). The arrowheads point to a ruptured follicle with acute inflammation.*
B. *Again, note the perifollicular inflammation. Perieccrine inflammation is seen here in horizontal section (arrowheads).*

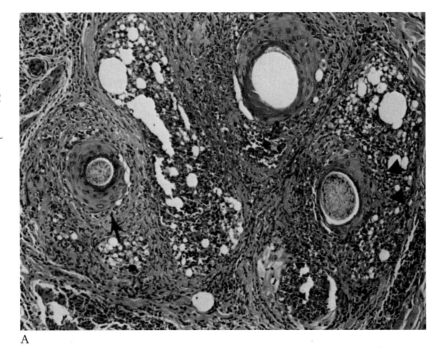

A

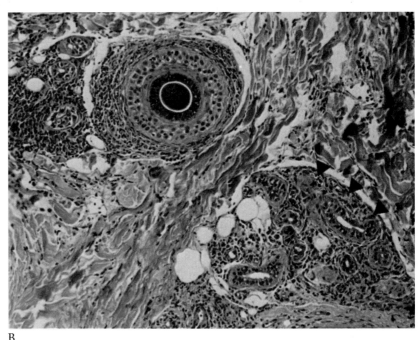

B

C. Pseudopelade of Brocq

1. Epidermis normal
2. Sebaceous glands diminished
3. Hair follicle changes vary with stage of disease
4. Perifollicular lymphocytic cell infiltration about the upper portion of the hair follicle
5. Thinning of follicular epithelium
6. Replacement of follicular epithelium by vertical fibrous tracts (stela) is late finding
7. Dilate keratin-filled follicular orifices

Special stains for elastic tissue highlight the fibrous tracts of advanced pseudopalade

D. Alopecia neoplastica

1. Dermal infiltrate of cytologically atypical cells representing a malignant neoplasm, usually metastatic
2. Expansion of the neoplastic cell population leads to eventual replacement of pilosebaceous structure due to pressure and ischemia

Any malignant neoplasm expanding within the skin may lead to alopecia

IV. Hyperplasia and neoplasms

A. Nevus sebaceus

1. Childhood

1. Epidermis irregularly and variably hyperplastic
2. Incompletely differentiated pilosebaceous structures with cores and buds of undifferentiated cells
3. Dermal collagen bundles often show irregular interlacing pattern

Characteristic histologic features of nevus sebaceus may occur in association with and adjacent to epidermal nevi

In some areas of a nevus sebaceus, the irregular epidermal hyperplasia may be the predominant histological finding; careful sampling may be required to establish the diagnosis

2. Adolescent and adult (Fig. 24-8)

1. Hyperkeratosis and **papillomatosis**
2. Large numbers of mature or nearly mature **sebaceus glands,** which may open directly to the surface rather than into a follicle
3. Small hair follicles
4. **Ectopic apocrine glands** in lower dermis
5. Dermis and subcutis show variable change in connective tissue organization

Nevus sebaceus and other epidermal nevi often show hamartomatous changes of the dermis and subcutaneous fat

Fig. **24-8.** A, B. Nevus *sebaceus.*
Papillary epidermal hyperplasia,
sebaceous hyperplasia, and numerous
ectopic apocrine glands constitute the
features of this hamartomatous disorder.
Before puberty, these features may be
less well developed.

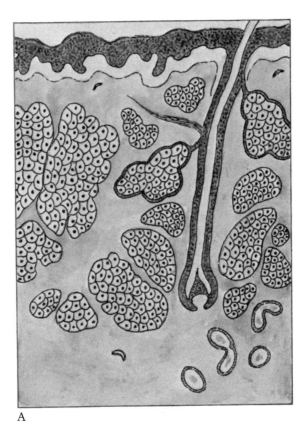

A

B

B. Sebaceus hyperplasia

One or more enlarged sebaceus glands, each composed of numerous lobules grouped around a central sebaceus duct

C. Sebaceus adenoma (Fig. 24-9)

1. Circumscribed lesion
2. Multiple lobules, irregular in shape and size, containing two types of cells:
   a. **Mature sebaceus cells** are located at the center of lobules, surrounded by:
   b. Undifferentiated germinative cells, indistinguishable from basal cells

Mature sebaceus cells usually predominate; a tumor with many basaloid cells and a few sebaceus cells is more likely to be a basal cell carcinoma with sebaceus differentiation or a sebaceus epithelioma

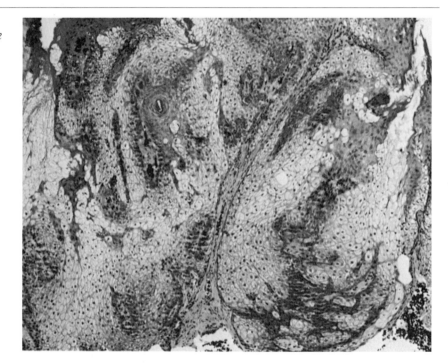

Fig. **24-9.** *Sebaceus adenoma. This tumor is composed of lobules of mature sebaceous cells.*

D. Sebaceus epithelioma .

1. Epidermis may appear normal or ulcerated
2. **Poorly circumscribed** proliferation of predominantly **basaloid cells** with focal differentiation toward sebaceus cells

MUIR–TORRE Syndrome:

1. Sebaceus tumors of classic types may appear but are often unclassifiable.
2. Some tumors are represented by extensive basaloid proliferative areas with some admixed sebaceus cells. Occasionally, lesions resemble basal cell carcinoma with marked areas of sebaceus maturation
3. Tumors may precede or may follow visceral carcinomas usually of the gastrointestinal tract
4. Other carcinomas, including laryngeal, genital urinary ovary, and uterus, may be observed

E. Sebaceoma

1. Composed of multiple nests of small basaloid cells in clusters
2. Basaloid cells in aggregates usually connected to the basal layer of the epidermis
3. Lesion sometimes dermal nodule
4. Striking cystlike or large ductular structure throughout the lesion
5. Foci of squamous differentiation toward center of the lesion
6. Infrequent mitoses

F. Sebaceus carcinoma
(Fig. 24-10)

1. Overlying epidermis may be normal
2. Tumor composed of irregular infiltrating aggregates of basaloid cells and **atypical sebaceous cells** with foamy cytoplasms and large hyperchromatic nuclei
3. Numerous mitoses; atypical forms may be present

G. Trichofolliculoma

1. **Large cystic spaces,** lined with squamous epithelium and containing keratinous material and hair shafts **surrounded** by groups of small hair follicles containing hair or keratin
2. Stroma rich with fibroblasts

Fig. **24-10.** *Sebaceus carcinoma. Irregular masses of sebaceus cells with pleomorphic hyperchromatic nuclei replace normal dermal structures.*

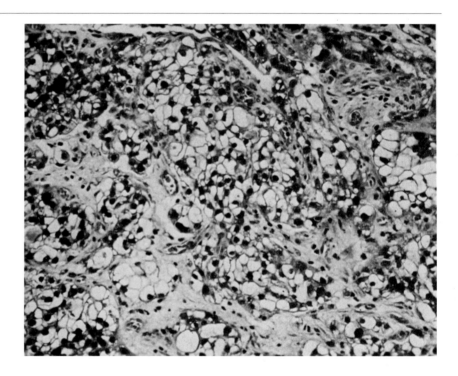

H. Pilar tumor of the scalp (proliferating trichilemmal cyst)

1. Interlacing **strands and lobules of squamous epithelium surround central keratinaceous areas**
2. Some nuclear anaplasia, squamous eddy formation with glassy keratinocytes, and individual cell keratinization
3. Circumscribed
4. Foreign-body giant cell response to extruded keratin common
5. **Calcification** common

This tumor is most commonly located on the scalp

Differential diagnosis: Squamous cell carcinoma

A rare variant the malignant pilar tumor shows extreme pleomorphism with extensive mitotic activity and heaping up of the peripheral wall of the pilar cystic component. It likewise shows extensive infiltrated invasion well away from the areas of rupture with keratinatious debris

I. Trichilemmoma
(Fig. 24-11)

1. Platelike or small lobular proliferation of epithelial cells connected to overlying epidermis or hair follicle
2. Superficial cells often vacuolated with coarse keratohyaline granules
3. Centrally located cells have **pale-staining or clear cytoplasm**
4. Peripheral cells exhibit **palisading**
5. Eosinophilic hyaline rim of compressed collagen frequently surrounds tumor

Differentiation toward glycogen-rich, clear cells as seen in outer root sheath of the hair follicle

The differential diagnosis desmoplastic trichilemmoma must be differentiated from squamous cell carcinoma

Malignant trichilemmal carcinoma, although rare, exhibits striking clear cell proliferative areas with marked atypia. There is often peripheral pallisading with some hyalinized basement membrane thickening and there are clearly areas of trichilemmal keratinization with hyalinized eosinophilic droplets in the cells. The lesions are mitotically active and show infiltrative features

Presence of PAS-positive diastase-resistant granules distinguishes lesion from eccrine carcinoma in which granules are diastase-sensitive

Fig. **24-11.** Trichilemmoma.
A. Continuity with the epidermis and/or hair follicle is usually apparent in these tumors, composed of cells with clear and eosinophilic (keratinizing) cytoplasm. Palisading of cells at the periphery of the tumor is usually present.
B. Cytologic features and a small hair are more apparent at this higher magnification.

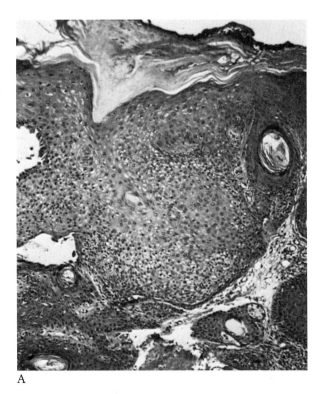

A

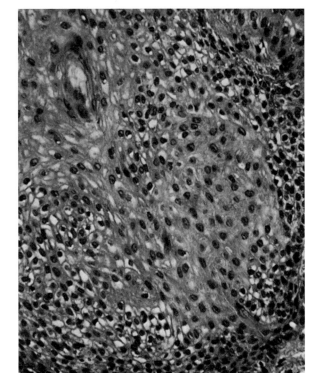

B

J. Trichoepithelioma
(Fig. 24-12)

1. Circumscribed tumor
2. **Horn cysts** with fully keratinized center surrounded by flattened basophilic cells
3. Reticulate or solid **aggregates of basaloid cells** with surrounding **cellular stroma**
4. Foreign-body giant cells and calcium deposits may be present
5. Melanin may be present within horn cysts and surrounding cells

Differential diagnosis:
Basal cell carcinoma

Desmoplastic trichoepithelioma is composed of variable numbers of horn cysts and very thin strands of basaloid cells separated by fibrous stroma

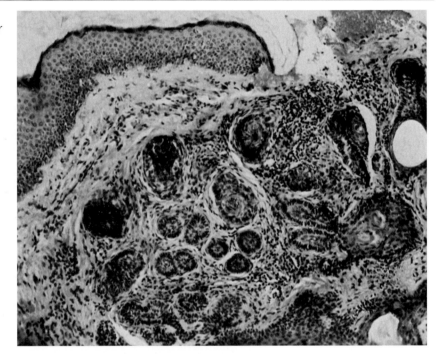

Fig. **24-12.** *Trichoepithelioma. Basaloid cells forming horn cysts and/or abortive hair follicles are seen surrounded by a fibromucinous stroma.*

K. Pilomatrixoma (calcifying epithelioma of Malherbe) (Fig. 24-13)

1. Circumscribed tumor located in the dermis, sometimes surrounded by a connective-tissue capsule
2. Irregular islands of cells made up of:
   a. *Basophilic cells*—cells with scanty cytoplasm, indistinct cell borders, and dark, round nuclei; mitotic rate often high
   b. *Ghost cells*—pale, eosinophilic cells with retained nuclear outlines (see Fig. 2-7)
3. Fibroblastic and inflammatory stroma, sometimes with foreign-body giant cells
4. Calcification often present; ossification occasionally occurs

Extensive infiltration of tumor may be a sign of aggressive behavior

Malignant pilomatrixoma shows extensive infiltration around the tumor nodule with pleomorphism of the infiltrating peripheral islands and mitotic activity. Sometimes the first sign of malignancy is recurrence of the tumor.

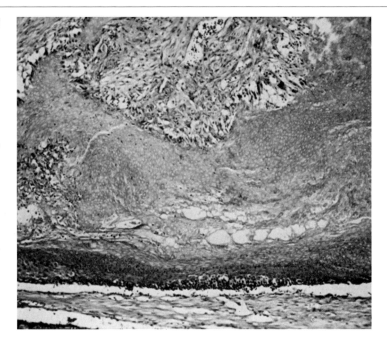

Fig. **24-13.** *Pilomatrixoma (calcifying epithelioma of Malherbe). Basaloid cells (here seen as a thin rim of darkly stained cells located near the base of the micrograph) and ghost cells (mummified cells with negative nuclear images located above the basaloid cells) are the distinctive components of this tumor. The amount of foreign-body inflammation (above the ghost cells), calcification, and fibrous stroma is variable.*

L. Trichoblastoma
(Fig. 24-14)

1. Dermal tumors with variable extension into the subcutis
2. Most without connection to the epidermis
3. Well-demarcated cords and nodules of basaloid cells
4. Palisading of columnar cells at periphery of lobules
5. Invaginations of spindle-shaped cells into tumor lobules (papillary mesenchymal bodies)
6. Occasional cases with abundant melanin pigment, abundant intervening fibrosis, or desmoplastic growth pattern

It is important to distinguish trichoblastoma, a benign follicular neoplasm, from basal cell carcinoma (Table 24-1)

Table **24-1.** *Histologic Features Distinguishing Trichoblastoma from Basal Cell Carcinoma*

Trichoblastoma	Basal Cell Carcinoma
Sharp circumscription	Variably circumscribed
No cleft artifact	Cleft artifact separating tumor from stroma
Papillary mesenchymal bodies	No papillary mesenchymal bodies
Densely cellular, fibrotic stroma	Variable stroma, often mucinous
Minimal tumor necrosis	Tumor necrosis common
Minimal host response	Common lymphocytic response
Extensive follicular differentiation	Variable follicular differentiation

Fig. **24-14.** Trichoblastoma.
A. Normal epidermis. Tumor nodules
   in the dermis and subcutis.
B. Cords and nodules of basaloid cells
   with peripheral palisading.
   Abundant melanin is present within
   the tumor nodules.

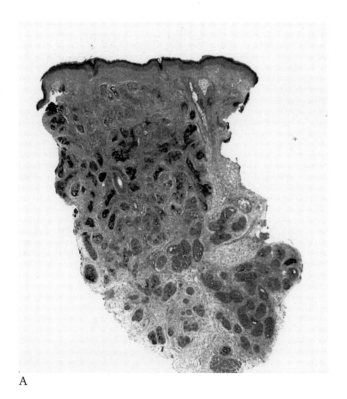

A

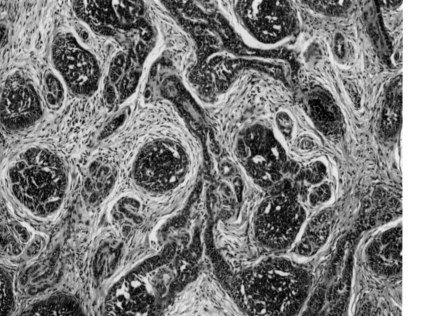

B

Suggested Reading

Folliculitis

Ofuji, S., and Uehara, M. Follicular eruptions of atopic dermatitis. *Arch. Dermatol.* 107:54, 1973.

Alopecia

Abell, E. Pathology male-pattern alopecia. *Arch. Dermatol.* 120:1607, 1984.

Elston, D. M., McCollough, M. L., Angeloni, V. L. Vertical and transverse sections of alopecia biopsy specimens: Combining the two to maximize diagnostic yield. *J. Am. Acad. Dermatol.* 32:454–457, 1995.

Gay Prieto, J. Pseudopalade of Broque: Its relationship to some forms of cicatricial alopecias and to lichen planus. *J. Invest. Dermatol.* 24:323, 1955.

Headington, J. T. Transverse microscopic anatomy of the human scalp. A basis for a morphometric approach to disorders of the hair follicle. *Arch. Dermatol.* 120:449–456, 1984.

Headington, J. T., Mitchell, A., and Swanson, N. New Histopathological findings in alopecia areata studied in transverse sections. *J. Invest. Dermatol.* 76:325, 1981.

Lattanand, A., and Johnson, W. C. Male pattern alopecia: A histopathologic and histochemical study. *J. Cutan. Pathol.* 2:58, 1975.

Mehregan, A. H. Histopathology of alopecias. *Cutis* 21:249, 1978.

Mehregan, A. H. Trichotillomania: A clinicopathologic study. *Arch. Dermatol.* 102:129, 1970.

Messenger, A. G., Slater, D. N., and Bueden, S. S. Alopecia areata: Alterations in the growth cycle and correlation with follicular pathology. *Br. J. Dermatol.* 114:337, 1986.

Pierard, G. E., and de la Brassinne, M. Cellular activity in the dermis surrounding the hair bulb in alopecia areata. *J. Cutan. Pathol.* 2:240, 1975.

Pinkus, H. Differential pattern of elastic fibers in scarring and nonscarring alopecias. *J. Cutan. Pathol.* 5:93, 1968.

Ronchese, F. Pseudopalade. *Arch. Dermatol.* 82:336, 1960.

Sperling L. C., and Lupton, G. P. Histopathology of non-scarring alopecia. *J. Cutan. Pathol.* 22:97–114, 1995.

Templeton, S. F., Sant Cruz, D. J., and Solomon, A. R. Alopecia: Histologic diagnosis by transverse sections. *Semin. Diagn. Pathol.* 13:2–18, 1996.

Van Scott, E. J. Morphologic changes in pilosebaceous units and anagen hairs in alopecia areata. *J. Invest. Dermatol.* 31:35, 1958.

Whiting, D. A. Diagnostic and predictive value of horizontal sections of scalp biopsy specimens in male pattern androgenetic alopecia. *J. Am. Acad. Dermatol.* 28:755–763, 1993.

Hyperplasias and Neoplasms

Berberian, B. J., Colonna, T. M., Battaglia, M., and Sulica, V. I. Multiple pilomatricomas in association with myotonic dystrophy and a family history of melanoma. *J. Am. Acad. Dermatol.* 37:268–269, 1997.

Binnick, A. N., Wax, F. D., and Clendenning, W. E. Alopecia mucinosa of the face associated with mycosis fungoides. *Arch. Dermatol.* 114:791, 1978.

Booth, J. C., Kramer, H., and Taylor, K. B. Pilomatrixoma: Calcifying epithelioma (Malherbe). *Pathology* 1:119, 1969.

Brownstein, M. H., and Shapiro, L. Desmoplastic trichoepithelioma. *Cancer* 40:2979, 1977.

Brownstein, M. H., and Shapiro, L. Trichilemmoma: Analysis of 40 new cases. *Arch. Dermatol.* 107:866, 1973.

Brownstein, M. H., Wolfe, M., and Bikowski, J. B. Cowden's disease: A cutaneous marker of breast cancer. *Cancer* 41:2393, 1978.

Cambiaghi, S., Ermacora, E., Brusasco, A., Canzi, L., and Caputo, R. Multiple pilomatricomas in Rubinstein–Taybi syndrome: A case report. *Pediatr. Dermatol.* 11:21–25, 1994.

Cohen, P. R., Kohn, S. R., and Kurzrock, R. Association of sebaceous gland neoplasms and internal malignancy: The Muire–Torre syndrome. *Am. J. Med.* 90:606–613, 1991.

Cohen, J. H., Lessin, S. R., Vowels, B. R., Benoit, B., Witmer, W. K., and Rook, A. H. The sign of Leser–Trelat in association with Sezary syndrome: Simultaneous disappearance of seborrheic keratoses and malignant T-cell clone during combined therapy with photopheresis and interferon alpha. *Arch. Dermatol.* 129:1213–1215, 1993.

Finan, M. C., and Connoly, S. M. Sebaceous gland tumors and systemic disease: A clinicopathologic analysis. *Medicine* 63:232–242, 1984.

Forbis, R., and Helwig, E. B. Pilomatrixoma (calcifying epithelioma). *Arch. Dermatol.* 83:606, 1961.

Graells, J., Servitje, O., Badell, A., Notario, J., and Peyri, J. Multiple familial pilomatricomas associated with myotonic dystrophy. *Int. J. Dermatol.* 35:732–733, 1996.

Gray, H. R., and Helwig, E. B. Epithelioma adenoides cysticum and solitary trichoepithelioma. *Arch. Dermatol.* 87:102, 1963.

Gray, H. R., and Helwig, E. B. Trichofolliculoma. *Arch. Dermatol.* 86:619, 1962.

Hashimoto, K., and Lever, W. F. *Appendage Tumors of the Skin.* Springfield, IL: Thomas, 1968.

Headington, J. T. Tumors of the hair follicle. *Am. J. Pathol.* 85:480, 1976.

Housholder, M. S., and Zeligman, I. Sebaceous neoplasms associated with visceral carcinomas. *Arch. Dermatol.* 116:61, 1980.

Manivel, C., Wick, M. R., and Muka, K. Pilomatrix carcinoma: An immunohistochemical comparison with benign pilomatrixoma and other benign cutaneous lesions of pilar origin. *J. Cutan. Pathol.* 13:22, 1986.

Miller, R. E., and White, J. J., Jr. Sebaceous gland carcinoma. *Am. J. Surg.* 114:958, 1967.

Moehlenbeck, F. W. Pilomatrixoma (calcifying epithelioma): A statistical study. *Arch. Dermatol.* 108:532, 1973.

Pujol, R. M., Casanova, J. M., Egido, R., Pujol, J., and de Moragas, J. M. Multiple familial pilomatricomas: A cutaneous marker for Gardner syndrome? *Pediatr. Dermatol.* 12:331–335, 1995.

Rongioletti, F., Hazini, R., Gianotti, G., and Rebora, A. Fibrofolliculomas, trichodiscomas and acrochordons (Birt–Hogg–Dube) associated with intestinal polyposis. *Clin. Exp. Dermatol.* 14:72–74, 1989.

Rulon, D. B., and Helwig, E. B. Cutaneous sebaceous neoplasms. *Cancer* 33:82, 1974.

Sciallis, G. F. and Winkelmann, R. K. Multiple sebaceous adenomas and gastrointestinal carcinoma. *Arch. Dermatol.* 110:913–916, 1974.

Wick, M. R., Goellner, J. R., Wolfe, J. T., et al. Adnexal carcinomas of the skin. II. Extraocular sebaceous carcinomas. *Cancer* 56:1163, 1985.

Wilson Jones, E., and Heyl, T. Nevus sebaceous: A report of 140 cases with special regard to the development of secondary malignant tumors. *Br. J. Dermatol.* 82:99, 1970.

Zackheim, H. S. The sebaceous epithelioma: A clinical and histologic study. *Arch. Dermatol.* 89:711, 1964.

Chapter 25

Disorders of the
Sweat Glands

I. Congenital absence of sweat glands
   A. Anhidrotic ectodermal dysplasia
II. Inflammatory reactions
   A. Miliaria
      1. Crystallina
      2. Rubra
      3. Profunda
   B. Neutrophilic eccrine hidradenitis
   C. Necrosis of eccrine gland: coma bulla
   D. Hidradenitis suppurativa
   E. Fox–Fordyce disease (apocrine miliaria)
III. Hyperplasia and neoplasms
   A. Syringoma
   B. Eccrine poroma
   C. Dermal duct tumor
   D. Porocarcinoma (malignant eccrine poroma)
   E. Pale (clear) cell hidradenoma
   F. Malignant nodular hidradenoma
   G. Eccrine spiradenoma
   H. Chondroid syringoma
   I. Malignant chondroid syringoma
   J. Syringocystadenoma papilliferum
   K. Hidradenoma papilliferum
   L. Cylindroma
   M. Apocrine adenoma
   N. Tubular apocrine adenoma
   O. Apocrine adenocarcinoma
   P. Sclerosing sweat duct carcinoma (microcystic adnexal carcinoma)
   Q. Mucinous eccrine carcinoma
   R. Aggressive digital papillary adenoma/adenocarcinoma
   S. Adenoid cystic carcinoma

Appendageal tumors exist within a characteristic stroma demarcated from the normal reticular dermis and usually containing increased spindled cells. The presence of this fibrocellular component of appendageal tumors helps to distinguish them from basal cell carcinomas.

There exist malignant epithelial tumors of the skin that resemble and are probably derived from appendages such as the *pilomatrix carcinoma* from the hair follicle and the *porocarcinoma* from the eccrine duct. These tumors are histologically characterized by anaplasia, infiltration, and a high mitotic rate. The histologic patterns of these tumors are complex and, we believe, beyond the scope of a primer. We refer interested readers to the Suggested Readings at the end of this chapter.

The Reactive Process and the Disease	Histopathology	Comments
I. Congenital absence of sweat glands		
A. Anhidrotic ectodermal dysplasia	1. Absent or severely diminished eccrine glands or ducts 2. Hair follicles may be diminished in number	
II. Inflammatory reactions		
A. Miliaria		
1. Crystallina	1. Subcorneal vesicle with slight spongiosis of the upper portion of the intraepidermal eccrine duct 2. Mild lymphocytic infiltrate present about and within affected ducts	See also Ch. 6, I.I
2. Rubra	1. Prominent spongiosis and vesiculation of the intra-epidermal and superficial dermal eccrine duct 2. Moderate perivascular lymphocytic infiltrate that extends into the affected epidermis	See also Ch. 6, II.G
3. Profunda	1. Intraepidermal intraductal hyperkeratosis 2. Spongiosis of intraepidermal duct and upper dermal duct 3. Rupture of intradermal sweat duct below dermoepidermal junction with marked lymphocytic infiltration of adjacent dermis	

B. Neutrophilic eccrine hidradenitis

1. Aggregates of neutrophils around eccrine coils
2. Variable necrosis of eccrine glandular and ductal epithelium
3. No associated dermal necrosis

Seen in association with induction chemotherapy

C. Necrosis of eccrine glands: coma bulla (Fig. 25-1)

See also Ch. 6, II.J

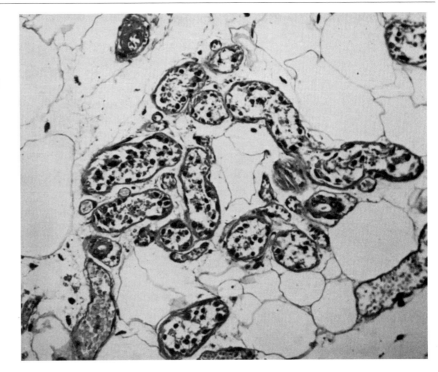

Fig. **25-1.** *Coma bulla (pressure necrosis). These eccrine glands exhibit nuclear pyknosis and cytoplasmic dissolution, which are changes of early necrosis. Note also the congested capillaries. The overlying epidermis had sloughed.*

D. Hidradenitis suppurativa (Fig. 25-2)

1. Polymorphous infiltrate throughout the dermis, with acute inflammation of apocrine glands
2. In late stages, inflammation around apocrine glands may be scant and fibrosis may be prominent

This disorder may be associated with:
Acne conglobata
Dissecting cellulitis of the scalp

The etiology of these disorders is unknown, and no clear relationship to sweat glands is established

E. Fox–Fordyce disease (apocrine miliaria)

1. Acute inflammation of apocrine glands associated with acute and chronic inflammation of the adjacent dermis and subcutaneous fat
2. Entrapment of secretion with dilation of apocrine glands
3. Chronic inflammation is associated with scarring in persistent lesions

Chronic lesions may exhibit only fibrosis and inflammation, without evidence of residual apocrine glands

III. Hyperplasias and neoplasms

A. Syringoma (Fig. 25-3)

1. Ducts, small cysts, and nests or strands of epithelial cells
2. Ducts and cysts lined with two layers of flat or cuboidal cells with eosinophilic, or clear pale cytoplasm

Syringomas usually present as multiple flesh-colored to yellowish papules around the eyes, or less commonly on the trunk

---

Fig. **25-2.** *Hidradenitis suppurativa. Acute and chronic inflammation in and about these apocrine glands is characteristic of early lesions. Fibrosis supervenes in end-stage or chronic disease.*

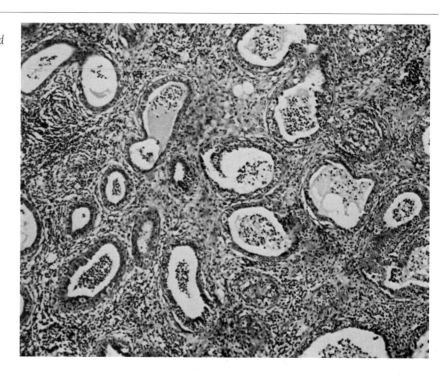

Fig. **25-3.** *Syringoma.*
A. *Tubules with tortuous configurations (when viewed in one plane of section) exhibit the irregular shapes seen in this micrograph. Some tubules allegedly resemble tadpoles* (arrow).
B. *Syringoma with clear cell differentiation.*

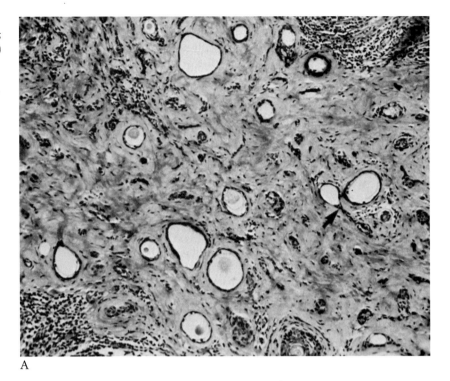

A

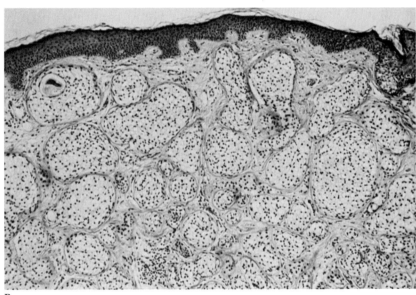

B

3. Cysts may contain keratin or amorphous material
4. Ducts and epithelial structures often have "tails," which give them the appearance of a **comma or tadpole**
5. Fibrous stroma in upper and mid dermis

Malignant syringoma shows focal areas of marked atypia, with marked pleomorphism, and numerous mitotic figures. Malignant syringoma shows an absence of the hyaline sheath, and often of the palisading of cells, in the periphery of the nodule

B. Eccrine poroma
(Fig. 25-4)

1. **Sharply dermarcated, wide, anastomosing bands of cells extend from epidermis** into the dermis
2. Basaloid or keratinizing tumor cells are uniform, small, and cuboidal, sometimes with intercellular bridges
3. Cells contain abundant glycogen
4. Tumor nodules contain small ducts with lumens lined by PAS-positive hyaline cuticle
5. Melanocytes and melanin usually unapparent
6. Edematous and inflamed fibrovascular stroma

Eccrine poromas characteristically present as a solitary nodule on the plantar surface of the foot but may occur anywhere

Intraepidermal eccrine poromas may be called *hidradenoma simplex*

C. Dermal duct tumor

Intradermal aggregates of basaloid cells with the same features as those of eccrine poroma (see B)

Fig. **25-4.** *Eccrine poroma.*
A. *Uniform, small epithelial cells in anastomosing bands connect to the epidermis. Inset: The glycogen-rich cytoplasm of these cells is PAS-positive and diastase-sensitive.*
B. *Photomicrograph for comparison.*

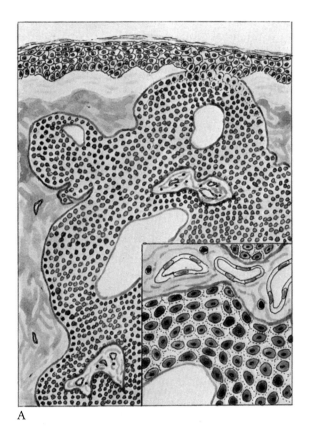

A

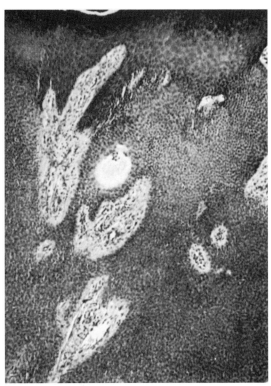

B

D. Porocarcinoma (Malignant eccrine poroma)

1. Extensive intraepidermal proliferation of severely atypical basaloid cells with squamous differentiation, focal clear cell areas and focal necrosis
2. Lesions sharply demarcated form adjacent keratinocytes
3. Cords infiltrate into the dermis with focal expansile nodule formation
4. Ductular structures frequently visible throughout tumor
5. Mitotic figures frequent in dermal component often with necrosis

E. Pale (clear) cell hidradenoma (Fig. 25-5)

1. This circumscribed tumor is located in the dermis, frequently extending to subcutaneous fat; epidermal connection is variable
2. Tumor is composed of **multiple lobules of epithelial cells containing ducts and cystic spaces**
3. Two cell types in solid portions consist of:
   a. Large polygonal cells with pale to **clear cytoplasm** and round nucleus
   b. Spindle and polygonal cells with eosinophilic cytoplasm and fusiform nuclei
4. Lumen of ducts lined by cuboidal or columnar cells
5. Ducts with PAS-positive inner hyaline cuticle may be seen
6. Cystic spaces, which may be quite large, contain eosinophilic amorphous material

Pale cell hidradenoma presents as a solitary, cystic, or nodular lesion on the face or trunk; the overlying epidermis may be smooth or ulcerated

Pale cells contain abundant glycogen, which is PAS-positive and diastase-digestible

The number of pale cells varies from few to numerous

Differential diagnosis:
Metastatic renal cell carcinoma
Sebaceous adenoma
Trichilemmoma

The term *eccrine acrospiroma* also is applied to a group of lesions that include:

Dermal duct tumor
Pale cell hidradenoma
Eccrine spiradenoma

Fig. **25-5.** *Pale (clear) cell hidradenoma. Basophilic and clear cells in large dermal masses with occasional ductlike spaces compose this tumor. Considerable variation in the number of clear cells present in this tumor is the rule but at times they may be absent.*

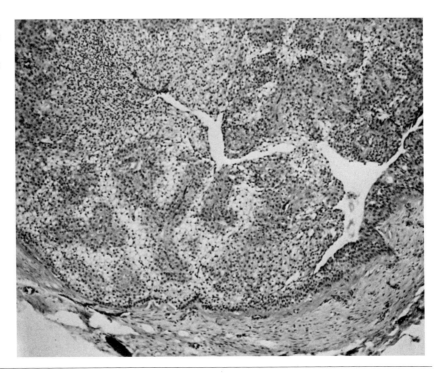

F. Malignant nodular hidradenoma

1. Large proliferative asymmetrical nodule, with extensive infiltration of the surrounding dermis and subcutaneous fat
2. Striking areas of syringomatous structures associated with other areas of chondroid or mucinous degeneration of the stroma
3. Quite prominent and striking nuclear atypia in some lesions, but variability within a given lesion commonly observed; mitotic activity frequent

G. Eccrine spiradenoma
(Fig. 25-6)

1. Normal epidermis
2. One or more well-circumscribed basophilic "balls" in the middle to lower reticular dermis
3. Tumor often composed of two distinct cell types:
   a. **Small cells** with scant clear cytoplasm and a round, dark, nucleus are located peripherally
   b. **Larger cells** with more abundant cytoplasm and a pale nucleus are located within the lobules and from anastomosing cords
4. The larger pale cells sometimes form small ducts lined by a PAS-positive, diastase-resistant, thin hyaline cuticle
5. Edematous stroma may contain many ectatic blood and lymph vessels

Eccrine spiradenomas present as painful, tender, red to blue nodules; they are *not* found on the palms, soles, axillae, or perineum

Eccrine spiradenomas may be observed in association with cylindromas

Malignant eccrine spiradenomas are usually large subcutaneous basaloid nodules with striking proliferative activity and multiple small glands with no evidence of a myoepithelial differentiation in the periphery of the glandular structures

This lesion often resembles the microcystic adnexal carcinoma with its deep penetration

Fig. **25-6.** *Eccrine spiradenoma.*
A. *The scanning picture is that of "blue balls in the dermis."*
B. *Two cell types can be recognized within the balls. Large cells forming ribbons and sometimes ducts are surrounded by smaller cells with dark nuclei and clear cytoplasm.*

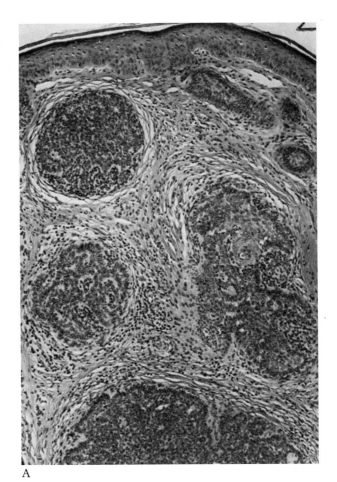

A

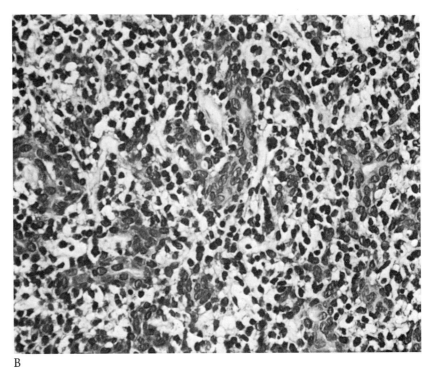

B

H. Chondroid syringoma (Fig. 25-7)

1. Normal epidermis
2. One or more dermal nodules composed of:
   a. Sheets, cords, and nests of epithelial cells
   b. Cuboidal cells that form tubular structures of varying size
3. Surrounding stroma may be fibrous, myxomatous, **cartilaginous,** and/or hyalinized

The chondroid syringoma is a solitary nodule, most commonly located on the head or neck

The differential diagnosis includes pleomorphic adenoma of salivary glands, which may extend to involve the skin

I. Malignant chondroid syringoma

1. Striking proliferation of glandular structures and sheets of squamous cells in a myxoid stroma
2. The chondroid zones noted are typically more prominent towards the center of the tumor
3. Stroma may show atypia in the fibroblastic component and in some of the chondroid areas

Malignant chondroid syringoma usually occurs in a preexisting lesion, present for many years, that suddenly changes

Fig. **25-7.** *Chondroid syringoma. Basaloid cells form a netlike pattern with numerous luminal spaces (A) and are closely associated with fibrous stroma, portions of which appear cartilaginous (B).*

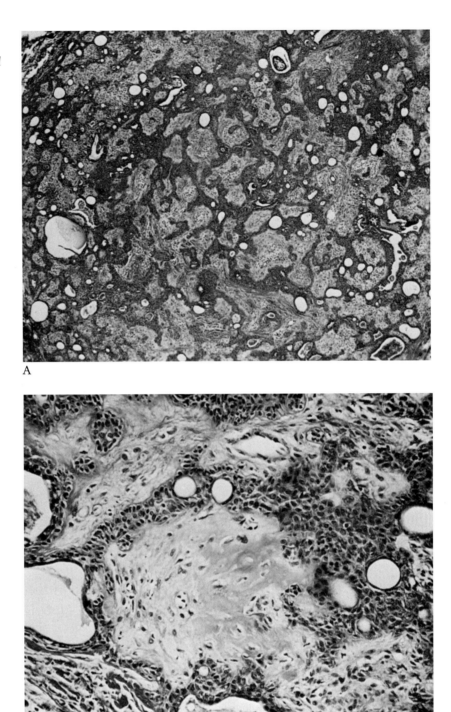

A

B

J. Syringocystadenoma papilliferum (Fig. 25-8)

1. Papillomatosis of epidermis with one or more porelike openings communicating with the dermal portion of the tumor
2. Beneath the porelike structure is a cystic, epithelial-lined invagination with papillary projections
3. **Papillary projections** are lined with:
   a. An outer (paraluminal) layer of columnar cells
   b. An inner (basal) layer of cuboidal cells
4. Columnar cells often exhibit decapitation secretion
5. Fibrous stroma contains numerous **plasma cells**

Most of these lesions arise in association with a nevus sebaceus and so are most commonly found on the head

Fig. **25-8.** *Syringocystadenoma papilliferum. This tumor exhibits the configuration of a papillary cystadenoma and communicates with the surface (A and B). The papillae are lined by a double layer of cells, and the stroma of the tumor characteristically contains numerous plasma cells (A, inset, and C).*

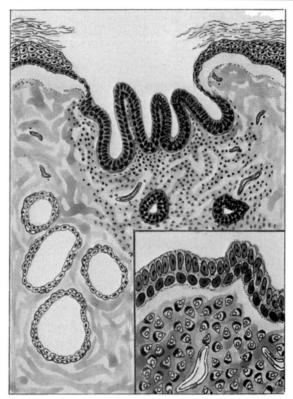

A

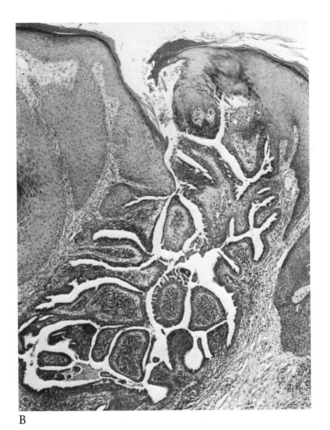

B

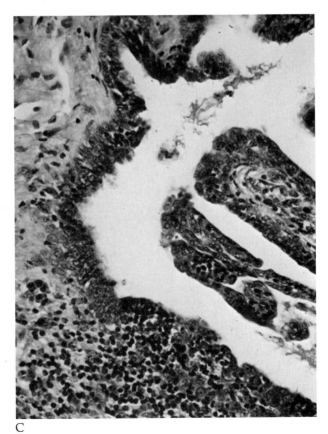

C

K. Hidradenoma papil-
liferum (Fig. 25-9)

1. One or more encapsulated
   intradermal nodules
2. Nodules composed of cystic
   spaces with complex folds and
   papillary projections, resulting
   in a delicate, mazelike
   appearance
3. Cystic spaces are lined by:
   a. A paraluminal layer of
      columnar cells with deca-
      pitation secretion
   b. A peripheral (basal) layer of
      cuboidal or flat cells
      sometimes
4. Stroma characteristically
   devoid of inflammatory cells

This hidradenoma typically presents as a slow-growing nodule
on the vulva

Fig. **25-9.** Hidradenoma papilliferum. This tumor is composed of anastomosing ducts (A) lined by basophilic cuboidal to columnar cells resting upon a layer of myoepithelial cells (B). It usually occurs on the vulva.

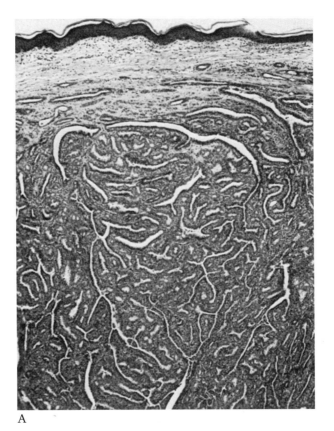

A

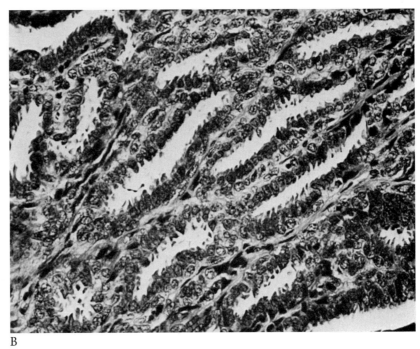

B

L. Cylindroma (Fig. 25-10)

1. One or more intradermal, basophilic nodules of varying size
2. Each nodule surrounded and outlined by an eosinophilic **hyaline band** of type IV collagen
3. The nodules lie in close approximation to each other and give a **jigsaw puzzle** appearance
4. Tumor nodules are composed of:
   a. **Peripheral small cells** with scant cytoplasm and a densely basophilic nucleus
   b. **Central large cells** with pale eosinophilic cytoplasm and a larger pale nucleus
5. Tubular lumens containing amorphous eosinophilic material may be present within the islands
6. Droplets of glassy eosinophilic hyaline material often deposited between cells

A cylindroma may be present as one or more flesh-colored to pink, firm nodules, usually on the head and neck; multiple lesions on the scalp may produce the "turban tumor"

The hyaline band around tumor islands and the eosinophilic hyaline droplets are PAS-positive and diastase-resistant

M. Apocrine adenoma

1. Dilated small vacuolar structures present in upper dermis
2. May show cystic dilations, but do not have tubular component
3. Cells lined by single layer of very brightly eosinophilic cytoplasm with decapitation secretion
4. Tumor is well-demarcated and not infiltrative
5. Myoepithelial cells are often visible when careful examination under high-power is carried

N. Tubular apocrine adenoma

1. Mid to upper dermis occupy the distinctive lobules containing dilated cystic structures
2. Lining of the cyst shows an inner layer of columnar like cells with apocrine secretion
3. Outer layer of flat cuboidal cells easily identified
4. Papillary projections extend into the cystic spaces often without a stromal component
5. Stroma is very delicate and fibrous and defines the entire adenomatous structure

These lesions occur commonly on the scalp and perirectal areas

Fig. **25-10.** *Cylindroma. Cell nests within the dermis, each surrounded by a hyaline sheath, fit together like a jigsaw puzzle. Darker cells are frequently located at the periphery of the nests, while lighter cells sit centrally.*

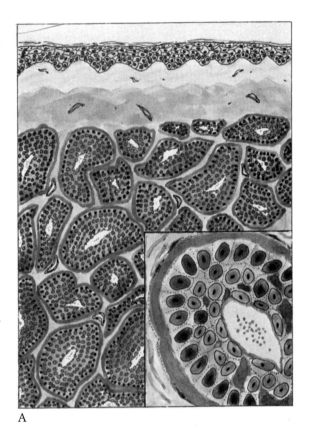

A

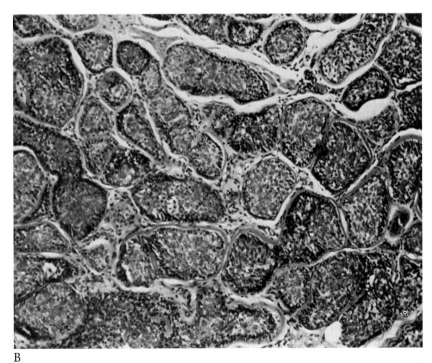

B

O. Apocrine adeno-
carcinoma

1. Variations between sheets of bright eosinophilic cells and cells with very complicated granular structures occur sometimes within the same tumor
2. In solid areas, small lumens are notable in more lingual areas
3. Papillary fronds can be observed in lumens
4. Pleomorphism is quite strikingly variable
5. Mitotic activity easily observed with atypical forms noted
6. Highly infiltrated tumor extending throughout the dermis and into subcutaneous fat
7. PAS-positive diastase-resistant granules present in cytoplasm
8. Hemosiderin present in cytoplasm in approximately one third of cases. Any cytokeratin usually expressed. S-100 positivity variable

P. Sclerosing sweat duct carcinoma (microcystic adnexal carcinoma)

1. Nests and **strands of epithelial cells in the reticular dermis,** some forming **cystic structures** resembling syringomas
2. Deep dermal penetration in an infiltrating pattern with **perineural invasion**
3. Cytologic features:
   Minimal cellular atypia
   Rare mitotic figures
   Variable cellular differentiation

These tumors typically occur on the mid-face; recurrence is common

Typical immunohistochemical profile includes positive staining for S-100, cytokeratin, and CEA

Q. Mucinous eccrine carcinoma

1. Striking appearance of small basaloid islands in areas of extensive mucinous replacement of dermis and subcutaneous fat
2. Mucinous zones separated by delicate fibrous strands
3. Nests of cells in islands are atypical, often with papillary configuration, and many with tubular lumens
4. Atypia variable, but mitotic figures frequent
5. Mucinous material, PAS-positive diastase-resistant, and positive for colloidal iron

Metastatic mucinous carcinoma—for example, of colonic origin, or breast—can be differentiated by the very large mucinous zones in the primary skin tumor which are the overwhelming predominant component of the carcinoma, but, of course, patients must always be evaluated for primary carcinomas elsewhere

R. Aggressive digital papillary adenoma/adenocarcinoma

1. Broad spectrum of changes from ductular structures to papillary projections into lumens, to tubular alveolar structures
2. Epithelial structures lie within dilated cystic lumens
3. More solid areas, composed of cellular zones, show ductular structures
4. Pleomorphism, necrosis, and numerous mitoses, characterize malignant forms
5. Metastatic behavior associated with high-grade malignant tumors

S. Adenoid cystic carcinoma

1. Dermal tumor lobules without epidermal attachment
2. Small basophilic cells organized in strands and cords within lobules (cribriform); rare mitotic figures
3. Some tumor lobules solid
4. Cystic areas contain mucin
5. Infiltrative growth pattern

A rare tumor usually present on the scalp

Suggested Reading

General Interest

Cooper, P. H. Mitotic figures in sweat gland adenomas. *J. Cutan. Pathol.* 14:10, 1987.

Santa Cruz, D. J. Sweat gland carcinomas: A comprehensive review. *Semin. Diagn. Pathol.* 4:38, 1987.

Miliaria

O'Brien, J. P. The etiology of poral closure: An experimental study of miliaria rubra, bullous impetigo and related diseases. *J. Invest. Dermatol.* 15:95, 1950.

Shelley, W. B., and Horvath, P. N. Experimental miliaria in man. II: Production of sweat retention anhidrosis and miliaria crystallina by various kinds of injury. *J. Invest. Dermatol.* 14:9, 1950.

Neutrophilic Eccrine Hidradenitis

Bachmeyer, C., Chaibi, P., and Aractingi, S. Neutrophilic eccrine hidradenitis induced by granulocyte colony-stimulating factor. *Br. J. Dermatol.* 139:354–355, 1998.

Beutner, K. R., Packman, C. H., and Markowitch, W. Neutrophilic eccrine hidradenitis associated with Hodgkin's disease and chemotherapy. *Arch. Dermatol.* 122:809, 1986.

Fitzpatrick, J. E., Bennion, S. D., Reed, O. M., et al. Neutrophilic eccrine hidradenitis associated with induction chemotherapy, *J. Cutan. Pathol.* 14:272, 1987.

Flynn, T. C., Harrist, T. J., Murphy, G. F., Loss, R. W., and Moschella, S. L. Neutrophilic eccrine hidradenitis: A distinctive rash associated with cytarabine therapy and acute leukemia. *J. Am. Acad. Dermatol.* 11:584–590, 1984.

Kuttner, B. J., and Kurban, R. S. Neutrophilic eccrine hidradenitis in the absence of underlrying malignancy. *Cutis* 41: 403–405, 1988.

Coma Bulla

Arndt, K. A., Mihm, M. C., and Parrish, J. A. Bullae: A cutaneous sign of a variety of neurologic diseases, *J. Invest. Dermatol.* 60:312, 1973.

Hidradenitis Suppurativa

Hyland, C. H., and Kheir, S. M. Follicular occlusion disease with elimination of abnormal elastic tissue. *Arch. Dermatol.* 116:925, 1980.

Shelley, W. B., and Chan, M. M. The pathogenesis of hidradenitis suppurativa in man. *Arch. Dermatol.* 72:562, 1955.

Fox–Fordyce Disease	Fox, G. H., and Fordyce, J. A. Two cases of a rare papular disease affecting the axillary region. J. *Cutan. Dis.* 20:1, 1902. Macmillan, D. C. Fox-Fordyce disease. *Br. J. Dermatol.* 84:181, 1971.
Syringoma	Hashimoto, K., Blum, D., Fukaya, T., et al. Familial syringoma: Case history and application of monoclonal anti-eccrine gland antibodies. *Arch. Dermatol.* 121:756, 1985. Headington, J. T., Koski, J., and Murphy, P. J. Clear cell glycogenenosis in multiple syringomas: Description and enzyme histochemistry. *Arch. Dermatol.* 116:353, 1972. Kudo, H., Yonezawa, I., Ieka, A., and Miyachi, Y., Generalized eruptive syringoma (letter). *Arch. Dermatol.* 125: 1716–1717, 1989.
Eccrine Poroma	Hashimoto, K., and Lever, W. F. Eccrine poroma: Histochemical and electron microscopic studies. J. *Invest. Dermatol.* 43:237, 1964. Holubar, K., and Wolff, K. Intraepidermal eccrine poroma: A histochemical and enzyme-histochemical study. *Cancer* 23:626, 1969.
Clear Cell Hidradenoma	Hashimoto, K., DiBella, R. J., and Lever, W. F. Clear cell hidradenoma: Histological, histochemical, and electron microscopic studies. *Arch. Dermatol.* 96:18, 1967.
Eccrine Spiradenoma	Castro, C., and Winkelmann, R. K. Spiradenoma: Histochemical and electron microscopic study. *Arch. Dermatol.* 109:40, 1974. Hashimoto, K., Gross, B. G., and Lever, W. F. Eccrine spiradenoma. Histochemical and electron microscopic studies. J. *Invest. Dermatol.* 46:347, 1966.
Chondroid Syringoma	Dardick, I., Van Nostrand, A. W. P., and Phillips, M. J. Histogenesis of salivary gland pleomorphic adenoma (mixed tumor) with an evaluation of the role of the myoepithelial cell. *Hum. Pathol.* 13:62, 1982. Mills, S. E., and Cooper, P. H. An ultrastructural study of cartilaginous zones and surround epithelium in mixed tumors of salivary glands and skin. *Lab. Invest.* 44:6, 1981.
Syringocystadenoma Papilliferum	Rostan, S. E., and Waller, J. D. Syringocystadenoma papilliferum in an unusual location. *Arch. Dermatol.* 1122:835, 1976.
Hidradenoma Papilliferum	Woodworth, H., Dockerty, M. D., Wilson, R. B., et al. Papillary hidradenoma of the vulva: A clinicopathologic study of 69 cases. *Am. J. Obstet. Gynecol.* 110:501, 1971.
Cylindroma	Cotton, D. N. K., and Braye, S. G. Dermal cylindromas originate from the eccrine sweat gland. *Br. J. Dermatol.* 111:53, 1984. Reynes, M., Puissant, A., Delanoe, J., et al. Ultrastructural study of cylindroma (Poncet–Spiegler tumor). J. *Cutan. Pathol.* 3:95, 1976.
Sclerosing Sweat Duct Carcinoma	Cooper, P. H., Mills, S. E., Leonard, D. D., et al. Sclerosing sweat duct (syringomatous) carcinoma. *Am. J. Surg. Pathol.* 9:422, 1985. Goldstein, D. J., Barr, R. J., and Santa Cruz, D. J. Microcystic adnexal carcinoma. A distinct clinicopathologic entity. *Cancer* 50:566, 1982.
Adenoid Cystic Carcinoma	Cooper, P. H., Adelson, G. L., and Holthaus, W. H. Primary cutaneous adenoid cystic carcinoma. *Arch. Dermatol.* 120:774, 1984. Wick, M. R., and Swanson, P. E. Primary adenoid cystic carcinoma of the skin. A clinical, histological, and immunocytochemical comparison with adenoid cystic carcinoma of salivary glands and adenoid basal cell carcinoma. *Am. J. Surg. Pathol.* 8:2, 1986.

Part **VI**

Panniculus

26. Diseases of the Subcutis

Chapter 26

Diseases of the Subcutis

I. Panniculitis
   A. Predominantly septal inflammation
      1. Erythema nodosum
      2. Other entities displaying septal inflammation
   B. Predominantly lobular inflammation
      1. Lupus profundus
      2. Pancreatic panniculitis
      3. Eosinophilic panniculitis
      4. Subcutaneous T-cell lymphoma
      5. Alpha(1)-antitrypsin deficiency panniculitis
      6. Lipodystrophy
      7. Subcutaneous fat necrosis of the newborn
      8. Sclerema neonatorum
      9. Cold panniculitis
      10. Injection granuloma
      11. Superficial thrombophlebitis
      12. Weber–Christian disease
      13. Calciphylaxis
      14. Benign cutaneous polyarteritis nodosa
      15. Crohn's disease
      16. Rosai–Dorfman disease
   C. Combined septal, lobular, and vascular involvement
      1. Nodular vasculitis (erythema induratum)
   D. Other disorders with occasional inflammation in the subcutis
II. Hyperplasias and neoplasms affecting the subcutis
   A. Benign
      1. Lipoma
      2. Angiolipoma
      3. Spindle cell lipoma
      4. Pleomorphic lipoma
      5. Hibernoma
   B. Malignant
      1. Liposarcoma
      2. Dermatofibrosarcoma protuberans
      3. Malignant fibrous histiocytoma
      4. Metastatic tumor

The subcutis or panniculus is a primary site of pathologic change in the disorders included in this chapter. The inflammatory disorders, panniculitides, are traditionally divided according to the site of inflammatory cell accumulation with erythema nodosum representing predominant "septal inflammation" and lupus profundus predominant "lobular inflammation." The specificity of the diagnosis of Weber–Christian syndrome is uncertain. All panniculitides may affect all structures in the subcutis. The classification is based upon the predominant site of involvement. In addition to inflammation, lobular panniculitis is usually characterized by fusion and loss of lipocytes as well as tissue necrosis. The end stage of panniculitis often results in fibrosis of subcutaneous fat.

The Reactive Process and the Disease	Histopathology	Comments

I. Panniculitis

  A. Predominantly septal inflammation

    1. Erythema nodosum (Fig.26-1)

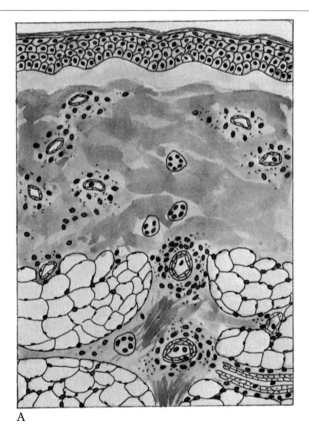

Fig. **26-1.** *Erythema nodosum.*
A. *Septal disease with sparing of lobules is characteristic. The septa may exhibit edema, acute and chronic inflammation, and multinucleate giant cells, as well as fibrosis, depending on the stage of the lesion. Large-vessel vasculitis and large granulomas are usually absent. Mild inflammation may be seen in the dermis overlying the lesion.*

A

B. *This micrograph illustrates the septal nature of the disease and the relative lobular sparing.*

C. *This higher magnification illustrates edema, lymphohistiocytic infiltrates with some angiocentricity, and multi-nucleate giant cells.*

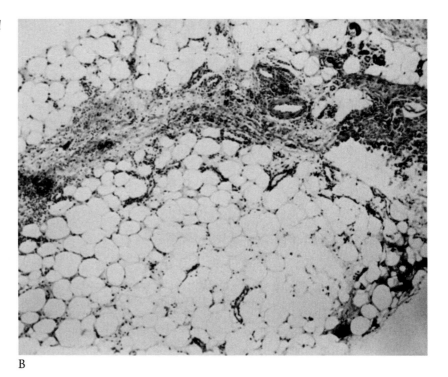

B

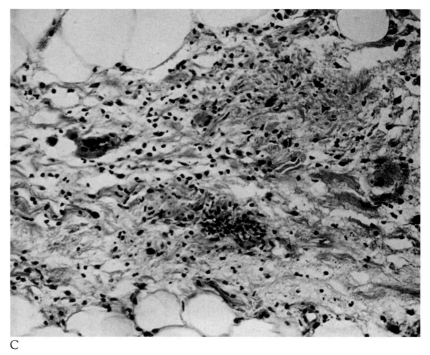

C

a. Early lesion

1. **Septal edema** with **polymorphous infiltrate** of variable intensity composed of lymphocytes histiocytic cells, neutrophils, multinucleate giant cells, and occasional eosinophils
2. Vasculitis with fibrinoid necrosis may be observed
3. Extravasation of erythrocytes.
4. Mild extension of inflammation between lipocytes peripherally located within the lobule

Dermal perivascular lymphocytic infiltrate is frequently observed

b. Late lesion

1. Septal fibrosis
2. Sparse inflammatory infiltrate with histiocytic cells and multinucleate giant cells common
3. **Paraseptal perivascular aggregates of lymphocytes** frequently observed (**Mieschner's nodules**)

2. Other entities displaying septal inflammation

Morphea/scleroderma
Necrobiosis lipoidica
Eosinophilic fasciitis
Migratory panniculitis of Vilanova and Piñol

B. Predominantly lobular inflammation

1. Lupus profundus (Fig. 26-2)

1. Lymphocytes, plasma cells, and histiocytic cells among the lipocytes
2. **Septal fibrosis** and **lobular hyalinized sclerosis** with loss of lipocytes and diminished lobule size
3. Variable superficial and deep dermal perivascular lymphocytic infiltrate
4. Lymphocytic vasculitis with **hyalinization of vessel walls** (onionskin appearance)
5. **Lymphoid follicles** often present

Characteristic epidermal and dermal features of lupus erythematosus may accompany lupus profundus or may be entirely absent
Direct immunofluorescence reveals granular deposits of immunoglobulin at the dermalepidermal junction
Dense lymphoid aggregate may be mistaken for lymphoma
Calcification may be observed

Fig. **26-2.** *Lupus profundus.*
A. *A diffuse lymphocytic infiltrate is present throughout the dermis and in the superficial subcutis.*
B. *A lobular panniculitis is illustrated here with coalescing fat cysts, foamy macrophages, and lymphocytes.*

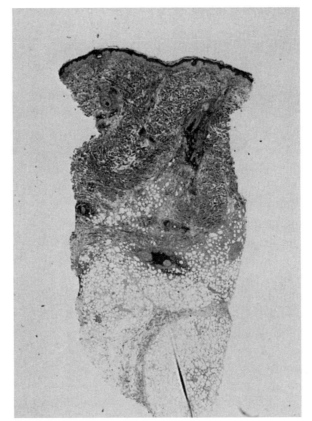

A

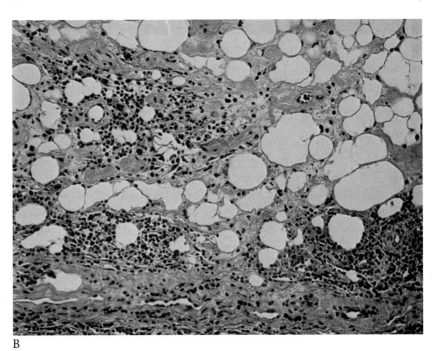

B

2. Pancreatic panniculitis (Fig. 26-3)	1. **Fat necrosis** with characteristic **"ghost cells"** in the lobules 2. Ghost cells have poorly defined, wispy outlines and no nuclei 3. **Calcium** (granular basophilic material) typically present in areas of surrounding fat necrosis 4. Variable infiltrate of neutrophils, lymphocytes, histiocytic cells, foam cells, and multinucleate giant cells	The associated pancreatic disorder may be inflammatory or neoplastic in nature
3. Eosinophilic panniculitis	1. Heavy infiltrate within the subcutis composed predominantly of eosinophils 2. Variable admixture of other inflammatory cells 3. Dermal perivascular infiltrate variable; may also be rich in eosinophils	Differential diagnosis: eosinophilic fasciitis Eosinophilic panniculitis is generally associated with other disorders. Among these disorders are Wells' syndrome, vasculitis, atopy, erythema nodosum, psychiatric illness, and pregnancy

Fig. **26-3.** *Panniculitis secondary to pancreatitis or pancreatic carcinoma. This highly magnified micrograph exhibits the characteristically ghostlike outlines of a nuclear necrotic lipocyte. Calcium deposits are present at the base of this micrograph as a dense linear band.*

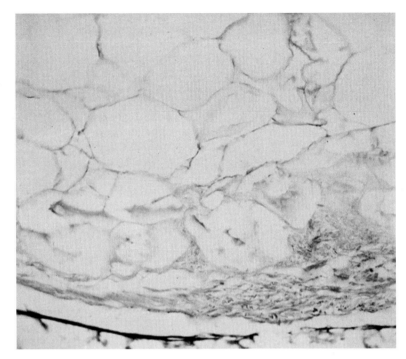

4. Subcutaneous T-cell lymphoma (Fig. 26-4)

1. Diffuse, heavy infiltrate of benign-appearing histiocytic cells with abundant amphophilic cytoplasms within the subcutis
2. Prominent **lymphophagocytosis** resulting in the so-called **bean-bag cell**
3. Erythrophagocytosis
4. Widespread fat necrosis with associated neutrophilic infiltrate may be present

Similar cytophagic histiocytic cells may be found in other organs

Erythrophagocytosis is seen infrequently in the skin and subcutis. It may be observed as an idiopathic finding or in association with other underlying illnesses, including leukemia and lymphoma, as part of a viral syndrome, sickle cell anemia, malaria, and Kaposi's sarcoma

5. Alpha(1)-antitrypsin deficiency panniculitis

1. Ulceration frequently present
2. Marked fat necrosis, often with inflammation in adjacent septa
3. Neutrophils at the margin of tissue necrosis, lymphocytes, histiocytic cells, and foam cells at the periphery
4. Septal leukocytoclastic vasculitis may be found

Panniculitis associated with alpha(1)-antitrypsin deficiency occurs in both homozygous and hemizygous patients. If this diagnosis is suspected, confirmation by determination of alpha(1)-antitrypsin blood level is recommended.

6. Lipodystrophy

1. Variable infiltrate of lymphocytes and histiocytic cells with phagocytized lipid within the lobules
2. Loss of lipocytes in more advanced cases
3. Inflammatory cells within the septa to some extent
4. Variable dermal perivascular infiltrate with lipid-containing phagocytes
5. Eosinophils and multinucleated giant cells occasionally observed

Although lipodystrophy is characteristically noninflammatory, inflammatory variants are recognized

Fig. **26-4.** *Subcutaneous T-cell lymphoma.*
A. *A dense infiltrate is present in the fat lobules.*
B. *The mononuclear cells display nuclear pleomorphism and cytophagia. Note the nuclear debris* (arrow) *phagocytosed by one cell ("bean-bag cell").*

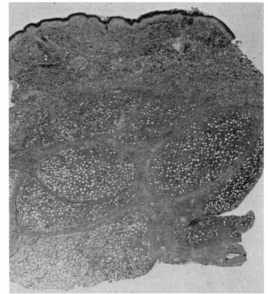

A

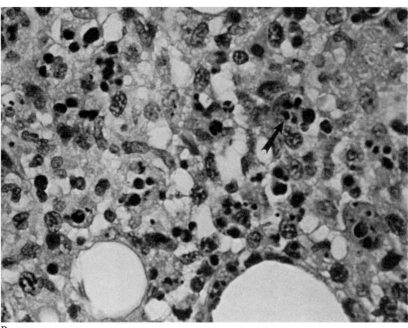

B

7. Subcutaneous fat necrosis of the newborn (Fig. 26-5)

1. **Fat necrosis** with a polymorphous infiltrate containing multinucleated giant cells
2. A variable number of lipocytes and giant cells contain **needle-shaped clefts in a radial array**
3. **Calcium** is deposited within the necrotic fat as basophilic granular material

In contrast to subcutaneous fat necrosis of the newborn, sclerema neonatorum displays fibrosis and widening of the septa and an absence of calcium deposition and of significant fat necrosis. Infants with sclerema neonatorum are generally gravely ill, whereas those with subcutaneous fat necrosis are generally well

8. Sclerema neonatorum

1. Lipocytes containing **needle-shaped clefts**
2. Little or no fat necrosis and inflammation
3. Fibrous bands extending through the subcutis

9. Cold panniculitis

a. Early lesion

Nonspecific lobular inflammation

b. Late (48 hours) lesion

Cystic spaces of variable size surrounded by acute and chronic inflammatory cells containing mucinous material

Fig. **26-5.** Subcutaneous fat necrosis of the newborn. Multinucleate giant cells are present within the fat lobules. These cells contain needle-like clefts.

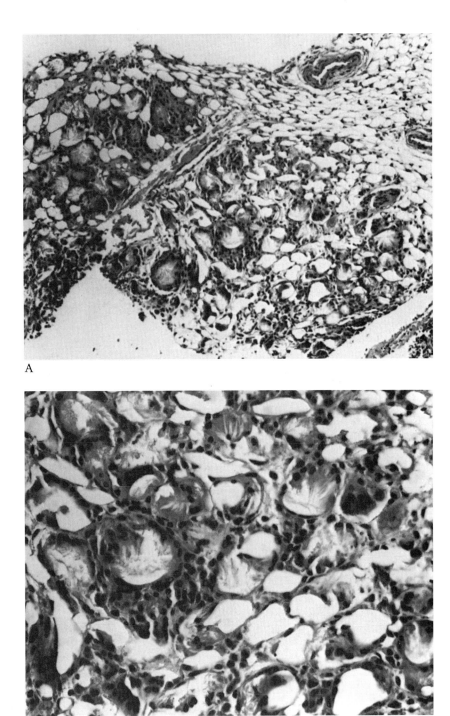

A

B

10. Injection granuloma (Fig. 26-6)	1. **Cystic spaces of variable size,** giving a "Swiss cheese" appearance to the subcutis 2. Marked **fat necrosis** 3. Infiltrate of lymphocytes and multinucleated giant cells of the foreign-body type 4. Extensive lobular fibrosis often admixed	The Swiss cheese appearance is due to the injection of various oils, most commonly mineral oil or paraffin; hence, the term *paraffinoma*. Factitial panniculitis also may result from injection of foreign substances into the subcutis. Polaroscopy is important to search for birefringent material.
11. Superficial thrombophlebitis	1. Inflammation around and within the wall of a large vein in the deep reticular dermis or subcutis; a vein may be identified by its oval or elongate cross-section; arteries tend to be round with smaller lumens 2. Occlusion of lumen by thrombus 3. Extension of the infiltrate into the surrounding subcutis may result in significant lobular panniculitis	See also Ch. 16, III.C.
12. Weber–Christian disease		
a. Early phase	Infiltration of lobules by neutrophils with focal lobular necrosis and abscess formation	Weber–Christian disease may be regarded as a syndrome consisting of tender erythematous nodules appearing in conjunction with fever. This diagnosis should be made only after consideration and exclusion of the other forms of lobular panniculitis.
b. Subacute phase	Numerous lipophages throughout the lobule; lipophages are recognized as histiocytic cells with abundant, foamy cytoplasm, which is phagocytosed lipid	

Fig. **26-6.** *Injection granuloma. Irregular ("Swiss cheese") spaces with marked acute and chronic inflammation are characteristic.*

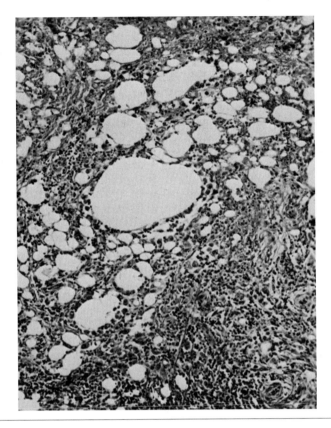

c. Late phase

Fibrosis of lobules with variable persistent fat necrosis and chronic inflammatory cells

As Weber–Christian disease becomes better understood, it appears that there are causes for this disorder, such as alpha (1)-antichymotrypsin deficiency. Therefore, Weber–Christian disease is a symptom complex for which there are probably many causes or at least several definable causes and an idiopathic type as well

The entity "panniculitis of Roth and Makai" is thought to be a type of idiopathic panniculitis, that is a subacute form of Weber–Christian disease. However, the nature of this lesion is not clear and most dermatopathologists do not use the term at the present time

13. Calciphylaxis (calci-fying panniculitis, consistent with calciphylaxis)

1. Small vessel thrombogenic vasculopathy
2. Early lesion shows fibrin thrombi with delicate speckled calcification of the thrombus
3. Later lesion shows intimal hyperplasia, with focal calcification and mural calcification
4. Extensive lobular necrosis associated with vasculopathy

Patients often have chronic renal failure. Peripheral calciphylaxis is associated with better prognosis; truncal calciphylaxis is associated with high mortality. The vessels of calciphylaxis should not be confused with the common Monckeberg's sclerosis, which affects larger vessels and shows medial calcification

14. Benign cutaneous polyarteritis nodosa

1. Small arteries exhibit inflam-mation, usually with mixed neutrophilic lymphocytic and eosinophylic infiltrate
2. Small veins are also involved by similar inflammatory infiltrate
3. The inflammatory infiltrate extends into the subcutaneous fat, and hence affects the lobule

Benign cutaneous polyarteritis nodosa is usually associated with arthralgias of the affected extremity. Recurrent episodes are common. The disorder has been associated with rheumatoid arthritis, hepatitis C, and ulcerative colitis

15. Crohn's disease

1. Granulomatous panniculitis, with epithelioid tubercles, predominantly present in the lobule and impinging at times on the dermis, and the septae
2. Lymphocytic infiltrate may be variable, with some infiltration present in some lesions, in others, no evidence of inflammation can be found

16. Rosai–Dorfman disease

1. Dense infiltrate involving dermis and subcutaneous fat, with prominent large lymphocytes, with abundant eosinophilic cytoplasm, are very characteristic
2. A polymorphous infiltrate including neutrophils and some eosinophils with some focal neutrophilic aggregates may be noted
3. **Emperipolesis** (phagocytosis of plasma cells and lymphocytes by large histiocytes) noted. Intravascular aggregates of large histiocytes with engulfed neutrophils are characteristic
4. Thick-walled venules cuffed by plasma cells at the periphery of lesions
5. Lymphoid aggregates and germinal centers at the periphery

Differential diagnosis:
Subcutaneous T-cell lymphoma with cytophagic histiocytic panniculitis (subcutaneous T-cell lymphomas, with hemophagocytic syndrome)
Histiocytes in Rosai–Dorfman disease stain with S-100, CD68, and CD1a

C. Combined septal, lobular, and vascular involvement

    1. Nodular vasculitis (erythema induratum) (Fig. 26-7)

1. Epidermal ulceration often present
2. Caseation necrosis (i.e., **granular necrosis of collagen** and fat) is characteristic and helpful when present but is frequently absent
3. **Granulomatous inflammation** consisting of epithelioid histiocytic cells and multinucleate giant cells is adjacent to necrotic areas; polymorphous infiltrate of neutrophils and lymphocytes may be intermixed
4. Necrotizing vasculitis of large and small vessels may be observed
5. Old lesions display fibrosis

Differential diagnosis:
  Tuberculosis cutis (including scrofuloderma)
  Syphilitic gumma
  Subcutaneous mycotic abscess
  Necrobiotic xanthogranuloma with paraproteinemia

D. Other disorders with occasional inflammation in the subcutis colon

Sarcoidosis
Granuloma annulare
Rheumatoid nodule
Periarteritis nodosa
Trauma
Leprosy
Deep fungal infection
Atypical mycobacterial infection
Deep folliculitis
Arthropod bite reaction

Fig. **26-7.** *Nodular vasculitis.*
A. *This panniculitis involves fat lobules and septae. Vascular thrombosis is present (arrows) within the septa.*
B. *The central vessel is surrounded by a lymphocytic infiltrate and displays fibrin degeneration.*

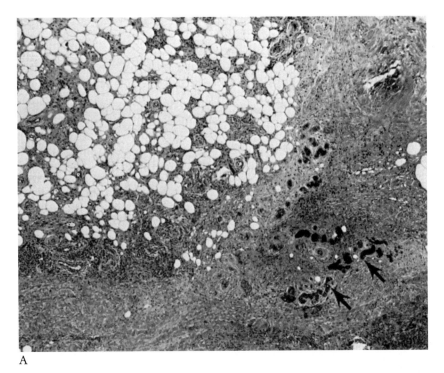

A

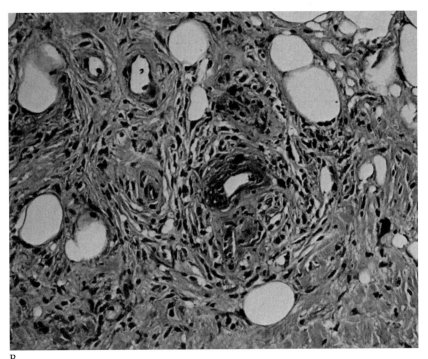

B

II. Hyperplasias and neoplasms
affecting the subcutis

    A. Benign

1. Lipoma (Fig. 26-8)	Proliferation of mature lipocytes within a thin connective tissue capsule	May be difficult to distinguish from normal subcutis
2. Angiolipoma (Fig. 26-9)	1. Proliferation of lipocytes 2. Proliferation of capillary-sized vessels at the periphery of the lobules and extending centrally to variable degrees 3. Fibrin thrombi	Normal fat lobules and lipomas contain vasculature most prominent at their peripheries. Recognition of vessel proliferation beyond normal is required to make the diagnosis of an angiolipoma
3. Spindle cell lipoma	1. Variable amounts of lipocytes and spindled cells admixed 2. Spindled cells are fairly uniform in size and shape, without numerous mitotic figures, and usually lie at the periphery of the lobule	

Fig. **26-8.** *Lipoma, Mature adipose tissue is present.*

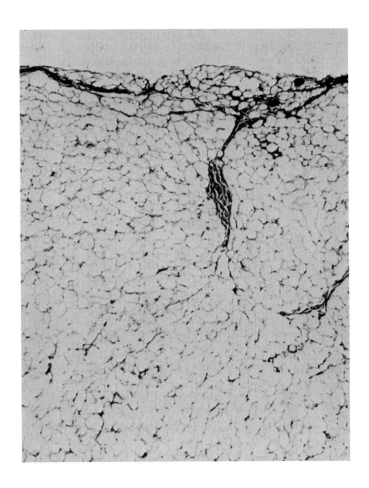

Fig. **26-9.** *Angiolipoma. A proliferation of capillary-sized vessels is present in addition to the adipose tissue.*

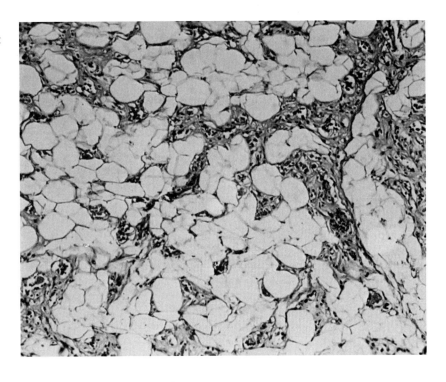

4. Pleomorphic lipoma

1. Circumscribed tumor with smooth borders that compress normal adjacent fat
2. Variable amounts of mature adipose and myxoid tissue admixed with collagen bundles
3. Cellular portion composed of mature adipocyte and **floret-type multinucleated giant cells**

A pleomorphic lipoma exists that has some features of a spindle cell lipoma but also displays multinucleate giant cells with a peripheral wreath of nuclei in an overlapping arrangement, resembling the petals of a flower—hence, the term *floret-type giant cells*. Spindle cell and pleomorphic lipomas are generally found on the upper back of adult men

5. Hibernoma (Fig. 26-10)

Encapsulated proliferation of immature round fat cells with vacuolated cytoplasm and central nucleus

These tumors are grossly brown on cut section. The individual cells are filled with mitochondria. These tumors tend to occur on the upper back of young adults

B. Malignant

1. Liposarcoma (Fig. 26-11)

1. Variable numbers of lipoblasts, the characteristic cell of all liposarcomas; lipoblasts are cells with large, hyperchromatic nuclei and single or multiple lipid droplets, which indent the nuclear contour.
2. Proliferation of lipocytes of varying degrees with protean accompanying connective tissue elements (see Comment)
3. The low power pattern may be that of an infiltrating, pleomorphic tumor, very suggestive of a malignant neoplasm or of a well-circumscribed tumor without notable cellular atypia
4. A diffuse, reticulated vascular pattern may be appreciated at low power
5. Number of mitotic figures is variable

Four basic patterns are recognized: well-differentiated liposarcoma, myxoid liposarcoma, round cell liposarcoma, and pleomorphic liposarcoma. A diligent search for lipoblasts is crucial in establishing the diagnosis

2. Dermatofibrosarcoma protuberans

While this fibrous tumor is generally centered in the dermis, it produces a pattern of delicate infiltration of the fat or replacement of the fat

See also Ch. 22, I.M

3. Malignant fibrous histiocytoma

This tumor often invades the fat lobules with its spindled cells and bizarre multinucleate giant cells

See also Ch. 22, I.N

4. Metastatic tumor

1. Metastatic lesions are usually located in the dermis but may involve the subcutis secondarily
2. Leukemia and lymphoma may involve only the subcutis

See also Ch. 22, V.A

Fig. **26-10.** Hibernoma. This benign tumor of adipose tissue is composed of cells of varying sizes. The cytoplasm of these cells contains fine to coarse vacuoles. Some of the larger cells have clear, nonvacuolated cytoplasm.

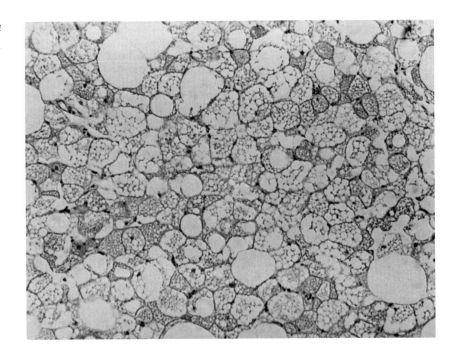

Fig. **26-11.** Liposarcoma. Lipoblasts are present, with markedly enlarged and bizarre nuclei.

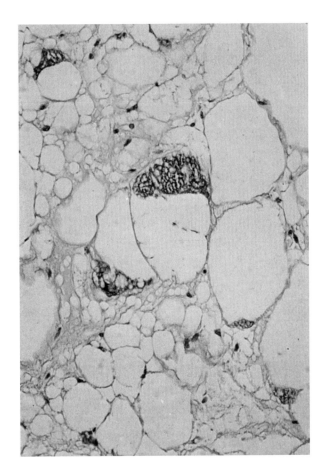

Selected Reading

Panniculitis

Beacham, B. F., Cooper, P. H., Buchanan, C. S., et al. Equestrian cold panniculitis in women. *Arch. Dermatol.* 116:1025, 1980.

Berman, B., Conteas, C., Smith, B., Leong, S., and Hornveck, L., 3rd, Fatal pancreatitis presenting with subcutaneous fat necrosis. *J. Am. Acad. Dermatol.* 17: 359–364, 1987.

Billings, J. K., Milgraum, S. S., Gupta, A. K., et al. Lipotrophic panniculitis: A possible autoimmune inflammatory disease of fat. *Arch. Dermatol.* 123:1662, 1987.

Bohn, S., Buchner, S., and Itin, P. Erythema nodosum: 112 cases. Epidemiology, clinical aspects and histopathology. *Schweiz. Med. Wochenschr.* 127:1168–1176, 1997.

Cannon, J. R., Pitha, J. V., and Everett, M. A., Subcutaneous fat necrosis in pancreatitis. *J. Cutan. Pathol.* 6:501–506, 1979.

Chen, T. H., Shewmake, S. W., Hansen, D. D., et al. Subcutaneous fat necrosis of the newborn. *Arch. Dermatol.* 117:36, 1981.

Chun, S. I., Su, W. P. D., Lee, S., and Rogers, R. S. I. Erythema nodosum-like lesions in Behcet's syndrome: A histopathologic study of 30 cases. *J. Cutan. Pathol.* 16:259–265, 1989.

Cribier, B., Caille, A., Heid, E., and Grosshans, E. Erythema nodosum and associated diseases. A study of 129 cases. *Int. J. Dermatol.* 37: 667–672, 1998.

Crotty, C. P., and Winkelmann, R. K. Cytophagic histiocytic panniculitis with fever, cytopenia, liver failure, and terminal hemorrhagic diathesis. *J. Am. Acad. Dermatol.* 4:181, 1981.

Forstrom, L., and Winkelmann, R. K. Acute panniculitis: A clinical and histopathologic study of 34 cases. *Arch. Dermatol.* 113:909, 1977.

Horn, T. D., Hines, H. C., and Farmer, E. R. Erythrophagocytosis in the skin: A case report. *J. Cutan. Pathol.* 15:399, 1988.

Hughes, P. S. H., Apisarntharax, P., and Mullins, J. F. Subcutaneous fat necrosis associated with pancreatic disease. *Arch. Dermatol.* 111:506–510, 1975.

Labbe, L., Perel, Y., Maleville, J., and Taieb, A. Erythema nodosum in children: A study of 27 patients. *Pediatr. Dermatol.* 13: 447–450, 1996.

Milligan, A., Chen, K., and Graham-Brown, R. A. C. Two tuberculids in one patient: A case report of papulonecrotic tuberculid and erythema induratum occurring together. *Clin. Exp. Dermatol.* 15:21–23, 1990.

Ollert, M. W., Thomas, P., Korting, H. C., Schraut, W., and Braun-Falco, O. Erythema induratum of Bazin. Evidence of T-lymphocyte hyperresponsiveness to purified protein derivative of tuberculin: Report of two cases and treatment. *Arch. Dermatol.* 129:469–473, 1993.

Sanchez Yus, E., Sanz Vico, D., and de Diego, V. Miescher's radial granuloma. A characteristic marker of erythema nodosum. *Am. J. Dermatopathol.* 11:434–442, 1989.

Schneider, J. W., and Jordaan, H. F. The histopathologic spectrum of erythema induratum of Bazin. *Am. J. Dermatopathol.* 19:323–333, 1997.

Schneider, J. W., Jordaan, H. F., Geiger, D. H., Victor, T., Van Helden, P. D., and Rossouw, D. F. Erythema induratum of Bazin. A clinicopathological study of 20 cases and detection of mycobacterium tuberculosis, DNA in skin lesions by polymerase chain reaction. *Am. J. Dermatopathol.* 17:350–356, 1995.

Smith, K. C., Pittelkow, M. R., and Su, W. P. D. Panniculitis associated with severe alpha(1)-antitrypsin deficiency. *Arch. Dermatol.* 123:1655, 1987.

Snow, J. L., and Su, W. P. D. Lipomembranous (membranocystic) fat necrosis. Clinicopathologic correlation of 38 cases. *Am. J. Dermatopathol.* 18:151–155, 1996.

Su, W. P. D., Smith, K. C., Pittelkow, M. R., et al. Alpha(1)-antitrypsin deficiency panniculitis: A histopathologic and immunopathologic study of four cases. *Am. J. Dermatopathol.* 9:483, 1987.

Winkelmann, R. K., and Frigas, E. Eosinophilic panniculitis: A clinicopathologic study. *J. Cutan. Pathol.* 13:1, 1986.

Hyperplasias and Neoplasms Affected in the Subcutis

Arbabi, L., and Warhol, M. J. Pleomorphic liposarcoma following radiotherapy for breast carcinoma. *Cancer* 49:878, 1982.

Bolen, J. W., and Thorning, D. Benign lipoblastoma and myxoid liposarcoma: A comparative light- and electron-microscopic study. *Am. J. Surg. Pathol.* 4:163, 1980.

Shmookler, B. M., and Enzinger, F. M. Pleomorphic lipoma: A benign tumor simulating liposarcoma. A clinicopathologic analysis of 48 cases. *Cancer* 47:126, 1981.

Snover, D. C., Sumner, H. W., and Dehner, L. P. Variability of histologic pattern in recurrent soft tissue sarcomas originally diagnosed as liposarcoma. *Cancer* 49:1005, 1982.

Index